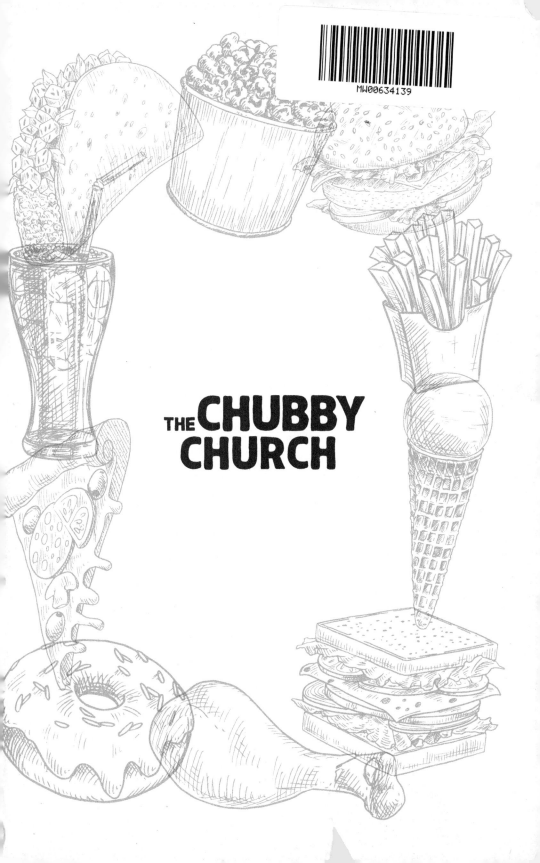

THE CHUBBY CHURCH

THE CHUBBY CHURCH

AN ORDER TO WIN THE
7 BATTLES OF THE WEIGHT & EATING WAR
FOR GOOD!

JENDAYI HARRIS
Emotional Fitness Trainer

WHOLE & FREE PRESS

The Chubby Church [Book 2]
An Order to Win the 7 Battles of the Weight & Eating War for Good!

© 2021 by Jendayi Harris

ISBN: 978-0-9971867-4-1 (paperback)
978-0-9971867-7-2 (ebook)
978-0-9971867-8-9 (audio)

LCC RM 222.2. H37 2021 DDC 613.2 dc23
© 2021 by Jendayi Harris

Front Cover: Vanessa Mendozzi & Sunil Kargwal
Back Cover: Najdan Mancic
Interior: Wordzworth
Editor: Sarah Hayhurst

Published by:
Whole & Free Press
P. O. Box 371391
Denver, CO 80237

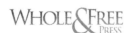

DEDICATION

With Great Love To:

My Heavenly Father, my All,
Words cannot express my love and gratitude.

To My Fathers

Grandpop Harris, Thank you for filling the gap.
You were my favorite eating buddy.

Grandpop Bunyon, You were the first author I knew.
Thank you for your teaching legacy.

Pastor Tayo, My spiritual father from heaven,
thank you for your prayers, wisdom, and warfare.

Dexter, Your loving kindness has changed my life.
Pastor Angelo, Your prayers always come at the time of need.

In Loving Memory and Honor

My father, Ellis E. Harris, Junior

Thank you for making me feel so special in the limited time we had.
Your winning coaching spirit and love for health
and fitness lives in me and this book.

DISCLAIMER

**Jendayi Harris, Whole & Free Press, Next Level Therapy, Llc.
Disclaimer for The Chubby Church Book Contents.**

This book, its content and any linked material are presented for informational purposes only and are not a substitute for medical advice, diagnosis, treatment, or prescribing. Nothing contained in or accessible from this book should be considered to be medical advice, diagnosis, treatment, or prescribing, or a promise of benefits, claim of cure, legal warranty, or guarantee of results to be achieved. Never disregard medical advice or delay in seeking it because of something you have read in this book. Neither Jendayi Harris, nor Whole & Free Press, nor Next Level Therapy Llc is a medical doctor or other licensed healthcare practitioner or provider. Consult with a licensed healthcare professional before altering or discontinuing any current medications, treatment or care, or starting any diet, exercise or supplementation program, or if you have or suspect you might have a health condition that requires medical attention. The United States Food and Drug Administration has not evaluated any statement, claim, or representation made in or accessible from this book or any linked material. The content of this book is not guaranteed to be correct, complete, or up-to-date. The Chubby Church e-book especially may contain links to other resources on the Internet. These links are provided as citations and aids to help you identify and locate other Internet resources that may be of interest, and are not intended to state or imply that Jendayi Harris or Next Level Therapy, Llc or Whole and Free Press recommends, endorses, supports, sponsors, or is in any way affiliated or associated with any person or entity associated with the linked material, or is legally authorized to use any trade name, registered trademark, logo, legal or official seal, or copyrighted symbol that may be reflected in the linked material. If you would like to communicate with us, please email *info@wholeandfreepress.com*.

Note: All references to diabetes refer to type 2 diabetes, not type 1 diabetes.

Disclosure: Remember to consider all advice with a medical doctor. The author and any affiliation with this book are not held liable for health recommendations.

TABLE OF VICTORY

Chapters in Book 2 are an extension of The Chubby Church Book 1, 1-20

Join the mailing list at
www.TheChubbyChurch.com

INTRODUCTION

Welcome to Book 2! I'm dancing like David, and you know why? It's because you're overcoming the weight and eating mountain! I'm so happy you've decided to get Book 2. I assume you've read Book 1, but if you haven't that's okay. You can still read Book 2 for practical advice on how to Win the *7 Battles of the Weight & Eating War for Good!*

And you'll still want to read Book 1 because there are several foundational points in Book 1 that will lead you to Whole & Free health and well-being in Body, Soul, and Spirit. There are also several references back to Book 1 throughout Book 2 which is why I started this book at Chapter 21. When I refer to Chapter 3 or 15, you'll know it's referencing Book 1.

As you know, nothing will change until you apply what you learn in Books 1 and 2. The two books must be read and applied together in order for you to breakthrough for life and overcome the weight and eating mountain that will lead you to prosperous health according to 3 John 1:2, Beloved, I pray that you may prosper in all things and be in health, just as your soul prospers.

It's normal for your weight to fluctuate as you learn to apply the Body H.A.B.I.T.S. You're also learning how to fit into your soul first and the skinny jeans will follow.

Remember Inner Transformation brings Outer Revelation.

In this book you're going to get my best advice to heal your relationship with food, eating behaviors, and your body. We're breaking free of all shame to manifest our most awesome, abundant life in Christ Jesus

Grab a few friends to read together and answer the Reflect & Share questions at the end of each chapter. Go now to *www.TheChubbyChurch. com* to join my mailing list for encouragement on your healing journey.

Thank you so much for being a reader!

———

We're going over a mountain, from a place of bondage to a place of freedom. Like the children of Israel, we'll move out of our weight and eating Egypt to our weight and eating promised land—as illustrated in Scripture. In this quest, you can't go halfway and win: you've got to go the whole way.

Each of *The Chubby Church* books represents half of the mountain we're to conquer. Let's walk through how this journey to win the weight and eating battle is structured.

Book 1: *A Call to Break Free of Weight and Eating Bondage* starts with us leaving our bondage behind, and then we ascend to the top of the mountain to gain our freedom. We're laying a foundation for freedom. This book covers the basics of body care, soul care, and spirit care.

Book 2: *A Call to Win the 7 Battles of the Weight & Eating War for Good!* descends down the other side of the mountain to reach the promised land. We're aiming for total victory to manifest our weight and eating freedom, health corrections, and lifestyle changes. We will reach and embrace wholeness and enjoy our promised land.

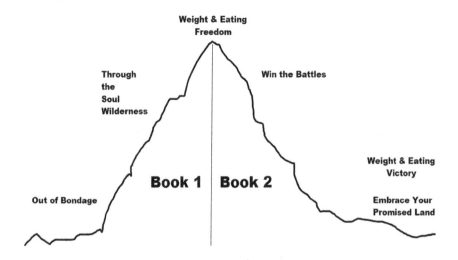

Out of Bondage

The children of Israel cried out to God to deliver them from the harsh conditions of enslavement by the Egyptians. They were desperate, and their desperation made them willing to change and embrace something different.

Are you desperate?

As they humbled themselves, God gave grace to be led by a chosen deliverer, Moses. Even though the Egyptians in our case may resemble chocolate-chip cookies or chips, God has heard our cry. Praise the Lord!

After hundreds of years of enslavement, the bondage expiration date came due.

How long have you struggled with weight and eating?

It's time for this struggle to end in your life.

Moses was as ready as anyone could be, given the circumstances. He said, "Yes, God," in spite of all of his own insecurities, like his lack of confidence in speaking, to lead the people out of their bondage.

The Israelites only had to obey and say, "Yes," when it was time to put blood on the doorposts, to collect goods, or to cross the Red Sea. And they did.

There was no turning back.

If they turned back, it would've been an early death sentence.

Pharaoh and his cohorts were blind to God's truth. Pharaoh only saw red when it came to God's people. As an oppressor, he was ruthless, without an iota of mercy in his enslavement of the Israelites. Pharaoh refused to let God's people go, even after ten plagues.

Ten. Plagues.

How much has your health or life been plagued by body image, medical threats, and eating struggles?

For Pharaoh, it took his firstborn son to die in order for him to let the people go. And when he did finally release them, he attempted to pursue them again.

Relentless.

How relentless has food temptation been in your life? Or the desire to diet? Binge? Criticize your body? Hide from mirrors? Or base your happiness on numbers on the scale?

Every Israelite had a decision to make. Do I trust the man of God leading us? Do I leave everything I've known and go? Or do I risk death?

At the moment of commitment, each thought, I either cross the Red Sea now or I'll be bound, killed, or drowned.

Freedom was the only life-giving alternative to bondage.

In one of the greatest miracles ever reported, the Red Sea parted, and the Israelites were free. A shout of victory could be heard in the heavens.

To be set free from weight and eating bondage, we cry out. It's time to move forward and get out of this place of turmoil with food, body image, eating, and weight.

In the first few chapters, we'll do that as we lay the foundation for freedom in body, soul, and spirit. In the next chapter, we'll complete a quiz to check how much weight and eating bondage grips us. I'll share more of my story to help you connect with your own weight and eating story. We'll cover the basics of body, soul, and spirit functions and how they relate to holistic healing.

We'll make a conscious decision to get free from weight and eating bondage for good—for life, and we'll complete **The Call to Weight and Eating Freedom Action Plan** to help us persevere up and over the mountain. Download yours and join the mailing list online at *www.thechubbychurch.com*. This commitment to freedom must be front and center as we move out of bondage and into our personal promised land.

Through the Soul Wilderness

The wilderness was a transition time from bondage to freedom. The Israelites had developed a bondage mindset across generations. I'm sure it was tough to eat the same food every day, wear the same clothes, and be around the same people.

Bondage was broken in the physical realm—they were away from Pharaoh and they were free from harsh physical labor. But, a sense of bondage lived in their hearts and minds. This was evidenced by their golden calf, complaints, and rebellion.

God delivered perfect instructions for living. But their longings for bondage overcame them. They didn't understand.

While they wanted to inherit the promised land flowing with milk and honey, or silk and money in modern terms, and slim and mobile in ours, many couldn't get there because their bondage mentality hadn't been broken. They weren't willing to do what was required to attain their freedom.

The goal of our wilderness is to root out the spirit of bondage based in fear, doubt, bad habits, and rebellion. We do so with deeper under-standing—in body, soul, and spirit.

In the same way, if we drop weight with the latest diet fad, the bondage will still be alive on the inside, and we'll be challenged again. That's why 90 to 95 percent of people who lose weight regain it and then some.[1] The soul wasn't addressed. Bondage still lives. Idols weren't demolished. Instructions weren't obeyed.

We'll face our truth on why we use food, like others use liquor or cigarettes.

Freedom comes with an investment of time to work on our mind-sets, character, identity—it's the soul work, the body work, and the spirit work that takes change, sacrifice, and shifts.

We'll walk through freedom strategies for body, soul, and spirit. We'll need to understand how we got here, and why, and the chains jerking us backward and keeping us stuck in the wilderness.

Chains like Body Neglect, The Dieter's Mindset, Soul Wounds, and Spiritual Chub. If we are unwilling to break the chains, chances are we'll be stuck in weight and eating bondage for life.

To counteract the chains, we'll Habitize Body Stewardship, Adopt the Freedom Mindset, Enact an Emotional Strength Training Plan, and Supersize Our Power Source.

We'll also gain an understanding of our soul's psychology in weight and eating bondage. You'll learn the psychological reasons that you self-protect with weight in Chubbology. We'll understand the *Inner Glutton* and our personal Grubbology. This insight helps us find the hidden reasons we sabotage progress, eat like there's no food supply, and beat ourselves up over the damage.

Win the Battles

Those who made it through the wilderness were confronted with the giants that inhabited their promised land. Out of a team of twelve scouts, only Joshua and Caleb believed they'd win. With God they knew they would take down the giants. But doubt paralyzed the Israelites. It was difficult for some to move beyond the wilderness to press through to the promised land.

The purpose of giants is to grow into the identity of who God says we are and what God says we can do. We defeat giants so that we can stay free. If giants overran the land, then the Israelites would be subject to future enslavement. There was no way to skip the battles. They had to not only be fought but won.

When we know who we are, there's no giant too big. When we understand who God is, we know we've already won.

We'll deal with the seven behaviors that keep this stronghold in place. With a strategy to win the battles we face, we can defeat them. To win these battles is to win the war.

Like the seven enemies the Israelites had to face, we'll have seven battles, too. They are compulsive overeating, food addiction, fleshy fasting, body shame, isolation, unclean eating, and generational yokes. When we go after our giant enemies and take a rightful position as a warrior of the Most High God—Ruler of all creation, we can be like Caleb and Joshua—zealous to overcome.

Embrace Your Promised Land

The Israelites experienced peace and rest for many years as they enjoyed the promised land. I want you to see this through, until you have the life in Christ that is promised to you of health and wholeness in body, soul, and spirit.

In the promised land is where you will experience your heart's desires. You get to enjoy all of the desires you've cultivated on why you wanted weight and eating freedom. Your victory is calling. And there's significant rewards for those who work for it and believe for it.

So today, I'm asking you, on behalf of the Lord, to commit to your freedom and to cultivate your desire to be free—no matter what ups and downs you face on the journey.

Freedom is bigger than weight and eating because on the journey to freedom from weight and eating a more abundant life in Christ will be gained.

We'll find antidotes for specific obstacles, unexpected treasures, and ruts along the way for you to embrace wholeness and defeat this stronghold for life. In this section, we'll review how to embrace and love your whole self, discern the red flags of recapture into weight and eating bondage again, be encouraged as you restore your health over time, and embrace the whole and free you.

Why I Relate to Moses

I flipped on the television to the Day Star network. The anointed Bishop T. D. Jakes of The Potter's House Church in Dallas was preaching. The next thing I knew I jumped out of bed and started praising God, like never before.

Overtaken by the glory of His presence in my bedroom, I fell to my knees with my arms spread wide.

"Hallelujah!" all of my heart, mind, and soul yelled out, in adoration. "Hallelujah! Hallelujah! Hallelujah!" A hundred times.

The Lord had spoken to my spirit. He said, "You are called to lift the bondage off the people and establish the kingdom of God."

My soul vibrated as glory intensified in the atmosphere. A powerful surge of His Spirit moved through me, and it held my arms in the air. TV church was still on in the background, but a full-on revival was happening right there in my bedroom in Denver, Colorado.

I felt the call. I felt it in every fiber of my body. I was called to lift bondage! My purpose of why I was here on the earth, why I had read countless books on psychological growth, and why I went through deep healing and agonizing pruning to heal my past, my character, personality, and my pain like my life depended on it. Why I had been trained in a wide variety of areas in life, health, business, finance, family, and marriage. And why I had testimonies for days on end.

Now, it all made perfect sense why anyone would have to do that depth of soul work. It was because I'm a believer on a mission to equip the body of Christ with practical and psychological wisdom. I'm to provide practical strategies and advice to do life in Christ well.

I knew my calling would manifest itself as an author to write books that help free people from their bondages—all kinds of bondages. But I had to start by overcoming my own biggest, hardest, most grueling, and primary battle—the one I call Weight and Eating Bondage.

This inkling to write was already in me. But like when the Lord called Moses to free the children of Israel out of their Egypt, I too felt incredibly inadequate, flabby, and not good enough. I relate to

Moses because I'm far from perfect, but my answer is always, "Yes, God!"

As you turn the pages of this book, know that I care deeply and resonate with the struggle with food, body image, weight gain, dieting, and binge eating.

I know what it's like to feel absolutely hopeless that my weight would ever change, that my mind would be forever held hostage by its obsession with my next meal, or wonder if I'd ever really like kale. I know what it's like to be a slave to food, a slave to cultural body image, a slave to the scale's report, and a slave to fear.

You too are an overcomer by the blood of the Lamb and the testimony of Jesus Christ (Revelation 12:11). Are you willing to do what it takes to overcome your weight and eating battle for good? *Will you commit to your freedom? Just go ahead and tell the Lord, "Yes!"*

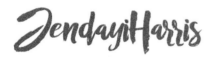

Soul Freedom Author & Teacher
Emotional Fitness Trainer
Lover of the True and Living God
Friend of the People
xoxoxo

Additional resources to help you in your journey,
such as courses and book clubs, can be accessed online at
www.TheChubbyChurch.com

CHAPTER 21

AN ORDER TO WIN

"Have I not commanded you? Be strong and of good courage; do not be afraid, nor be dismayed, for the Lord your God is with you wherever you go"

–JOSHUA 1:9 NKJV

Jesus saved your soul, but it's up to you to save your health.

ayi, Dayi," my brother yelled my childhood nickname as he trampled into the house out of breath, "You've got to help me. Come beat up this girl! Please, come on! Hurry!"

He tugged my arm.

Nervous, I followed out of pride.

We ran outside to the fight scene. Several neighborhood kids in my grandparent's suburban town gathered on the expansive, green front lawn. Everyone waited to see who was going to fight—Resthbutha.

Well, her name wasn't Resthbutha, but it should've been.

I was about ten years old, tough and tall. However, had I known I was about to fight a thirteen-year-old, seven-foot, wild renegade with lumberjack hands, I wouldn't have been so quick to run outside.

I shook with fear like Scooby-Doo as my opponent growled her giant teeth at me.[1] My eyes were like saucers. I didn't want to look bad in front of my baby brother, so I went into battle.

1

My dukes went up, and I must've gone down because I don't remember what happened. I'm pretty sure I was on the ground for a second before I booked it into my barely five-foot granny's arms of protection with the sound of evil chuckles of a flat-out victory for Resthbutha.

I went into a battle unprepared with an enemy I didn't know. In fact, it wasn't my enemy.

More damaging, what if we've been fighting the Weight & Eating War without understanding our enemy?

We need to understand the real enemies behind the Weight & Eating War.

And we need battle plans to take them down.

Prayerfully, we'll defeat our giants and win the battles that have hindered our success for far more than slimmer waistlines but for the advancement of the kingdom of God for good, His good.

> **Because health is our most valuable asset to progressing the kingdom of God, it's no wonder it's under attack.**

Because health is our most valuable asset to progressing the kingdom of God, it's no wonder it's under attack. In Book 1, we did the foundational body, soul, and spirit work to be Whole & Free.

To gain the victory, in this book I'm going deeper into our relationship with food, body shame, and eating because these things reveal your body and your destiny the most.

My goal is to clear up the world's confusion and bring us back to truth.

This book supports you to manifest your same level of anointed spiritual fitness in areas of emotional, mental, and physical fitness as well to embrace the Whole & Free you in Christ. Are you ready to know your enemies, win the battles, and overcome?

Why We Must Win

Our battles are the emotional, physiological, spiritual, or mental fights within us in the Weight & Eating War. Obesity and other chronic diseases are the outcome of unhandled weight and eating bondage. We're in bondage to the Standard American Diet of mostly processed foods and fatty, bacteria-laden meats, and we miss what God said about food.

> *Obesity and other chronic diseases are the outcome of unhandled weight and eating bondage.*

What is kindled as an innocent sweet tooth takes over the whole body. What starts as a few extra pounds grows into a chubby suit that feels impossible to get out of. Then, we're at a greater risk for chronic diseases, lethargy, and early death.

In the United States of America, obesity rates have climbed over 35 percent in nine states.[2] In thirty-one states, obesity has reached over 30 percent, and is over 20 percent in all states.[3] For perspective, in 1985 only twenty-two states had 5 to 10 percent of their populations that were obese.[4]

That's an alarming growth rate that affects families, health, and national security.

A body mass index (BMI) greater than 25 is overweight, whereas a BMI greater than 30 is obese.[5] (See Chapter 23.) Today we have classes of obesity that didn't exist years ago.

Currently, two of every three of us are overweight or obese. And one in thirteen of us is morbidly obese.[6] Sadly, one in six children ages two to nineteen are obese and contracting adult-onset chronic diseases such as type 2 diabetes in childhood.[7]

To be normal weight is abnormal. This is an indication of how far from God's physical design of the body and healthful human diet we've strayed.

Obesity itself claims a minimum of 300,000 deaths each year.[8] Early death is the outcome of continuing to eat in a way that is out of alignment with God's ways.

See, death of the heart is called heart disease. Death of the mind is called dementia. Death of cells is called cancer. And death of the pancreas is called type 2 diabetes.

We're out of divine alignment in health, which is evident by our excess. We really do perish for lack of knowledge. We must win to get into divine alignment for a best destiny in Christ Jesus.

What's at Stake?

Look at the high stakes to *Win the 7 Battles of the Weight & Eating War for Good*.

You win back:

- Your destiny. Do you sense your health destiny may end up in a hospital bed?
- Your freedom. Do you feel tormented by your food, weight, and body image thoughts?
- Your mind. How many of your thoughts are about how fat you feel or ice-cream?
- Your family's health. Are your poor eating habits rubbing off on your children?
- Your authentic beauty. Do you feel like you're hiding your good looks?
- Your emotional health. Do you feel isolated because of weight or bingeing?
- Your energy. Could you do more good if you had more energy?
- Your integrity. Do you desire to be aligned with God's ideals regarding health?
- Your relationships. Could you deal with conflict with people instead of eating over it?

What else is at stake for you? What will you win? Why do you want to win? When you know your why behind your efforts, you keep your motivation to persist until the victory is won.

Connect to your list of reasons and desires to overcome from Book 1, Chapter 5. Or download the action plan at *www.thechubbychurch. com* to refresh your vision and desire to overcome for good.

Remember Jesus already won it all. It's up to us to take it by force. That force is the effort, not in striving but in surrendering. We'll need to let go of those things that no longer serve our highest calling.

David battled for the throne and his legacy. Jesus battled for eternity, and the establishment of His throne on earth. Keep your stakes in view because you battle for your destiny and the abundant life in Christ Jesus.

Destiny Drainers and Killers

We don't come out the womb obese nor eating fried chicken. Most get caught in the Weight & Eating War years down the line. So, it's important to consider how this struggle affects us over time and causes health risks or what I call destiny drainers and killers.

Weight is a symptom of poor health. Obesity is the natural outcome of not resolving weight and eating bondage. It steals health and energy, which steals destiny.

> *Weight is a symptom of poor health. Obesity is the natural outcome of not resolving weight and eating bondage.*

Think about it: if we spend our time obsessing over treats, our money on prescription drugs, and energy going to doctors, is that an effective use of time, energy, or money? Do we have a higher calling then causing and creating health concerns?

Heart disease is the leading killer in the United States. As body mass increases so does the risk of heart failure. Research shows a 5 to 7 percent increase of risk for every increased unit of body mass.[9] Yes, heart disease risk goes up for every burger and fries meal eaten.

Atrial fibrillation (AF), a form of chest pain with symptoms of shortness of breath, heart palpitations, and dizziness, is highest among the obese. Obesity increases risk by 49 percent.[10]

And 65 percent of hypertension cases are due to obesity, which can also lead to strokes.[11, 12]

I mentioned in Book 1 how a good family friend died on the way to church. It's sad to know that 325,000 people die from sudden cardiac arrest each year.[13] And someone with a BMI over 40 carries the risk of sudden death and high risk for cardiovascular diseases.[14]

Cancer risks are elevated with excess weight as well. Eight percent of all cancer cases are directly caused by excess body fat. Fat cells are extremely toxic because they hold toxins and other excess we consumed and didn't need.

Excess weight and poor diet accounts for 35 percent of all cancer cases.[15] The American Cancer Society reports, "The obese ... get breast cancer, endometrium, colon and rectum cancer, kidney, esophagus, and pancreatic cancer as well as cause cancers of the cervix and ovaries, gallbladder, liver, melanoma, non-Hodgkin lymphoma, and aggressive forms of prostate cancer."[16]

We order that mouthful whenever we get greasy takeout.

Do you want reduced medical bills? If so, it's important to win this battle.

Ninety percent of type 2 diabetes sufferers are overweight.[17] Diabetics are on medications for life if they don't change their habits. And so are asthma victims.

Asthma prevalence is 40 percent among the overweight and over 90 percent among the obese.[18]

Researchers report, "Obese patients get more acute attacks, need more asthma medication, more frequent visits to the ER, and have more hospital admissions than non-obese patients with asthma."[19]

Aren't we supposed to be fruitful and multiply? Several studies show obesity affects various reproductive health issues including the ability to get pregnant, stay pregnant, and have a healthy pregnancy.[20]

Twenty-five percent of infertility in men and women is due to excess weight as well as pregnancy problems such as "miscarriage, gestational diabetes, preeclampsia, and complications during labor and delivery."[21, 22] In men, obesity reduces sperm count and sperm mobility.[23]

Obesity is the primary cause of problems with challenged knees, backs, and hips. Harvard reports that 33 percent of joint replacements are a result of obesity.[24]

What's crazy is, despite the reality that many obese people will need hospitals, over 35 percent hate going to them because of small gowns, weigh-in embarrassment, biases of doctors and nurses, and narrow exam rooms.[25]

Other health concerns related to being overweight and obese are sleep apnea, kidney disease, and fatty liver disease.[26]

The list goes on.

Physical health conditions aren't the only problems though. Mental health such as mood and anxiety disorders are highly associated with obesity by at least a 25 percent increase in risk.[27]

And in a study of 9,125 participants, big body mass was highly correlated with major depression disorder, bipolar disorder, and panic disorder.[28]

When I was obese, I had several of these issues—pre-diabetes and heart arrythmia as well as depressive moods and panic attacks.

Diet matters.

These health outcomes are *not* your portion in Jesus Christ! You do not have to continue to choose foods that lead to poor health and mental anguish just because they're convenient, advertised, inexpensive, or super tasty.

We get obese from what we eat. Clearly, the Standard American Diet (S.A.D.) is in truth quite sad and costly.

7

The Costly Burden

Obesity is not just a burden on the bones, organs, and soul, but it's a burden to both our personal and national budgets.

Compared to non-obese individuals, health care costs were $1,429 higher.[29] Total obesity health care costs are estimated at $147 billion annually.[30] And the productivity cost to employers was an estimated $8.6 billion per year due to higher absenteeism from work.[31]

Obese or not, how is your weight and eating affecting your day to day? Does it add or subtract from your quality-of-life accounting?

Not only does weight and eating bondage cost more, but also those who struggle with obesity make less. Obese men are underrepresented in higher paying leadership positions and obese women are paid at least 12 percent less than non-obese women.[32]

Significant cultural weight biases affect obese people. I mentioned health care professionals, but the love life can also suffer in both mate selection from a dating perspective in adults and playmate selection in children.[33]

Weight and eating bondage is a serious epidemic with serious costs and devastating consequences. Not one of the food giants who confuse us by marketing nutritional additives in deceptive packages will choose to take responsibility. Huge sums of money can blind morality.

Tobacco companies made it look cool to smoke until finally all the reports caught up to the government to sanction them. Today we see smoking as the smoke and mirror of coolness that it is.

Eventually, society and the government will catch up to the cancer-causing damage of the Standard American Diet delectables, but we can stop participating in poor health outcomes today.

Are you ready to win?

The Seven Battles of the Weight & Eating War

To battle is to engage in a fight or struggle.[34] In them we go head-to-head with enemies. In a battle we rise to overcome things that are against us and within us to gain the victory. A war is a series of battles. Each of the seven battles of the Weight & Eating War, provides an opportunity for you to rise-up into the warrior you are in Christ.

The Holy Spirit empowers you to win each one.

Here they are:

Battle #1 – Food Addiction (the Standard American Diet—S.A.D.)

What do sugar, baked goods, diet soda, and chocolate have in common? They're irresistible and make us feel compulsive and out of control. Processed foods as well as specific ingredients stimulate excess eating, which causes excess weight and the food crazies.

So, we'll need to **Rebuke the Sugar Demon and her Cheesy Cousins and win our first battle with the primary physical root cause of weight and eating bondage, which is food addiction or the** Standard American Diet (S.A.D.).

In Chapter 22, I'll motivate you to let go of your problem foods and the S.A.D., which is actually a Satanic Addictive Deception (also S.A.D.). That's super sad and makes us sheep feel b-a-a-a-d. (Note: The S.A.D. acronym used throughout this book.)

Battle #2 – Overeating

Our second battle is overeating. We'll **Perform a Gluttonectomy, Stat.** We'll dig deeper into the behavior of overeating, its effects, and the meaning of gluttony. There is no condemnation here, but there will be healing and strategies to figure out how much food you need and the right types of foods.

A scientific approach works best to take down compulsive over-eating and bingeing. So, there you go: we'll deal with the taboo sin of gluttony in Chapter 23.

Battle #3 – Unclean Eating

Have you ever accidentally drunk a cola with ants in it and thought, **Eww, Spit It Out, That Wasn't Food?** I hope not. I made that mistake when I put a cola on the windowsill and then drank it hours later. It was nasty. But few things are nastier than eating what God never called food. We'll learn from our Master Dietician about biblically and naturally clean eating in Chapter 24.

Battle #4 – Undereating

Ever wake up and decide to fast? Usually after you've had, oh, I don't know, a huge burger meal, a bag of popcorn, and fudgy cake the night before? When we're in fear of fudgy pudgy, we want to fast after eating it. I call this fleshy fasting.

In Chapter 25, we'll learn about spiritual and healthful fasting but **Forgo Fleshy Fasting** for good. While fasting is a spiritual discipline, we'll defeat all or nothing restrictive undereating that causes weight regain, malnourishment, bingeing, and depression.

Battle #5 – Body Shame

What do you think about your body? Are you harassed by constant negative thoughts about it? Do you avoid photos and mirrors, or are you obsessed with them? No really, are you a selfie queen?

To have shame about your body is causal to poor eating, binge eating, and weight and eating bondage. I assure you; you'll want to **Jump Off the Body Shame Train** to manifest your best health and happiest self. You will not want to miss this insight.

Battle #6 – Soul Shame

Would you rather spend a night in with binge foods than people? Or does your weight feel so embarrassing that you decline events? Isolation is a byproduct of shame and guilt. Our soul shame also stunts us in relationship skills, which is why we eat over conflict or fill our voids with food more than friendships.

If you avoid others because you feel ashamed of your eating habits, your weight, or lack real relationship skills, Chapter 27 will help you to **Decline Dates with Icy Isolation as we deal with the core emotional root of Weight and Eating Bondage—Soul Shame.**

Battle #7 – Genetic Predisposition

You may be thinking, "Jendayi, my whole family is fat, so how in the world will I ever be different?" I hear you. But fatness is a state of being that can be altered. We make chubby choices because we've learned to make chubby choices.

And it's true that you, like me, may have genetic predispositions working against you. In Chapter 28 we'll **Resize Family Fat Genes** to get the advantage.

Which of the seven battles are you most excited to conquer? In Christ we overcome, we fall seven times, and we get up each and every one of them. Will you be unstoppable? Unrelenting? Determined?

Will you do whatever it takes to conquer these battles and get to your personal promised land in Christ Jesus—the land of your best energy and health? Will you win the Weight & Eating War for good?

Yes, my friend, yes you will.

An Order To Win

To win the Weight & Eating War is about much more than weight or eating.

It is an order.

A kingdom of God calling.

Our Commander has spoken.

He has instructed us on what to eat, how to live, and how to care for our bodies. I have sensed His presence in this book as a prophetic call. It's not just a book, it's a call and an order to support your divine destiny and align yourself with His ways.

Wrong foods stuff down truth, spiritual awakening, and spiritual maturity.

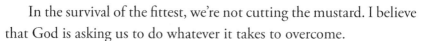

> It's not just a book, it's a call and an order to support your divine destiny and align yourself with His ways.

In the survival of the fittest, we're not cutting the mustard. I believe that God is asking us to do whatever it takes to overcome.

To persist until we have the victory.

To never give up.

To increase our knowledge, wisdom, and understanding in relationship to food for our sake and His.

Not because He doesn't love you but because He does.

God weeps over our struggles.

You have a right to life abundantly. And you deserve peace with yourself, your body, and your choices. Many poor health outcomes are preventable and several are reversible when we realign our ways with our Creator's ways, which will consequently realign our weight.

And since they (the big food and beverage companies, government, media, educational system, factory farmers, medical establishment, and pharmaceuticals) won't take responsibility, we must take it fully for ourselves.

We've Got To Change

The fact of the matter is it's time to change. Yes, you've got to change. God has given us the power to generate wealth, but He's also given us the power to generate health (Deuteronomy 8:18).

Personally, I had to look in the mirror and tell myself, "Jendayi, you must change." I told this to myself many times.

I didn't want to. But I needed to. We need to.

Say it, "I must change." It stings a bit, but you know it's true.

We're going to win, but to win we must make changes—the changes we've avoided up until now ... the changes that

> **God has given us the power to generate wealth, but He's also given us the power to generate health.**

are very uncomfortable but only for a short while. We're called to win the war that has taken casualties of organs, energy, confidence, accomplishment, and time.

> **We're called to win the war that has taken casualties of organs, energy, confidence, accomplishment, and time.**

Change is difficult. Change is scary. And change may not taste so good at first. Change may need to work up a sweat. Change may have to go out when it wants to sit at home. Change has to end bad relationships with foods. But change doesn't have to be hard.

We can decide to embrace change instead of kicking against it.

I mean, why wait? We wait for horrible health news that we intuitively know is coming, and then we change because a doctor tells us we need open heart surgery or have lumps in our breasts or testicles.

> **We can decide to embrace change instead of kicking against it.**

Let the Great Physician be your authority.

Let you be your authority. You're not a victim to poor health. No one is forcing you to woof down all that ice cream.

You are your own creator of your health destiny and outcomes.

Jesus saved your soul, but it's up to you to save your health.

So again, it's time to change.

And while you could quit, don't. I won't let you quit. I refuse to

> *Jesus saved your soul, but it's up to you to save your health.*

sit on the sidelines and watch you eat yourself to death.

So, persist until you win. Press on toward the prize. End the wishing, hoping, and wanting, and turn your passivity into action.

Embrace change. Choose life. Win the battles.

Lean into the discomfort. And be cheerfully willing to do whatever it takes to win your vitality, sanity, great looks, and best life outcomes.

The power of Jesus Christ lives in you.

You can let go of all weight that has easily beset you!

REFLECT & SHARE

1. Why do you want to win the Weight & Eating War for good?

2. What are you sick and tired of within the struggle?

3. Which battles are hardest for you to face?

PRAYER

Heavenly Father,

Thank you in advance for helping me to apply and practice what was shared in Book 1. I invite you to speak to me through Book 2. Help me to make the necessary changes I need to make.

I give you all of the stress and anxiety I feel when I think about what my weight and eating can do to me.

Open my mind and heart to receive changes.

Empower me to be unstoppable. Empower me to learn about the abundance of your ways in my eating. Help me to persist and persevere until I'm fully aligned with your will with foods, my body image, weight, and eating.

I cry out to you to align my choices to your perfect will.

Thank you for going before me and defeating my weight and eating giants once and for all. Thank you for guidance, wisdom, and joy in the process of becoming a new creation.

In Jesus's name we pray, amen.

CHAPTER 22

REBUKE THE SUGAR DEMON AND HER CHEESY COUSINS

Battle #1 – Food Addiction (the S.A.D.)

---

*"Wide is the gate and broad is the road that leads
to destruction, and many enter through it"*

–MATTHEW 7:13 NIV

---

*The Sugar High ... 100% Legal. 100% Fun.
—A Greeting Card*

Part One: Understanding Food Addiction

What do birthday parties, holidays, and weddings all have in common? Cake. And all sorts of other junk foods.

We love our junk, especially in the form of cake. But what if we enjoy our delicious foods a bit too much—like when we eat not just a piece but the whole cake? Remember my cookie story in Chapter 3? Well, it's about to get real.

As long as you have a sugar and junk problem, you'll have a weight problem.

Food addiction is a vicious battle with serious giants. So, we'll deal with it in three parts. In Part One I'll help you increase your understanding and awareness about food addiction. In Part Two we'll face

17

> " As long as you have a sugar and junk problem,
> you'll have a weight problem. "

your giants of problem foods and their addictive ingredients. And in Part Three we'll slay these giants to win the battle with food addiction for good.

Pay attention to any upset you experience as you read this chapter because it may be a sign of how much of a sacred cow some of your problem foods may be. Please don't shoot the messenger.

Oftentimes we want to blame emotions and psychological factors for our issues with food. Only it's the food we have in our systems that continues to create a problem with food. As we look at problem foods and their ingredients, we'll begin to see that bingeing, overeating, and emotional upsets that lead to emotional eating are caused by addictive processed foods and addictive ingredients, such as refined salt, oil, flour, sugar, and milk products like cheese.

The cause of poor health is poor diet. Poor diet is caused by addictive foods and beverages laden with chemicals urging us to continue to eat them and forgo healthier options.

> " Poor diet is caused by addictive foods and
> beverages laden with chemicals urging us to
> continue to eat them and forgo healthier options. "

Let me be clear, food addiction is the primary root cause of Weight & Eating Bondage and poor health; therefore, be open as we target the real idols hiding behind the struggle.

The Voice of Food Addiction

Certain ingredients are a lot like your favorite dance song. As I listen to Earth, Wind, and Fire's *September,* the beat gets in my brain, and before you know it, I'm dancing in my chair. Sugar, like the beat of the music, gets in your head and soon it's instructing your body to go eat more.

Certain foods and ingredients cause a voice of addiction to harass you with food thoughts.

Yes, addiction has a voice.

The voice of addiction is sneaky because it sounds like you.

Listen for it.

It convinces you to take that trip to Seven Eleven to get that two liter—*I'm so thirsty.*

Or to stop at the church bake sale—*It's for charity for goodness' sake.*

Buy six boxes of Girl Scout cookies—*Those girls are adorable; I have to buy.*

Or pick up a brownie mix from the grocery store—*The kids will love it.*

It lures you to say, "Yes, more peanuts, please."

It gives you all kinds of ideas for what to eat when you're not hungry and urges you to act immediately.

"Oh, a blueberry muffin sounds good," it says.

Then you're stuck, unable to move forward in your life, until you have that blueberry muffin. The voice activates a jury in your mind and rationalizes its points.

As its representative attorney, it sells you reason after reason of why you want that blueberry muffin and why you deserve it. It makes you think that you don't care about your health or weight goals or that you can worry about the consequences later—after you eat the muffin, of course.

One won't hurt. Many times, we buy what the voice of addiction is selling, which is itself—yup, more addictive foods. Like the salesman who keeps calling, it's persistent. It knocks on the door of your noggin to insist on a muffin solution for a feel-good time.

Addiction promotes more of the struggle, more of the depression, more of the hopelessness, more of the pain, more of the waiting for life to happen, more of the weight gain, more of the health problems, more isolation, more of the same ol' same.

Exhausting.

Do you really want to buy that?

Are you affected by the voice of food addiction? Let's see.

AM I A FOOD ADDICT? QUIZ

Mark each statement below that resonates with you:

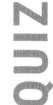

1. I become out of control with certain foods, ingredients, and/or beverages. ☐

2. I often overeat, binge, or stuff myself with food. ☐

3. I frequently crave specific foods and ingredients. ☐

4. I've taken food out of the trash and eaten it. ☐

5. I often eat when I'm not hungry. ☐

6. I eat to escape my feelings or tiredness. ☐

7. I'm preoccupied with food thoughts. ☐

8. I'm more interested in the food at social gatherings than the people. ☐

9. I eat differently when with others than alone. ☐

10. I've secretly taken other people's food. ☐

11. I know I should cut back on eating certain foods. ☐

12. Others are concerned about my eating, weight gain, or food choices. ☐

13. I experience fatigue, digestive distress, guilt, sadness, or anxiety after I've eaten certain foods, but I keep eating them. ☐

14. I find it difficult not to eat specific treats or drinks on a daily basis. ☐

15. I've struggled with food for a long time. ☐

16. I experience agitation, sadness, or anxiety when I cut back on certain foods. ☐

17. I feel hopeless in my relationship to food and weight. ☐

18. I can't seem to stop choosing foods I know aren't good for me, even though I try. ☐

19. I have an on-again, off-again relationship with certain foods or beverages. ☐

20. I worry that my food choices will cause health problems. ☐

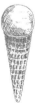

Total Checked: **Any statement marked is a sign of food addiction.**

_____

Defining Addiction

Before I define food addiction, let's talk about what addiction means. Addiction is having a conflicted desire to both keep and let go of a specific substance or behavior.

On one hand, you enjoy it immensely. On the other hand, it causes havoc in your life and well-being. At the heart of any addiction is an inability to stop something you want to stop.[1]

Addiction is described as a "chronic, relapsing behavior in the face of negative consequences and the overwhelming urge to continue something you know is bad for you."[2] In other words, you want the chips, but you don't want the chips because eating the chips will lead to the consequences of weight gain and upset with yourself.

If anything in your life causes this inner conflict, it's an addiction.

The Addiction Game

Another telltale symptom for addiction is if we play the Addiction Game. What's the Addiction Game? It's a game with three plays.[3]

- **Crave:** An overwhelming urge for something. Addicts phein.[4] An urban word that means to crave something greatly or until satisfied with their drug of choice—"I must get caffeine now."
- **Binge:** A compulsion to overindulgence in a fast-paced manner by the substances or behaviors we crave in objectively large amounts in a short period of time.
- **Withdrawal:** A chemical change happening in the brain due to removal of the addictive substance or behavior that has emotional and physical effects such as irritation, grief, headaches, or nausea.

Anytime we crave, binge, and have withdrawal from anything or anyone an addiction is present.[5] The Addiction Game continues every time we indulge our cravings to delay the uncomfortable withdrawal process.

We repeat the behavior and say to ourselves, "Just one more time."

Only 'one more time' nor moderation or limiting the ingredient seems to work.

Which foods cause you to play the Addiction Game?

Food Addiction Defined

Food addiction, and more accurately *processed food addiction,* isn't the type of addiction that would make one steal their neighbor's television or rob loved ones of cash, but it's an addiction, nonetheless.

Food addiction is an inability to stop consuming specific foods or ingredients. Typically, they are highly palatable foods and beverages loaded in explicit quantities of fat, salt, sugar, or flour that promote poor health, negative moods, and other life challenges.

I realize to some it can sound ridiculous to be addicted to foods, but to us, we know that food addiction is real.

> "Food addiction is an inability to stop consuming specific foods or ingredients."

How else can Sarah have explained her trips to the grocery store rushing through the aisles to buy her favorite snacks, inhale them in seconds when she returned to her car, and feel sick and depressed the rest of the night?

Or Liz's secret of gorging on pizza and chocolate, then hating herself the next day as she dealt with embarrassing gas?

Why would Mike eat from three different takeout places for dinner?

How do we explain why someone at risk for amputations from diabetes or a quadruple bypass still sips sweet tea?

The only explanation for the plump advancement of lifestyle diseases is our addictive diets.

Notice how you're not addicted to all foods, just specific foods.

There's no issue with cabbage.

If your doctor said, "You can never eat cabbage again," you'd say,

"Okay, have a great day." If your doctor said, "You can never eat *(insert favorite highly palatable food here)*," you'd say, "Oh my goodness! That's impossible!" You'd demand a second opinion and walk out offended.

See, highly palatable foods can be more addictive than drugs, so it's no wonder the overweight and obesity rate is expected to reach 86.3 percent by 2030.[6]

We don't phein for foods we need. To phein is to have an intense craving or urge that must be met by any means necessary. We phein for highly palatable foods loaded with intoxicating ingredients—the chocolate bar, pizza, and birthday cake.

Research helps us to understand that despite the fat pride movement, no one wishes to be overfat.

In a study of forty-seven obese people, all of them would rather be a normal weight, even if given multimillions of dollars to stay obese.[7] Obesity is difficult to bear. In the same study, all would rather be a normal weight with an amputated leg than remain obese.[8]

Because I've been there, my heart breaks for the stuffed down cries of a food addict banging to get out of the chubby cage. I wished someone were as direct with me about food addiction as I am with you. Even so, we want to keep our addictive foods, but we know we must choose to overcome.

In our right minds, we wouldn't choose to eat this way and create an abnormal, unhealthy body. But we're drugged by our addictive foods and not in our right minds. And it certainly doesn't help that our dealers are on every street corner and our drugs are socially acceptable. Haven't you gotten the stink eye from loved ones when we decline their tempting treats?

In our right minds, we wouldn't choose to eat this way and create an abnormal, unhealthy body. But we're drugged by our addictive foods and not in our right minds.

If you've felt hopeless around food, food addiction begs to be accepted as the most logical, physical root cause of weight and eating struggles in your life.

Kay Sheppard, expert and author of *Food Addiction: The Body Knows*, said, "Food addiction is a chronic, progressive, and ultimately fatal disease. It is chronic because the condition never goes away, progressive because the symptoms always get worse over time, and fatal because those who persist in the disease will die an early death due to its complications."[9]

Food addiction has stages, and if not corrected, it only gets worse.

Stages of Food Addiction

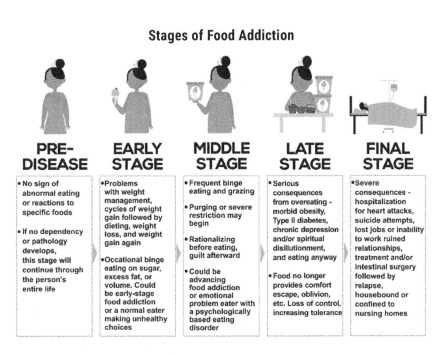

PRE-DISEASE	EARLY STAGE	MIDDLE STAGE	LATE STAGE	FINAL STAGE
• No sign of abnormal eating or reactions to specific foods • If no dependency or pathology develops, this stage will continue through the person's entire life	• Problems with weight management, cycles of weight gain followed by dieting, weight loss, and weight gain again • Occasional binge eating on sugar, excess fat, or volume. Could be early-stage food addiction or a normal eater making unhealthy choices	• Frequent binge eating and grazing • Purging or severe restriction may begin • Rationalizing before eating, guilt afterward • Could be advancing food addiction or emotional problem eater with a psychologically based eating disorder	• Serious consequences from overeating - morbid obesity, Type II diabetes, chronic depression and/or spiritual disillutionment, and eating anyway • Food no longer provides comfort escape, oblivion, etc. Loss of control, increasing tolerance	• Severe consequences - hospitalization for heart attacks, suicide attempts, lost jobs or inability to work ruined relationships, treatment and/or intestinal surgery followed by relapse, housebound or confined to nursing homes

Illustration 22.1   The Progressive, Pervasive Stages of Food Addiction[10, 11]

Reflection Question: Which stage represents where you are with food addiction best?

It's important to know our degree of food addiction severity as well.

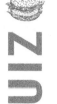

QUIZ

SEVERITY LEVEL OF FOOD ADDICTION

Check the number of severity points to identify your food addiction severity level.

1. My parents are or have been addicted (i.e., nicotine, alcohol, drugs, processed foods, sodas, or pain pills). ☐

2. I've struggled with food since I was a child. ☐

3. I've been addicted to substances other than food. ☐

4. I've engaged in risky behavioral addictions (i.e., sex, gambling, pornography, speeding tickets, or road rage). ☐

5. I have a family history of addiction. ☐

6. I have a chronic illness due to poor diet. ☐

7. I have undergone surgery for weight loss. ☐

8. I have difficulty admitting that I'm a food addict. ☐

9. I have attended food addiction recovery groups. ☐

Total Checked:

_____

Severity level is stronger for each box checked. And the more boxes checked, the stronger the boundaries around food and your environment may be needed to overcome a genetic predisposition. Please finish reading each chapter and may finishing this book be a sign to you that you will overcome.

No matter the stage or severity level, it's not too late because you're still here! You can, and I believe you will, decide to let go of problem foods and behaviors for your highest good!

Your Brain, Hormones, and Food Addiction

In the brain, compulsive eaters have every bit of the battle that drug addicts do from brain scans that compare processed foods to alcohol, heroin, and cocaine.[12]

Anna Katherine, author of *Anatomy of a Food Addiction* describes it as chemical warfare. Several chemicals in the brain are responsible for helping us to feel pleasure over pain.

All addiction works with the reward pathways in the brain that seek pleasure and reward. It's well researched that most who struggle with addiction are low in reward seeking and emotionally soothing neurotransmitters, dopamine and serotonin.[13]

Certain ingredients in foods, such as sugar, salt, flour, or oil, create an addictive voice in the brain due to the nature of their deep, pain-numbing, immediate mood-altering pleasure that they offer. These highly palatable foods give our brains a surge of opioid and dopamine release that comes with an inevitable drop and the search for more of them.[14] Therein lies what health authors Douglas Lisle and Alan Goldhamer call *The Pleasure Trap*. This is cycle or trap we can't get out of if we continue to eat certain ingredients.

It's also no secret that food giants intentionally addict us, looking for the cravability of their edible creations.[15]

Highly palatable delights increase insulin levels. Insulin levels are the strongest promoter of obesity, heart disease, diabetes, cancer, and more.[16] (See Chapter 12.) And when insulin is up, so is cortisol. Both insulin resistance and cortisol spikes keep our bodies in a chronic state of inflammation, which promotes disease.

Leptin is the satiation and fullness hormone. These tasty creations create an inability to feel satiated, so we eat more.[17] The brain and hormonal imbalances created by addictive ingredients makes obesity an easy win and normal weight an Olympian feat as food addiction persists.

Furthermore, eating machine-made foods that exploit our brain and body chemistry deadens the desire for the earth-made foods God intended for us to eat in His second instruction to human beings (Genesis 1:29–30), which is to eat fruits and vegetables.

And God said, "See, I have given you every herb that yields seed which is on the face of all the earth, and every tree whose fruit yields seed; to you it shall be for food. Also, to every beast of the earth, to every bird of the air, and to everything that creeps on the earth, in which there is life, I have given every green herb for food"; and it was so (Genesis 1:29–30 NKJV).

Pray for your taste buds' redemption!

The most logical explanation for the food crazies and chronic health epidemic is the addictive Standard American Diet or the S.A.D., which is also the opposite of what God said to eat to avoid the need constant for prayer lines for health matters.

Public Enemy Number One – The Standard American Diet (S.A.D.)

We've been eating with the enemy. The Standard American Diet is a way of eating and living dominated by processed and ultra-processed foods and their effects.

We eat at least 70 percent of our calories from processed foods and only 16 percent from whole fruits and vegetables.[18] This caloric make up, makes for a constipation nation. But we're not only backed up, we're drugged up with a collective of addictive ingredients.

In Genesis 1:29–30, God instructs us to get most of our calories from plants. That is a variety of His abundant supply of fruits, seeds, and vegetables—mostly green.

Herein lies the problem.

> The most logical explanation for the food crazies and chronic health epidemic is the addictive Standard American Diet or the S.A.D., which is also the opposite of what God said to eat to avoid the need constant for prayer lines for health matters.

We overconsume meat, dairy, refined carbohydrates, and refined fats, which leads to all sorts of deadness. We're to choose life by eating as we're designed to eat, which is mostly or at least half of our daily calories from nature's loving supply of fruits, seeds, legumes, whole grains, and vegetables.

Those who eat all God's way report being more spiritually connected, clear in thinking, focused, peaceful, in tune with nature, and emotionally open.[19]

If we continue to accept the Standard American Diet way of eating, we're being disobedient to God's Life Abundantly Standard (L.A.S.). Because when we choose dead foods over living ones, we're also choosing death over life.

> " Those who eat all God's way report being more spiritually connected, clear in thinking, focused, peaceful, in tune with nature, and emotionally open. "

Our lifestyles—inclusive of processed, ultra-processed highly palatable foods, horrifically treated animals for meat and dairy products, fast foods, eating on the go, lots of dining out, countless entertainment hours, over- and under-eating, and dieting on-again and off-again behaviors—isn't just about food or eating.

It's a philosophy—a culture of disconnection from God.

I feel like Jesus when I say, "Those who have ears let them hear."

If we look at the fruit of the Standard American Diet, we can see our rich, dead food lifestyles make us vulnerable to Satan's Agenda of Death (also S.A.D.).

Look at the number of people currently suffering from largely preventable diseases related to the Standard American Diet according to the Centers for Disease Control (CDC):

- 34,200,000 have type 2 diabetes, 87,000 die annually [20, 21]
- 88,000,000 have pre-diabetes[22]

- 135,000,000 are obese, at least 300,000 die annually[23, 24, 25]
- 121,000,000 have heart disease, 659,000 die annually[26, 27]
- 16,900,000 have or have had some form of cancer that are alive today, 599,000 die annually[28, 29]

In 2016, 1.9 billion were affected by obesity and overweight around the globe according to the World Health Organization.[30] Worldwide rates of obesity due to western dietary practices have tripled since 1975, along with astronomical rates of chronic diseases.[31]

The Standard American Diet is interchangeable with its truth as a Satanic Addictive Deception and Satan's Agenda of Death to kill, steal, and destroy (John 10:10). The acronym S.A.D. represents all three because they are one and the same.

Standard American Diet (S.A.D.) = Satanic Addictive Deception (S.A.D.) = Satan's Agenda of Death (S.A.D.).

The spiritual agenda is to deaden your spirit, numb your emotional body, and hijack your heart to stay fixed on food idols.

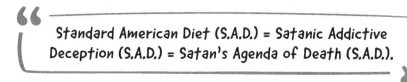

> Standard American Diet (S.A.D.) = Satanic Addictive Deception (S.A.D.) = Satan's Agenda of Death (S.A.D.).

If you buy into the deception, you'll want more entertainment, less of God, less of the Word, and less of His Spirit. You'll do less for the kingdom than you know you could be doing. You may not see your kids marry or be around to impart a legacy of Christ.

Instead of completing projects or helping others, your focus will go to lethargy and ailments. You'll end up in disease treatment versus the cure, which is always God's food truth at the foundation.

See, if something is evil, wouldn't it make sense for it to disguise itself as something good? Evil at its worst appears good and even normal but instead creates confusion to distract from truth.

Real evil is sneaky, and it gets on the inside.

Real evil embezzles money right under your nose or sexually molests your child next door. Real evil is disguised as something white and pure, sweet and celebratory, but it burglarizes priceless nutrients from your sacred temple (body). Anything that can cause at least 59 percent of deaths each year and delusion on what to do with your life sustenance (food) is wicked.[32]

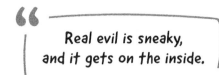

Real evil is sneaky, and it gets on the inside.

This is what I mean by eating with the enemy.

How many times have you played on again, off again with your problem foods?

Will you love yourself enough to let abusive food lovers go?

Wouldn't the best answer for health be to stop eating them altogether?

We intuitively know that the S.A.D. is the biggest root source of weight and eating bondage.

It's the broad way.

"Wide is the gate and broad is the way that leads to destruction ... narrow is the gate and difficult is the way which leads to life, and there are few who find it" (Matthew 7:13–14).

We must reject the Standard American Diet if we want true freedom.

Let's set a new standard and take back our families from poor health. Let's be determined to stop creating disease in our bodies today.

I'm not suggesting any diet. I'm suggesting the truth of nature's food.

Will you take heed to God's instructions in this critical area of life and remove yourself from the broad way?

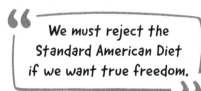

We must reject the Standard American Diet if we want true freedom.

A Note on Food Politics

Food addiction is a term that food giants know well, but they want society at large to be dazed and confused by their slick tactics.

Both big food and big tobacco target children first to hook them from an early age.[33] They advertise to everyone around the globe. After that, they sit back, refresh marketing efforts, and reap in the profits.

Meanwhile, we foolishly rejoice in the brands of these big food and beverage companies, believing they care about our health.

Several Scriptures warn of deception. We're not to trust wolves in sheep's advertising. And one great deception is our consumption.

We see that we're getting sicker, larger, and more tired. We must question our consumption and the powerful forces against our ability to choose well—the forces of marketing, research, and ingredients.

Our human minds are easily conditioned and persuaded.

When cereal brand ads were broadcasted, sales skyrocketed.[34] And we watch more than fifty hours of television per week filled with fast-food commercials.[35] Our minds influence our mouths to eat what we see advertised.

If kale were advertised, we'd eat more of it.

But honest foods don't need to be advertised, do they?

An apple is nutritious and doesn't need a special label or a commercial to let us know. However, packaged products are like flashing neon lights in a casino town that shout their benefits throughout grocery aisles, aren't they?

As a result of marketing, eating these foods has become socially preferred and acceptable; however, in truth these problem foods are an abomination to our bodies and insane—just like cohabitation, fornication, pornography, gender confusion, divorce, and swearing are socially acceptable but not God's best for our lives.

And the staggering amount of research, most of it conflicting or contradicting, only reinforces the marketing by creating food and health confusion. We feel the need to research the benefits of this or that super-food or to supplement when we'll recover our health best by eating an abundance of simple, real foods.

Let's dive into the ingredients that work together as part of the S.A.D. to get you out of this mess.

Part Two: Facing Problem Food Giants

A Breakup Story

I think you know what your problems foods are, but sometimes it's hard to pinpoint the ingredients posing the addictive problem. When I looked at the foods I struggled with, they all contained refined wheat flour, refined sugar, and refined fat (oils/butter).

It was an epiphany for me to realize that I didn't like the flour alone, but it had to come with fat and sugar to make it worthwhile, you know?

Other foods such as chocolate chips, popcorn, or tortilla chips were fine when controlled, such as a smaller portion size or not keeping them in the house.

But cake—that relationship had to end. I mean, it beat me up in every possible way. If I could've called 911 for its domestic brutality, I would've.

Cake physically abused me with stiffness in muscles, gastrointestinal emergencies, instant fatness, and bronchial wheezing. It mentally abused me by battering me with condemnation. It emotionally abused me by making me wallow in shame and guilt after indulging. And it spiritually abused me by demanding I obey it, rejecting God's voice every time I gave in.

What a nightmare that relationship was! As with most abusive relationships, it took time to muster the courage to leave. I had to gain the courage that I can stand in the world, cake free. That I could love God, myself, freedom, and energy more than the cake. I mean, what had cake done for me lately? Nothing. Nothing at all.

This relationship fraught with disorder, struggle, and pain had to end. No one knew I was in such an abusive relationship. My weight seemed to be an obvious indicator, but it was my secret. I didn't want to rat out my lover, especially because I was dependent on cake for my happiness.

Little did I know that letting go of cake opened an amazing new beginning. I made room for real love. I chose foods that loved my whole body and brain back, not just my taste buds, and foods that gave me joy, nourishment, and energy instead of depletion. My weight released, sanity returned, and productivity boosted. I began to live.

For a while, cake tried to win me back. I'd have some of it in small amounts like when my cousin baked pound cakes for holidays. But even a little cake perked up the addictive voice.

And if I didn't intentionally cleanse it out of my system, I'd fall into eating it daily again. It stopped being worth it when I grew my worth. I got too smart to obey its stupid suggestion to play the Addiction Game. I learned to love my freedom more than even a taste.

So, I slammed the door shut. I stood strong without talking about it and without worrying about what others would think when I said, "No, I don't want any." And I don't give cake any attention when I see it at a party. Cake has no power over the new me. Our past is history.

Some of your problem foods may have lesser problematic variations. For me, certain wheats like semolina pasta or spelt didn't pose a problem—mostly because those types of wheat aren't sprinkled with chocolate chips or lavished in frosting.

There's also a difference between refined flour versions of the product and non-refined versions. All of this was a discovery of what worked for me, my brain, and my body. I realized that I needed to eat in a way that was aligned with who I was, where I wanted to go in life, and my values.

> **Food is the fuel for your destiny, highest calling, and purpose.**

Enter a discovery of learning and choosing what's best for you. As you learn your body, mind, and foods, you'll find what works and what doesn't work to support your highest vision for your life.

Food is the fuel for your destiny, highest calling, and purpose. And the food you pick determines the quality of your life.

Find Your Problem Ingredients

What are your problem foods? What foods can't be controlled or eaten in moderation?

EXERCISE

On a sheet of paper, make a list of all your problem foods. Then, use the Problem Ingredients Chart to find the ingredients that hook you.

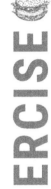

Chart 22.2 Problem Ingredients Chart

	EXAMPLE	PROBLEM FOOD	PROBLEM FOOD	PROBLEM FOOD
List the name of your problem food, then make a check mark for each ingredient it contains.	Chocolate Chip Cookies			
1 Refined sugar (added sugars, HFCS)	x			
2 Artificial sweeteners				
3 Natural sugars (whole fruit/dried fruit/ alternative versions of sugars like raw honey, raw agave, maple syrup, coconut sugar)				
4 Cheese or milk	x			
5 Wheat based	x			
6 Refined flour (all versions)	x			
7 Natural/whole flour				
8 High sodium				
9 High fat	x			
10 Alcohol				
11 Caffeine	x			
12 Chocolate	x			

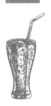

What do your problem foods have in common? What specific ingredients or ingredient combinations are you addicted to?

As you let go of your problem foods, a new abundant, supportive relationship with food can begin.

If I can do it, so can you. With God all things are possible (Matthew 19:26).

You're Not Alone

There's no need to feel ashamed of food addiction because you're not alone and it's not your fault. In a study of 398 participants who marked their addictive foods, processed foods won. Are any of your problem foods on the addictive foods chart below?

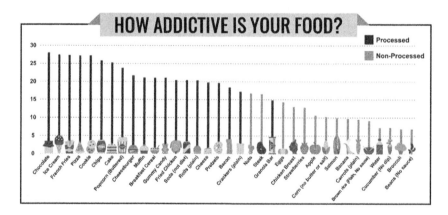

Chart 22.3   Common Addictive Foods[36]

What foods did you have in common with the participants in the study? I'm guessing you were good with cucumbers, am I right? It's no surprise processed foods have addictive, drug-like qualities.

Let's dig into the ingredients that addict us.

The Ingredients That Addict Us

While it's easy to demonize one ingredient, which I did by labeling this chapter 'Sugar Demon,' I don't want us to do that.

The Standard American Diet utilizes refined natural and chemical ingredients that work together as butt and gut fertilizer. So, let's not discriminate.

We'll look at exploited natural ingredients here and a few chemical ingredients in Chapter 24.

> " The Standard American Diet utilizes refined natural and chemical ingredients that work together as butt and gut fertilizer. "

Dr. Howard Moskowitz PhD, a Harvard psychophysicist, was given credit for these drug-like qualities in foods, called the "bliss point."[37]

The "bliss point" was unique for each type of processed food or beverage.[38] It's a scientific formula of the exact amount of sugar (usually refined High Fructose Corn Syrup HFCS), fat (refined oils), and refined salt that would make an edible creation craveable so that the customer, us, would buy it again.[39]

Moskowitz was hired by top food companies around the world for his genius in increasing the sales of many products from sauces to soft drinks.[40] In other words, he and many other food engineers, hooked millions of consumers to drive trillions in sales for companies, which drives trillions in medical bills for us.

Most of our problem foods are like science projects or edible chemical concoctions that leave us filled with shame, guilt, and regret—as they should since they're built on a foundation of greed.

So, how do we know this bliss point or that the Sugar Demon and her Cheesy Cousins have taken over?

- Your plate no longer welcomes vegetables.
- Your meals are imbalanced.
- You don't seem to cook or prepare your own food.
- You've neglected grocery stores for weeks.
- The convenient store knows you by name.
- The only thing you desire to eat is either doughy, gooey, saucy, cheesy, chocolatey, or crunchy (i.e., sandwiches, ice cream, pretzels, chips, burgers, fries, donuts, milkshakes, gravy-laden mashed potatoes, and candy all fall into the sugar category).
- Your body acts out (i.e., fatigue, moodiness, gas, bloating, yeast infections, joint aches, constipation, impotence in males, colds, and cravings).
- You feel on edge, irritable, agitated, impatient, and short-fused.

Refined foods are stripped. The sugar cane plant or beet is crystallized into a granule. Dense corn is processed into high fructose corn syrup (HFCS). Mineral rich salt is turned into table salt. Hearty brown wheat becomes white flour. Cow's milk becomes cheese. And the bitter cocoa tree becomes sweet chocolate.

Anything refined can become drug-like because it no longer has the foods' bulk nutrients and fiber to slow down metabolism. With such fast absorption and a rapid rush of chemical responses within the body, it takes over the brain.[41]

> **When we let go of problem foods, we get our food power back.**

When we let go of problem foods, we get our food power back. Food power is the willpower that's been lost because of refined ingredients and chemicals in your system. Basically, you can't say no to the chocolate bar because the chocolate bar ingredients are dominating your system.

No matter how you slice it, we're going to need to look at these foods differently—not as delectable goodies but as deleterious non-foods. They're not delicious; they're engineered. They're not loving our friends or children; they're promoting disease, depression, and an inability to focus.

Again, processed foods raise inflammation in the body, which raises insulin. High insulin levels cause all chronic diseases—obesity, diabetes, heart disease, cancer, dementia, and Alzheimer's.[42]

Read through the addictive ingredients of the S.A.D. Each one is described over the next several pages.

Here we go.

Get To Know the Sugar Demon

A poem for you. Sugar is fun. Sugar is sweet. Sugar at a party can't be beat. And sugar, my friend, is at least eight to fourteen times more addictive than cocaine.[43,44] It's a legally approved drug that affects the brain like the illegal drugs of cocaine and heroin and as much as alcoholism.[45]

At the nucleus of the sugar family is refined sugar or high fructose corn syrup (HFCS), but it has extended family. Uncles of white rice, aunts of pretzels, and those stubborn cousins' white bread, potato chips, cookies, sandwiches, and French fries are a part of this big family tree, sharing its tasty, toxic DNA.

Like that welcoming church mother who knows everybody, the sugar family is inclusive, inviting, comforting, and always available with the families' around-the-clock, open-door policy. It's just a convenient store or cupboard away.

On one hand, we like it a lot. On the other hand, we hate the impact it has on our mood, shape, mind, and spirit. Like an abusive lover is that addiction of any kind. But this lover is a family friend we can't shut the door on because she keeps showing up, especially at special occasions, offering sweetness to our desperate need for a pick me up.

The glycemic load is the amount of time it takes for a food to surge blood sugar. All of the sugar family has a high glycemic load and will promote insulin resistance, the key factor for chronic diseases and problematic weight. Processed foods high in fat and high in glycemic load (sugar) is a recipe for all major diseases.[46]

It's time to slam the door.

Sugar offers no benefits to the body except for taste. And that taste is a high.

A sugar high.

Our eyes gloss over, a sudden glee fills us, our bad day fades away, and all with only one bite of the stuff. As with any high, an inevitable low comes when blood sugar drops, making us reach again for the packet of regret.

The World Health Organization as well as the American Heart Association recommends no more than about 25 grams total of sugar per day.[47] That's six teaspoons for women (25 grams or 100 calories), nine teaspoons for men (37.5 grams or 150 calories), and less for children. But 82 percent of Americans are consuming more than 10 percent of calories from sugar.[48] That is about 77 grams or twenty teaspoons.[49]

In a household of three, Americans get a deadly 171 pounds per year of refined sugar.[50] If we add HFCS and sugar aliases, that number easily doubles per person.

Children get hooked on sugar from an early age, which promotes attention disorders, lowered intelligence quotients (IQ), and earlier onset of lifestyle diseases.[51]

Data clears denial and deception.

It helps to reduce consumption since added sugars are reported on nutrition labels in recent years.[52]

Listed or not, zero refined sugar is required for health, and none is recommended to thrive in health.

It's no secret that sugar has been named responsible for our obesity and diabetes epidemic.[53] In 1958, 1.6 million Americans were diagnosed with diabetes.[54] In 2018, that number was 34.2 million.[55]

But, unlike the Coronavirus where the Centers for Disease Control are on the job monitoring the outbreak, they don't do enough to end processed food consumption because it's our own personal choice to consume.[56]

I hope I've driven this message home: to sell more, people need to want more to buy more. The way to get people to buy more is if they can't stop eating it.

It wasn't easy for sugar to first be added to foods.

It required much labor.

See, it was our addictive appetites for sugar that led the dramatic abuse of a people in the Transatlantic Slave Trade to get that labor.[57] I validated this on a trip to the African American Museum in Washington, D.C.

At the start of the tragic slave trade was sugar.

Only an insatiable appetite for sin can drive mass wicked behavior.

Like pornography and gross sexual appetites drive human trafficking, food porn drives the onset of diet-related diseases.

See, slavery was a necessary evil in the eyes of the greedy because it took much work to turn an over ten-foot-tall sugarcane, juicy, nutrient-rich plant to a tiny, dry granule with no nutritional benefits at all.

The manufacturing ease and lessened cost of sugar beets and eventually high fructose corn syrup (HFCS) accelerated sugar's worldwide fame and co-starring chronic diseases.[58]

Sugar's Effects on the Body

After a plethora of medical tests, hospital visits, and several days of migraines with no answers, William Dufty saw a pamphlet that said, "If you're sick, it's your own [dang] fault. Pain is the final warning. You know better than anyone else how you have been abusing your body. Stop it. Sugar is poison, more lethal than opium, and more dangerous than an atomic fallout."[59]

Appalled, he cleared his kitchen and ate only real whole foods. After many a sugar bender, Dufty came to the truth: it's best to abstain from all celebrated ingredients of the Standard American Diet altogether.

He described his withdrawal symptoms, which included sweating, tremors, nausea, and the like, as agonizing. But after a few days, he felt a splurge of joy and taste bud redemption. He thanked God for the deliciousness of vegetables and grains that nourished like sugar never could.

He also eliminated sugar ailments, such as hemorrhoids, bleeding gums, fatigue, excess body fat, and skin rashes to name a few.

William Dufty's book *Sugar Blues* has helped millions since the '70s to remove sugar from their diets in exchange for a better mind, body, and mood.

In the *Case Against Sugar*, author Gary Taubes finds that it wasn't until after cigarettes were laced with sugar that cigarette sales went through the roof.[60] Prior to sugar additives the smoke was intolerable, and smoking wasn't popular. But sugar made inhaling easier just like it makes the medicine go down and everything easier to eat.[61]

Taubes quotes the Sugar Research Foundation who said, "It was 'the marriage of tobacco and sugar' that made possible both the astounding success of the American cigarettes worldwide and the lung cancer epidemics that followed."[62]

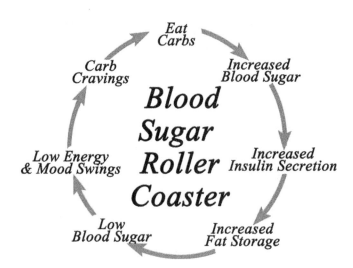

Illustration 22.4   Blood Sugar Roller Coaster[63]
[*Carbs refer to refined/processed foods]

Dr. Nancy Appleton, PhD, in her book *Lick the Sugar Habit*, explains the chemical imbalance of the S.A.D. and lists sugar's 146 damages to our health. (See Victory Morsels.) She emphasized sugar's 'unbalancing act' to the body, its systems, and organs when we consume this toxin.

Obesity and other chronic diseases are an effect of malnourishment. Chronic disease has a chronic nutrient thief called sugar and other ingredients of the S.A.D. Both obese and diabetic patients have major deficiencies in vitamin D, omega 3, chromium, magnesium, B3, B6, B7, B12, C, K, zinc, iodine, and iron.[64,65]

Chromium is a trace mineral necessary in insulin and glucose metabolism regulation.[66] Our bodies need chromium to digest sugar, but high sugar intake depletes chromium. And sadly, a chromium deficiency also causes sugar cravings, making for a cycle of malnourishment.

A chromium deficit is also strongly correlated to diabetes, obesity, and mental states of confusion.[67] In coronary artery disease deaths, patients had no chromium at all in their largest vein.[68]

Was it depleted by a high sugar diet?

Our teeth are also trying to tell us something. Another example of sugar's unbalancing act in the body is calcium-phosphorus balance, which affects plaque in the teeth and arteries.[69]

Does your dentist get on your case for plaque buildup? Is your enamel worn? Do you have your own teeth? Or did cavities take them out?

By the time I was twenty-three years old, I had thirteen fillings. See, the food addiction signs were there the whole time. Chinese medicine gives other signs of our mineral deficiencies such as nails with dark lines and ridges.[70]

Sugar, which includes high fructose corn syrup, white rice, white breads, fried potatoes, and white flours, causes inflammation, insulin-resistance, impaired glucose function, and health issues, such as osteoporosis, arthritis, erectile dysfunction, and cancer. Mentally, sugar can impact and cause anxiety, depression, mood, and attention disorders.[71]

> " Think of sugar like a moocher living with you
> who eats up all your food and doesn't pay rent,
> month after month after month. "

Sugar offers no nutrition and robs our bodies of nutrition. Think of sugar like a moocher living with you who eats up all your food and doesn't pay rent, month after month after month.

To be Whole & Free, any relationship that's all take and no give in your life must go.

Dr. Appleton says, "If you don't stop doing the things that make your body sick, all the medicine, vitamins, and nutritional supplements in the world won't make you well."[72]

And I say, "Amen."

The Taste Bud Rebellion Effects of Artificial Sweeteners

Do you consume artificial sweeteners? Notice how you cut down on calories by using artificial sweeteners, but these sweeteners cause us to eat more and gain more. Artificial sweetener consumers eat more cake because their brains crave more sweetness.[73]

How? Well, the hyper-sweetness of artificial sweeteners can be as high as 200 times the sweetness of sugar, which makes taste buds rebellious to the lesser sweet tastes of fruits and vegetables.[74]

In other words, these chemicalized sweeteners are like little, tap-dancing devils on your taste buds that stomp away any desire for fruits and vegetables.

> " Chemicalized sweeteners are like little,
> tap-dancing devils on your taste buds that stomp
> away any desire for fruits and vegetables. "

Studies of rats prove what my health coaching clients experienced with the addictive nature of diet soda likened unto cocaine addiction as well.[75] A study of diet soda drinkers who drank at least twenty-one cans each week were more likely to be overweight or obese.[76]

Numerous studies show that artificial sweeteners pose other problems, including thyroid hormone imbalance, insulin resistance, headaches, migraines, mood disorders, and fibromyalgia.[77]

Other side effects include visual impairment, headaches, dizziness, visual impairment, disorientation, and ear buzzing to name a few.[78] It's best to take these chemicalized taste bud rebels out of your daily consumption and test your tolerance and responses to an alternative real sweetener option like monk fruit, cassava root, or stevia.

The Best Sweet Replacement

We're wired for sweet. Our tastes buds have sweet receptors in abundance compared to other tastes.[79]

There are plenty of natural sweeteners that may work for you as an alternative, such as agave nectar, dark maple syrup, or monk fruit. But part of the Standard Addictive Deception is a complete rejection of the right type of sweet, which are fruits because people think that they're too much sugar or too many carbs.

God's candy is fruit.

Fruit is abundant in fiber, vitamins, and minerals. Unlike candy and junk foods where we always want more because we're never satisfied or nourished, fruit is a sweet that satisfies.

Whole-carbohydrate forms of energy such as fruit support proper digestive health because of their binding agents of minerals, fiber, and glucose to aid it to metabolize well. Definitely get the high fructose corn syrup out because it metabolizes directly to fat. It's discussed already in Chapters 7, 8, and 12.

Researchers say, "Low fruit consumption is considered to be the fourth leading contributor to the global disease burden, and thus one of the major attributable risk factors for diseases, such as being overweight, hyperglycemia, and hypercholesterolemia (high cholesterol) ... Due to their anti-obesity effects as well as their vitamin and mineral contents, health organizations are suggesting the consumption of fruit for weight reduction purposes "[80]

How easy is it to chop up watermelon, grab a banana, or munch on an apple? Make a switch to eat fruit as your dessert. It's magical for our energy, health, and body mass.

The Bible says that it's not good to eat too much honey and now you know why (Proverbs 25:27).

Got a Salty Tooth?

Lord knows, some folks are more salty than sweet. Salt addiction is as strong as sugar addiction. We often go back and forth between the two.

Refined salt—and more often it's chemicalized version Monosodium Glutamate (MSG)—affects reward centers and various opioid receptors in our brains.[81] Several studies have proven refined salt and MSG to be addictive.[82]

> Lord knows, some folks are more salty than sweet. Salt addiction is as strong as sugar addiction.

In a study of chimps, who usually eat only fruits and vegetables, once they were introduced to salty biscuits, they only wanted more salty biscuits.[83]

Now, who does that sound like? Us, right?

Once we eat salt, we prefer it because it's flavorful, especially when combined with fat (potato chips) and refined starch (pretzels), which makes it drug-like. At least 77 percent of our salt intake comes from processed foods, which would otherwise taste like cardboard.[84]

Bread and pizza are our top foods for excess dietary salt, followed by chicken, canned soups, microwave dinners, movie popcorn, and processed meats.[85, 86]

We know we eat more when salt is in the ingredients. Consider a bag of nuts. Plain, raw nuts—a few are fine. A bag of salty nuts? Well, the serving size can be the whole bag, can't it?

We also eat 11 percent more daily calories when we consume refined salt.[87] A study of Russian cosmonauts preparing for a long mission showed they wanted more food on the increased sodium diet.[88] Sugar steals the binge limelight, but salt is an official contender.

A study by Psy Tech showed over 2,800 binge eaters chose salty-crunchy snacks like pretzels or corn chips to be three times more addictive than chocolate.[89]

Dr. Michael Gerber, MD, author of *How Not To Die* quotes research that says, "Humans are genetically programmed to eat ten times less sodium than we do now."[90]

Unlike sugar, sodium (40 percent of salt) is a necessary mineral with a daily requirement of 2,300 mg, more if you're an athlete, and less (1,500 mg) if you have hypertension or risk factors for heart disease.[91]

However, 90 percent of us eat 3,400 mg per day.[92] Children need less but eat 2,900 mg per day, putting them at risk for disease sooner.

Health authorities consider high blood pressure the main risk factor for early death in our modern world; many call it our top killer.[93]

If we continue to eat excess sodium without enough potassium and other mineral rich vegetables and fruits, blood pressure won't regulate, and lifelong medications will be necessary.

Since 1937 studies showed that an optimal blood pressure is 110/65 throughout the lifespan.[94] Our standard blood pressure metric of 120/80 may already be elevated at baseline and has been raised to a new normal to accommodate the S.A.D. effects as we age.[95]

Anytime we eat salt, our blood pressure rises for up to three hours.[96] And since 1929, extensive studies have demonstrated blood pressure is reduced if less salt is consumed.[97, 98]

In the largest study of modern human diets, researchers found that as veggie and fruit intake went up, blood pressure went down.[99]

This is to be expected because fruits and vegetables have large stores of potassium whereas processed foods have very little. See, it's the imbalance of sodium and potassium and other minerals in the body that matters for health.[100]

A potassium rich diet can cure high blood pressure.[101] We need 4,700 mg of potassium each day to maximize health and feel slimmer. We get half of that which explains hypertension and bloat.

A high sodium diet chronically elevates high blood pressure triggers: thirst without wanting to drink water, imbalanced blood sugar, fatigue, migraines, and nausea.[102]

Dr. John Dinicolantonio, PhD, cardiologist research scientist and author of *The Salt Fix,* makes the case that sugar is just as much, if not more, at fault for hypertension and heart disease as salt.[103] Studies show that after just one night of eating refined sugar, blood pressure increased more than salt.[104] This is because too much HFCS and refined carbohydrates creates too much insulin, which causes blood pressure to rise.

So, what should we do?

What God said: eat more fruits and vegetables.

Salt cravings indicate that our stress managing adrenal glands may be maxed out.[105] If you struggle to put the saltshaker down, do an experiment: add mineral rich sources of sodium and potassium. Increase celery, beets, carrots, oranges, cantaloupes, dates, potatoes, cabbage, and a variety of dark leafy greens.

I've studied several diets to find food truth. Sodium is not something we need to be concerned about if we eat lots of real food. Do your best to eliminate excess sodium, but if it's needed in recipes, try the unrefined gray or pink salt as discussed in Chapter 7.

Remember that we're supposed to be the salt, not eat it all (Matthew 5:13).

We've got more ingredients to explore that drive the weight and eating bondage bus. Let's deal with the cookies, crackers, and cakes.

Frankenwheat and Its Starchy Floury Friends

I don't have to tell you that flour and refined carbs are addictive, but, of course, I will. These foods have been the bane of our healthy eating for a long time.

Let's be real. How many times have you overindulged on pizza, packaged baked goods, or pasta?

Alone, flours and potato products are rather bland from any taste at all. If the crispy wings weren't deep fried and salty, they wouldn't get as much tasty attention.

Let's talk about the main flour we use today.

Frankenwheat is a genetically altered version of wheat in baked goods, pizza dough, and pasta.[106] It's a featured ingredient in many processed foods.[107] Food manufactures use frankenwheat or hybridized, genetically altered versions because it binds to opiate receptors in the brain that cause appetite to increase, which makes us eat more of their products.[108] Americans eat 133 pounds per year or half a loaf of white bread per day.[109] It's addictive. This explained my cake addiction, and it also explains your bread addiction. All wheat isn't bad; in fact, our body is made to digest it.[110] But refined, hybridized wheat and any other refined flour (even gluten free versions) is asking for disease, fatness, and depressive moods.

Dr. William Davis, MD, author of *Wheat Belly*, found that these new strands of wheat led to leaky gut and over 200 medical conditions in the body.[111] Frankenwheat intake is also correlated to the mass epidemic of diabetes.[112]

On average his patients lost about twenty-seven pounds in under six months by eliminating wheat.[113] Gluten, the addictive, opioid-triggering protein, has high concentrations in wheat and contributes to gastrointestinal issues. Many signs of sensitivity to gluten exist, such as brain fog, bloating, diarrhea, constipation, cramping, cravings, anxiety, and any chronic diseases.[114]

Dr. Davis said, "The amazing thing about wheat elimination is that removing this food that triggers appetite and addictive behavior forges a brand-new relationship with food."[115]

To pass on the food crazies and depression, you may need to pass the breadbasket.

Commercial baked-goods eaters are 38 percent more depressed than non-baked good eaters.[116]

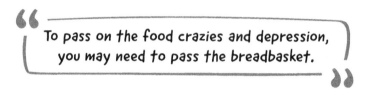

To pass on the food crazies and depression, you may need to pass the breadbasket.

To get happier, add whole grains like millet, brown rice, or barley to your diet because the benefits are tremendous. They provide fiber, an abundance of nutrients including energy giving vitamins, and are highly satiating. All whole grains, including whole wheat sources such as kamut or spelt, do have significant benefits to reduce disease—namely diabetes.[117]

Also test which flour alternatives don't excite your addictive voice. Oat flour can be made by blending rolled or steal cut oats. Brown rice or almond flour are worth a try as well.

Refined carbohydrates—grains and starches—convert right from starch to glucose in the metabolism, spiking both blood glucose and blood fat as well.[118] So even though crackers, bread, and fried potatoes don't taste like sugar, this doesn't mean that they don't react as sugar.[119]

On the flipside, Dr. John McDougall, author of *The Starch Solution*, has proven that healthful starchy vegetables promote disease reversal and weight reduction. He recommends that we eat real starch, which reduces blood sugars and blood fat, instead of the refined versions that addict us. Sweet potatoes, beans, squash, and peas are low in calories and quite satiating.

Many parts of the world like China and Latin America have diets high in starch, yet they haven't struggled with weight like Americans. In the past I was a carbophobe, one who fears all carbs. But adding whole carbohydrates and beans has only helped my health and well-being.

A carbophobe will struggle until she learns how to work with foods that have been avoided due to nutritional inaccuracy. If you struggle with bread, lean on Jesus. He is the Bread of life, and I guarantee that His bread doesn't create food crazies (John 6:35).

Over the next two chapters we'll clear all lies and understand foods better to continue to break free from problem foods.

The Slippery Slope of Oils and Fats

The reason Lay's prophesied that we couldn't eat just one chip is because they deep fried them and drenched them in refined salt.

It's not rocket science.

> " The reason Lay's prophesied that we couldn't eat just one chip is because they deep fried them and drenched them in refined salt. "

The salt and oil combination in chips or fried chicken is just as addictive as the sugar and fats in mini donuts.

When we eat refined oils that are processed and then heated at high temperatures, we get free radical damage at a cellular level. Free radicals are unstable molecules that create oxidative stress.[120] Oxidative stress has enormous dangers for every disease.[121]

In human brains, fat is preferred to ease pain and contributes to opioid levels that soothe us. Since oil is a smooth operator and has no fiber, we can easily eat a lot of it. But at 100 calories per teaspoon, we can see why it doesn't help our cause. And it may be obvious, but non-essential excess fat in our diets will store as fat quickly on our bodies.

Like a marbled steak, fatty diets feed into organs and muscles like the liver and heart. And big food can't sell oils alone. Recall that 'bliss point' because these oils and fats must be paired with other addictive ingredients for it to do its damage.

For food addicts, refined oils in processed, fried, and fast foods are troublesome because they stimulate eating more and addiction.[122]

The body needs a variety of fats—only not much.

The S.A.D. is over-weighted in saturated fats and under-weighted in vital anti-disease fats, namely omega 3s, found in chia seeds, salmon, walnuts, and ground flax seeds. Three walnuts or a teaspoon of chia seeds contains all the omega-3 we need for the whole day.

But Americans eat 40 to 50 percent of daily calories from the types of fat that cause disease—saturated and trans fats. Saturated fats are found mostly in animal foods, such as meats, eggs, cheese, and milk, and trans fats are found in deep-fried selections and packaged products.

To wrap your mind around how much saturated fat we eat, a cup of diced chicken has 25 percent of our daily intake for saturated fat. And a quarter pounder with cheese meal from McDonalds? A whopping 82 percent.[123]

Oh, harken thee, angels, and block our paths from fast food!

Does your problem food have trans-fat?

Watch for hydrogenated oil or partially hydrogenated oil on labels. These oils add hydrogen to make them solid at room temperature. It lengthens the shelf-life in stores and your arteries.[124] Trans fats are both natural and processed, and only recently, after many sudden deaths, has the amount been required to be reported on nutrition labels.

Deep-fried anything does make for a mighty fine dining experience. However, anytime you go to a restaurant, you unwittingly increase your intake of oils.

Chef AJ knew firsthand the extreme use of oils in restaurant foods and its effects on food addicts like herself. So, she took out oils of her and her husbands' diet. She has skills so he didn't taste the difference, and after two months he lost all eight of his excess pounds.[125]

I love that she teaches food addicts how to prepare their favorite problem foods to be free from their addictive ingredients. You can find her mouth-watering recipes without S.O.F.A.S.— sugar, oil, flour, alcohol, and salt—on YouTube. Funny, when we take these ingredients out, we'll get off the sofa since real health promotes activity.

Reducing oils and fats reduces inflammation and insulin levels.[126]

World-renowned nutrition educators recommend 10 to 15 percent of total calorie intake should be from fat for optimal health and energy and not to exceed 20 percent of total calorie intake.[127]

How much fat do you eat per day?

How much is refined versus whole source fat?

Dr. Dean Ornish, MD, an esteemed heart doctor and author, and co-author Anne Ornish wrote *Undo It!* They share how a holistic health plan that includes dietary fat intake of 10 to 15 percent has reversed heart disease in thousands of hopeless cases.

Dr. Cyrus Khambatta, PhD, and Robbie Barbaro in their best-seller *Mastering Diabetes*, help others reverse all types of diabetes by rejecting the Standard American Diet as well as eating an abundance of fruits and vegetables to keep dietary fat at 10 to 15 percent of total calories per day.

Ketogenic lifestyles recommend 50 to 75 percent of calories from fat and 5 percent of calories from carbohydrates. Only there's inadequate proof that a high fat, low sugar diet can prevent or reverse chronic diseases and lacks sustainability. If you want to eat high fat, do so in a non-Standard American Diet way by using quality sources like avocados or olives.

A recipe for chronic diseases is any diet high in both sugar and fat.

Focus on the right amount of healthy fats for your body.

Eat nuts, seeds, and avocados in the proper portion—the size of a thumb or ¼ cup. Per our previous conversations, avoid salty nuts and stick with raw or roasted to avoid nutty cravings.

Use low-sodium broths for sautéing or balsamic vinegars for dressings to positively impact your health and the waistline.

Oil is good. It's a blessing and has many uses. Let's use it to anoint ourselves and others for healing and reduce guzzling the refined kind, deal? (Mark 6:13).

Does Milk Really Do a Body Good?

John Robbins, heir to his father Irv Robbins, who founded Baskin-Robbins, grew up in the luxury of wealth. He speaks of his childhood memories of an ice-cream cone shaped swimming pool and ice cream for breakfast.[128]

John questioned his health and diet when his uncle Burt Baskins suddenly died of a heart attack. Burt was just over fifty years old, obese, and ate a whole lot of ice cream.[129]

John broached the subject to his father and said, "Do you think there could be any connection between his heart attack and the amount of ice cream he would eat?"[130]

Irv said, "No! No! No! His ticker just got tired and stopped working."

Irv's piercing response reflected the denial that his beloved food idol caused early deaths. It served as a catalyst for John to reject the S.A.D. and discover the path to health for himself and others at large. John saw how obese, unhappy, and unhealthy his family was a result of their poor diet, and he wanted nothing of that lifestyle or outcome for his life or ours.[131]

So, he left wealth in the Baskin-Robbins empire to stand for health. An empire that was the first multi-billion-dollar, global ice cream company. He also went on to write *Diet for a New America* becoming a celebrated food, animal rights, and environmental health advocate.

Later Irv's health was threatened by diabetic amputation. Open to John's health advice, Irv also rejected the S.A.D. His cholesterol went from 280 to 150, his diabetes went into remission, he never had the amputation, and ultimately extended his life by twenty years.[132]

It's not too late.

Some may care less about ice cream but wrestle with letting go of cheese. Cheese is not only high in saturated fat and sodium per slice or ounce but also in calories that are difficult to burn off. I feel the cheese puff immediately if I eat it.

In a study by the University of Michigan with 500 participants, the highly processed taste bud rock star was proven to create food addiction tendencies.[133] So much so, that even a bite of cheese can lead to an order for pizza.[134]

President of the Physicians Committee for Responsible Medicine and author of *The Cheese Trap*, Dr. Neal Bernard said, "Casomorphins attach to the brain's opiate receptors to cause a calming effect in much the same way heroin and morphine do."[135]

Cheese is most addictive because of its morphine containing proteins called casomorphines built from casein. Compared to human milk, dairy has ten times as much casein per liter or 2.6 casein proteins per liter in human milk versus 26 per liter in cow's milk.[136] We eat 646 pounds of dairy per capita in the U.S. from mostly sick, stressed cows, which makes for a serious cheese high.[137]

Are you a big kid like me and appreciate milk and cookies? Milk and cookies are a profoundly nurturing combo. Dr. Julie Wei, MD, an award-winning pediatric ear, nose, and throat doctor, treated thousands of children with a disturbance she called milk and cookie disease.[138]

She said, "Sugar is the nicotine and alcohol addiction that has already occurred in America to very young children, and this is a problem we have to save our children from."[139]

She testifies of miraculous healing from eliminating dairy.

A variety of symptoms are produced by allergenic foods, such as:

- Cough and croup (a barking cough)
- Allergy like symptoms (runny nose and itchy eyes)
- Asthma like symptoms (wheezing, tight chest, and trouble breathing)
- Excess mucous
- Eczema
- Congestion and a host of others

This is because adding acidic sugar to acidic fat to acidic dairy (body heat raises acid-levels of milk) makes for a chronically inflamed body.

Whole milk has benefits. But 75 percent of the world is lactose intolerant and unable to receive any of milk's benefits.[140]

If you have allergies, digestive problems, fertility, hormonal, or respiratory issues, dairy is a problem food. Its estrogen hormones are a risk factor for infertility and cancers, especially prostate cancer and asthma.[141]

Dairy has been marketed to us as a great source of calcium for the bones. Yet, research has proven that too much calcium and calcium itself is not enough to prevent osteoporosis.[142]

In fact, cow's milk is attributed to the greatest number of fractures.[143] With so much milk and cheese consumption in the United States, it's a wonder why the number of hip replacements has increased 205 percent from 2000–2010 in the middle aged.[144]

Funny, I was on the plane with two middle-aged men next to me, and the topic was their recent hip replacements. I think I did a praise dance when I got off that plane.

A better idea is a holistic vitamin and mineral profile. Vitamin D, K, A, and others are more directly related to better bone health.[145] You can find great nutrition for all the body's systems in fruits and vegetables, going back to Genesis 1:29–30.

Kale has 150 mg of calcium versus milk at 125 mg. Kale provides true nourishment to the bones and all other systems, whereas dairy may provide calcium but robs lung capacity. Take dairy out of the diet and the skin clears up too. Personally, I needed allergy medicine a few times a month for years. After eliminating dairy, I haven't needed any allergy medicine.

God's best foods add health without sorrow.

Thankfully, we can substitute with creamy avocado, nut milks, and amazing vegan cheese spreads.

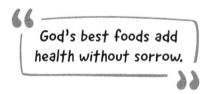

God's best foods add health without sorrow.

Have you tried nice cream? You can get the texture and flavor of ice cream with frozen bananas in a variety of fun flavors. Just unpeel, freeze, and blend bananas for a delicious substitute.

We've eaten dairy products for a long time, but the quality of dairy has diminished. As a child, it was super fun to go to the dairy farm with my grandfather. But where are those dairy cows now? I'll answer that in Chapter 24.

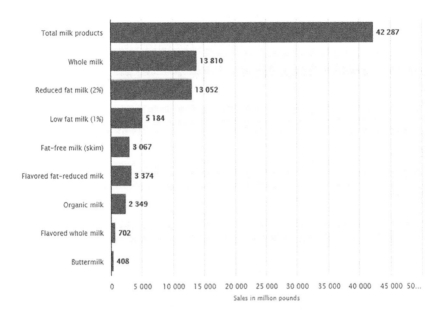

Chart 22.5   Milk Product Sales in the US[146]

Per the chart, if everyone's buying it, it's probably best to pass. Milk and milk-based products are the highest selling foods in the United States.[147]

The promise of a land flowing with milk and honey did motivate the Israelites to get to their promised land (Exodus 3:17). Your personal promised land free from weight and eating bondage may flow with almond milk and maple syrup, but it'll be yours, nonetheless.

Remember that we want to avoid the broad way, which is the highway to hospitals, as much as possible.

Chocoholics

Chocoholics are self-identified food addicts who can't get enough chocolate. Did you notice in the addictive foods chart that chocolate is number one? Cacao is packed with nutrition. In one bar there's 59 percent magnesium, 70 percent iron, and 25 percent of potassium daily needs.

Chocolate is the ultimate food for an emotional hug because it elevates serotonin due to its tryptophan contents and can provide feelings of love and affection because of its oxytocin content. Oxytocin is a powerful neurotransmitter stimulated by emotional bonding, such as a mother and her child or a husband and wife.

Confession: I once ate four large chocolate bars in one setting. And that was only part of the problem, the other part was that it was only 9 a.m.

I was looking for mother love. See, the week I gorged on chocolate my mom had ignored me, emotionally cutting me off. I told you my dad story in Chapter 3, but my mom story needed a couple books of its own. Namely, *Undiagnosed* a memoir and *How To Not Suck as a Mom: An 8 Step Action Plan To Win Back the Heart of Your Adult Child and Find Your Joy*. As you can tell from the titles, I needed motherly love and comfort that chocolate was rather equipped to provide.

Chocolate is a powerful thing to help feel some love when you need it. So, I can't argue that it didn't comfort.

It's just not a good treatment for sad moods or emotional issues because it creates emotional roller coasters due to its other components of sugar and dairy.

And Lord knows I needed therapy, not chocolate.

Components of sugar, refined fats (in cheaper brands), and milk powder make it irresistible and addictive.

Cacao powder, chocolate in the raw form, is a great alternative for baking and hot chocolate. It's loaded with minerals, but it's difficult to overindulge on cacao when used with alternative natural sweeteners like agave or stevia and nut milk.

If our diets are low in fruits and vegetables, especially dark green, leafy ones, we'll continue to crave. But chocolate also contains caffeine.

And yes, caffeine is addictive too.

Running on Coffee and Jesus

Are you struggling with coffee, chocolate, soda, or energy drinks? We don't have processed foods anonymous yet, but caffeine has made it. And most adults drink a cup daily. Unlike processed food addiction, *The Diagnostic and Statistical Manual of Mental Disorders* officially recognizes Caffeine Use Disorder as a substance addiction.

Several studies have knocked out the fantasy that it's not. In four studies, 30 to 93 percent of participants met criteria for Caffeine Use Disorder.[148]

For a Caffeine Use Disorder diagnosis, all three of the following criteria need to be endorsed:[149]

1. a persistent desire or unsuccessful effort to control use,

2. use despite harm, and

3. withdrawal.

Caffeine has its own addiction centers just like alcohol. Caffeine is another highly socially accepted drug of choice.

Coffee does have antioxidant powers and nutrients and can ward off disease. In combined studies with over 450,000 participants, those who drank one cup daily reduced diabetes type 2 risk by 7 percent per cup.[150] Studies show that coffee may also support prevention of dementia, Alzheimer's, Parkinson's, liver damage, and other risks.[151]

But the best benefits are from decaf not regular.

However, if you struggle with sleep per Chapter 10, caffeine will further hinder rest. Poor sleep is a direct assault to our waistlines and makes us vulnerable to problem foods and overeating.[152]

Also, most pair coffee with other addictions like sugar, artificial sweeteners, and/or heavy cream. Research does also show that the weight and eating struggle will continue to be a struggle for those who consume caffeine.[153]

Sadly, not much competes with coffee but Jesus, apparently, on some T-shirts I've seen. Yerba matte, carob drinks, or plain old water may eliminate the need for a fix.

Alcohol Is Processed Food Too

Alcohol takes grains like rye and beats it into Grey Goose to order at the bar.

Besides chronic diseases, the number of fatalities from alcohol use is our third leading preventable cause of death, right after tobacco and poor diet.[154] People are sobering up as sales of mocktails are increasing while beer is decreasing.[155]

Tiny benefits of red wine are offset by the numerous subtractions to health. And you're better off just eating grapes to get the same benefits.[156]

Alcohol is toxic to every system of the body, like refined sugar and refined oils. Alcohol is addictive and causes binge drinking that contributes to 75 percent of alcohol burden costs on society, which includes car accidents and injuries.[157]

Several medical professionals and establishments suggest that alcohol be removed from the diet for optimum health. In one of the largest studies on alcohol usage in 195 countries, researchers said this: "The widely held view of the health benefits of alcohol needs revising ... [all data] continued to show how much alcohol use contributes to global death and disability. Our results show that the safest level of drinking is none."[158]

Like sugar, we need zero alcohol for health.

The National Cancer Institute says the removal of alcohol may prevent a variety of cancers.[159] Studies show that alcohol intake puts us at risk for "mouth, throat, colon, and liver" cancers.[160] And one daily drink increases mouth and throat cancer by 20 percent.[161]

> **Like sugar, we need zero alcohol for health.**

The Breast Cancer Prevention organization warns that women who drink three glasses of wine or alcohol per day increase their chances of cancer by 15 percent, which increases by 10 percent for each additional drink.[162]

And the beer belly isn't a fallacy. Obesity, weight problems, and alcohol consumption are highly correlated in several studies.[163]

A large set of research shows that those who've had bariatric surgery often become alcoholics.[164] Wine and alcohol may be tasty, but besides excess weight, dehydration, or more life troubles, it causes sooner than desired wrinkles that Botox cannot fix.[165]

> " The beer belly isn't a fallacy. Obesity, weight problems, and alcohol consumption are highly correlated in several studies. "

Several Scriptures speak to sobriety: 1 Peter 1:13, 1 Peter 5:8, 1 Thessalonians 5:6–8, Romans 13:13, Galatians 5:19–21, and several more.

No judgment, but as believers it's a good goal to reduce or eliminate alcohol for several reasons but mostly for our mental sobriety as God's army.

And what are you doing at the bar anyway? Go home.

Letting Go

Problem foods are like cigarettes. The tides are changing as we get smarter, but it took thousands of studies, twenty-five years of research, and many people to die from cancer before the tobacco industry was sanctioned.[166]

Despite thousands of studies with clear evidence on the dangers of processed foods and addictive, toxic ingredients discussed, we still may have a long way to go.

Abortion is another free choice I liken unto problem foods. I am pro-life. Most people who choose abortion don't realize they're taking their own child's life.

Did you see *Unplanned*? If not, check it out. That movie sums up deception quite well.

I had an abortion when I was a teenager. And I wish I hadn't. In a deep healing prayer session with the Holy Spirit, I lamented about who I was to do such a heinous act. How much could I have hated myself to not regard my own child's budding life? If I had known who I was and whose I was, I wouldn't have done such a hateful act to myself or that child. But that's the power of deception for you.

Problem foods are pro-life or pro-choice murder too—only more slowly. But the results are in. Problematic processed foods and ingredients kill the arteries, organs, quality of life, and ultimately cut your life short. Clearly, it's best to happily let them go, grieve if you must, and eat foods made by nature.

> **Problematic processed foods and ingredients kill the arteries, organs, quality of life, and ultimately cut your life short.**

I want you to think about your identity for a moment.

Who are you to continue to live your life around your problem foods?

Who are you to be willing to damage your body, increase chances of risk, stay in the food crazy camp, or carry around the heaviness of excess weight? What does eating fake foods say about you spiritually? Mentally? Emotionally?

What does it mean about who you are spiritually to willingly take part in the Satanic Addictive Deception?

Let's not keep buying bigger sizes to accommodate for our self-harm. We're not created to play small. God hasn't called us to fit in. He's called us to stand out and to stand up to the unloving, unhealthy, false nutrition of the Standard American Diet.

Allow your Whole & Free identity in Christ to emerge—an identity beyond weight and eating struggles.

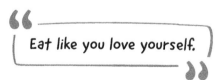

> **Eat like you love yourself.**

Eat like you love yourself.

Eat to love and honor God.

Only you can commit to healing yourself. What you'll find when you reduce your addictive ingredients and shut the door on problem foods is that you'll feel amazing. You'll discover how easy it can be to live and eat healthfully.

You'll find it easy to plan meals, exercise, finish projects, and clean your house. Your confident self, healthiest body, and food power returns. Everything gets better when these foods exit your psyche. Let's let them go, shall we?

Part Three: Win the Food Addiction Battle

How to Rebuke the Sugar Demon and Her Cheesy Cousins for Good!

Right before God told us what to eat, He said, "Be fruitful and multiply, replenish the earth and subdue it. Have dominion over every living thing" (Genesis 1:28).

The way we eat is supposed to fuel a greater purpose of fruitfulness, and we have God-given dominion over food. To get our food power back, it's important to get the addictive foods out.

There are two main models for treating addiction. The first is the disease model that has infiltrated our society. This model says that you cannot control your addiction because it's a disease. It tells you to attend recovery groups or expensive rehabilitation programs for life to survive the disease. Food addiction rehabilitation programs can be upwards of thirty thousand dollars.

However, after much research, there is no evidence of the disease model in the Word of God. Although there are benefits, the disease model has a questionable success rate, is very expensive to treat, and continues dependency on the disease model to stay intact.

And yes, certain substances will always interact with the brain in the same way. Any working brain exploited by an unnatural or refined substance can cause it to be enslaved to that substance.

The second model of addiction says that if we commit to abstinence despite any reason to partake, we're free from the addiction. This is the habit choice model of addiction that's fully aligned with the Word of God.

This model has an extremely high success rate, costs nothing to treat, and gives you back your God-given food power.

In other words, if you binge on chocolate, it's your responsibility to end your relationship with chocolate, for good.

Chocoholism, solved.

Once solved, you won't have to worry about addiction because you won't consume it ever again. You become a normal person who simply doesn't eat chocolate.

Do alcoholics continue to drink a little?

No, because the way we become unaddicted is by not ever engaging in the thing we're addicted to again. Not ever. You're uncomfortable with that, but I'll share with you why as we go.

The way we become unaddicted is by not ever engaging in the thing we're addicted to again.

Battle Strategy #1 – Apply Supernatural Self-Talk

Jack Trimpey was a social worker who tried everything to defeat his chronic alcohol addiction. Well, he did, and he's helped countless alcoholics, food addicts, and drug addicts since with his methods for *Rational Recovery*.

He teaches how to recognize and externalize the voice of addiction and then disobey it. I've taken these principles and applied them with the Word of God in a book called *Supernatural Self-Talk*.

Self-talk comes from a variety of places. For food addiction, self-talk comes from the midbrain, a primitive, carnal, survival part of our brains. This midbrain is all about survival and carries our core human wiring for procreation (sex) and food.

Essentially, we have two brains: the intelligent and the animal.

Our best thinking is done in the neo or pre-frontal cortex of the brain. This is the part of us that wants to stop our poor relationship with food.

Our primitive thinking is done in the midbrain, what we call our beast, and only wants to eat highly palatable foods.

It has no other desires or aspirations.

You (the neocortex) can gain power over 'it' the beast (the midbrain).

In the images of the structural model of the brain, you can see that the beast brain is a part of an innate intelligent survival system that drives primitive behaviors for pleasure.

The only reason we want highly palatable foods is for deep pleasure.

The Two-Part Brain

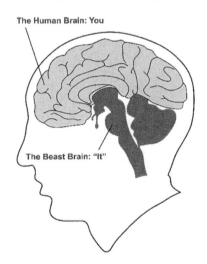

The Structural Model of Addiction

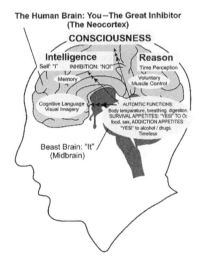

Illustration 22.6   Image of the Brain [167] Note: Our brains are complex, but the simplicity of two parts is helpful for the purpose of ending addictions with problem foods via the steps below.

Follow the steps below to apply *Supernatural Self-Talk*.

Step One: Name and Externalize the Addictive Voice

Jack Trimpey and his wife Lois Trimpey call the addictive voice the Feast Beast for food addicts. In *Rational Recovery*, they call it the Beast, for alcoholics and substance users.

Dr. Glenn Livingston, PhD, author of *Never Binge Again*, calls it, rather appropriately, the Pig. In Dr. Livingston's work with the Pig, he provides detailed support to end binges in his coaching programs. He describes binges as eating problem foods or anything you don't want on your food plan, which we'll discuss.

Marsha calls her beast the Sugar Demon as it represents to her the nature of what her beast calls her to do—harass her to eat sugar.

In Genesis 4:7, God warned Cain that *sin* was crouching at the door, waiting to devour him.

God externalized and named the voice that was driving Cain to sinful behavior, Sin. Sin is another name for the beast.

Pick out a name for your beast to separate your beast (the voice of addiction) from your truth.

Step Two: Recognize When the Beast Speaks

Jack Trimpey termed the skill of recognizing the addictive voice the Addictive Voice Recognition Technique (AVRT®). You can hear your addictive voice clearly when you say to yourself, *I don't eat chocolate ever.*

Doubtful thoughts as well as suggestive thoughts to eat the addictive food will provide you with a bounty of comments from the addictive voice or Beast Baloney—or as Dr Livingston calls it, Pig Squeal®.

Thoughts like, *That's impossible! I can't do that! I'll feel so deprived! That's crazy!* and *Everyone eats chocolate from time to time,* are all examples of Beast Baloney or the voice of addiction that cons us into fatness, lethargy, unhappiness, poor health, food crazies, prescription drugs, and bingeing.

The more you recognize its persuasive vocabulary, the more you can disarm its power. It's tricky because your beast uses language that sounds like you and even uses the pronoun "I" to deceive you.

Let's practice.

You hear in your head: "I've read a long chapter. My head hurts. I really deserve this (problem food or ingredient)."

Is it you or your beast? If you've guessed beast, you're right! It's the beast trying to start some food trouble. See, you can learn this skill.

We can recognize who's talking when we consider where the suggestion will lead us. So, ask yourself, "What does this suggestion want me to do?" If the suggestion leads you off track in your eating, then you know it's your beast, not you.

Remember your beast has one goal—to get into food trouble.

Step Three: Disarm your Beast's Power

Your beast can only suggest what it wants you to do because it has no arms, legs, or hands to do it itself. The suggestion is only powerful when your physically do what it suggests.

The beast has no power at all.

It cannot do anything, only you can.

You have all the power.

You're the one with a physical body to: get your car keys off the counter, open the door, walk to your car, open the car door, start the car, drive to the fast-food joint, order a cheeseburger, go to the window, pay, drive away, unwrap the package, eat the cheeseburger, and pull up to your home.

God provides many points to escape temptation (1 Corinthians 10:13). Each point from thought to action is an escape.

Cain also didn't see the impulsive nature of the beast. God let Cain know that he didn't have to listen to the voice of sin. It was Cain's choice to obey sin. You can disobey your beast. You can stop the impulse to act because your beast has no hands, legs, or car keys—it only has suggestive words in a fictitious mouth.

It cannot act.

Therefore, it's completely disarmed upon recognition of its lack of power and your ownership of yours.

Step Four: Realize Your Beast Only Wants One Thing

Your beast doesn't care about you. Not even a little bit. All it wants is the donut. It doesn't care that you have prediabetes, your pants don't fit, you hate your body, or you've struggled to get free from donuts for years.

It just wants the donut.

So, think about this: where will you end up if you keep obeying your beast's suggestions? Where will you be next year if you listen to the beast instead of your truth? How will you handle another five years of the same food mistakes and their consequences? How will God feel if you keep choosing your beast over Him?

And which of your heart's desires will be delayed?

Your beast will lead you far from the abundant life.

So, say the cold, hard, truth about your beast out loud: "My beast is ruthless. It doesn't care about me, my health, my marriage, my spiritual life, my obedience to God, my love for my family, or anything else that matters. It wants what it wants to my detriment and ultimately my demise. It wants to eat junk, bring me to poverty, keep me stuck, never complete my project, sabotage my marriage, and ultimately kill, steal, and destroy me and my family line, destiny, and mission for the kingdom of God" (John 10:10).

"It's absolutely true. You caught me. I just want to binge on my problem foods! Can we get a donut now?"—your beast.

Repeat the cold, hard, truth about your beast one more time.

Let the words go deep. Sobering, isn't it?

This beast, if obeyed, can cause you to end up with amputated legs, on medications for life, and bitter with many regrets of not recognizing its stupid antics sooner.

Step Five: Create Your Problem Food Plan

The best way to know the voice of your beast is with a clearly written, black-and-white plan.

If you have no plan or strategy for the future use of your problem foods, a taste could turn into a month-long binge.

Remember, I'm not the food police.

You get to decide what you want to eat and do with your life. I'm your coach to empower you to choose God's best for yourself.

Problem Food Plan Example

A problem food elimination plan sounds like this: I will never eat (insert problem foods and ingredients) again. Not ever, not when (your usual excuses). I don't want it for any reason whatsoever for the rest of my life, through eternity.

You may need to specify conditions that you can agree to, but once the plan is created, write it down.

Your plan must be black and white so that you know if your beast is suggesting otherwise or not. If someone offers you a KitKat bar, you can say with confidence, "No thanks. I don't want sugar."

A law or plan promotes freedom. God created the Ten Commandments so that we would know who He is and how to honor His ways.

To love Him is to obey Him. It's a good thing that thou shall not murder, covet, or dishonor parents. It's a great thing that we should love the Lord our God with all our hearts, minds, and souls and love our neighbors as ourselves as the primary laws in the kingdom of God.

These laws are health to our bones, life-giving, and promote goodness on the Earth. Without laws or guidelines there's too much gray. And your beast has a hay day with gray! It thrives on food confusion and ambiguity.

Never is the only language that makes sure your beast doesn't have any loopholes to pervert your choices. If it thinks it will have fun after your twenty-one-day vegan cleanse, your seven-day sugar fast, or after you've lost thirty pounds, it will wait patiently to pounce on you then.

So never is the best language for it and establishes your future for success. Never also helps you quickly recognize when the beast speaks so that you can target the lies and doubts.

Never can be renewed every day. Take it one day at a time. Develop your confidence that you can let go of your problem foods for the rest of your life. Just like you'll never slap your grandmother or rob a bank, you can plant the seed of never engaging with certain problem foods again.

Without a clearly defined plan for our problem foods, your Sugar Demon or Cheesy Chucky will plot on sabotaging you.

Susie struggled with fried chicken. She went through the drive through at least three times a week.

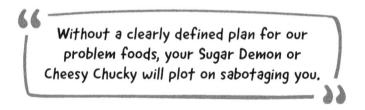

> Without a clearly defined plan for our problem foods, your Sugar Demon or Cheesy Chucky will plot on sabotaging you.

Her plan: "I will never eat fried chicken again—not ever, not when I'm tired, lonely, upset, or don't feel like cooking. I won't eat it for any reason whatsoever for the rest of my life through eternity."

When tempted to get fried chicken, Susie rebuked her beast like follows.

Susie's Beast: "Yeah, right you'll be headed to get your usual fried chicken place tonight. Who wants to live without fried chicken? That's no fun."

Susie: "No, I'm never eating fried chicken or any wheat products or refined flours ever again. You can't do anything, only I can. I have the power here, not you. I don't really want fried chicken; it's not healthy, and it's not helping me. So that's that."

Susie went on to release weight and gain back her sanity. It's also helpful to specify an alternative. Susie opted baked, unbreaded chicken as desired. Her alternative supported her to break free of fried versions.

Since problem foods have already done such damage to your life, as well as all the people pleasing, accept your plan and its wisdom unapologetically.

No need to explain, argue, or rationalize with others or your beast about it.

Any doubt isn't you—it's the beast.

Any food pushers (friends and family) who insist you eat food you don't want is their beast trying to seduce yours.

Use your best thinking to create a fool-proof problem foods plan. Add alternatives and usage instructions for them, such as Susie's commitment to eat baked instead of fried chicken.

Step Six: Analyze How to Prevent Going Off Plan

If you do go off your plan, it's important to know how to prevent it in the future. The foundation was laid in Book 1 for you to be a strong analyst to prevent overeating and poor food choices to avoid breaking your food plan.

Relapsing isn't a problem in this method because you're committed to never consume the problem foods or beverages again. But if you're off plan, you know the beast is out of its lair.

So, if you eat off plan, first figure out what triggered a taste of your old problem foods and what you can do to prevent it in the future. Then, decide right then and there never to eat or drink it again. Finally, silence your beast for good by telling it, "I am never eating (problem food/ingredient) ever again."

Susie met her friends for dinner and was so famished that she took a bite out of the chicken finger appetizer once she sat down.

When she realized that her beast got her, she figured she was vulnerable due to hunger. Going forward, she'll drink more water and pack a piece of fruit.

Susie cuffed her sneaky beast, recommitted to her freedom from fried chicken, and joined the dinner conversation.

And while there are lots of reasons for entertaining your beast, such as lack of sleep, dehydration, hormones, emotional upset, and spiritual neglect, don't allow any to be an excuse to eat off plan.

But if you have a taste, don't waste a second condemning yourself.

Another principle of *Supernatural Self-Talk* is never to condemn yourself. Jesus didn't, and you don't need to either.

Your beast loves your condemnation because in the past it used your bad feelings to get you to binge. Now that you can see it for what it is, you can analyze, recommit, and move on with your life.

I know your beast is nervous right now because its master is picking up her lost dominion and using it. Get good at this skill; it's a simple solution to a lifelong problem.

Many have broken their food addiction from their unshakeable decision to never engage with their problem food again.

And while your beast only seeks pleasure, isn't your biggest pleasure the peace, sanity, joy, and much easier slimness that comes from finally owning your power?

You can do it without making a big fuss, attending meetings, or winning tokens. You don't need to tell anyone, explain, or track the number of days free from your problem foods. You just need to mean business by taking back your power from a truly powerless, smack-talking beast.

Battle Strategy # 2 – Go Cold Turkey

Jesus said, "If your right eye causes you to sin, pluck it out and cast it from you; for it is more profitable for you that one of your members perish, than for your whole body to be cast into hell" (Matthew 5:29).

Let's turn this into a situational success verse: If my problem food causes me to sin (self-harm), I need to stop eating it and get it out of my system completely, for it is more profitable for me that I reject the problem ingredient than for my whole body to be cast into disease, sickness, and turmoil.

I think He was trying to tell us not to believe the moderation of the junk food lie.

I do. I really do.

Many can attest to the fact that it's easier to stop eating sugar and junk food altogether than it is to attempt moderation again and fail.

With moderation the substance is still in your system, which sparks the Addictive Game anytime you're vulnerable and further delays the benefits of food freedom by another five, ten, or thirty years.

We don't have time for that.

In Part One, I emphasized that food addiction is a pervasive and progressive disease.

Dr. Vera Tarman, author of *Food Junkies: Recovery from Food Addiction*, proves the best and most successful plan for us is abstinence from problem foods. You know your problem food history, and when you abstain completely, you won't repeat the history.

Moderation is not an option for problem foods. Have you tried it successfully? Haven't you felt your best in periods of abstinence? Is it time to sustain that abstinence for life? I hope so because we thrive when we let these foods go and replace them with alternatives that don't cause the same struggles.

Abstinence brings rewards that are deep and profound. (See Victory Morsels.)

Here are some tips for going Cold Turkey:

Boldly Face Withdrawal

There are two things that going cold turkey does for you: gets your brain unhooked and your taste buds back in order. You can start now or pick a date.

Undoubtedly the first couple days you'll hear Beast Baloney saying things like, "I can eat a little. Just one bite won't hurt. Do I really need to let sugar go?" But you already know what to do.

With the tips below withdrawal can be surprisingly easy:

- Have simple, balanced meals, and food supplies ready
- Decide alternatives options to have on hand
- Dedicate time to making new healthful recipes
- Watch videos about the benefits of going problem ingredient free
- Keep your schedule full
- Avoid tempting places and environments
- Clean up the kitchen and refrigerator from problem foods
- Get at least seven hours of sleep each night
- Hydrate

Withdrawal doesn't last long, but the benefits are lifelong.

The acute withdrawal period for a problem food or ingredient can last anywhere from three to ten days, but total withdrawal can take up to a month. Use water to flush your system and support your body's natural healing processes.

Cold-like symptoms, headaches, nausea, irritability, or down feelings are all positive signs your body is cleansing.

When you say no to problem foods, you say yes to finishing what you start.

You say yes to your dreams.

You say yes to more of God.

As you let go of your problem foods for good, you'll gain back your belief in yourself, confidence in your food power, and restore your taste buds to sanity.

> As you let go of your problem foods for good, you'll gain back your belief in yourself, confidence in your food power, and restore your taste buds to sanity.

And, while you may still have problems and trauma to deal with to make you a better you, it's all easier when your problem foods aren't there to delay transformation. You can move forward freely to grow, heal, and prosper.

Don't delay withdrawal because you're afraid to make changes overnight. It was overnight that I stopped eating fast food three times per day.

You can be an overnight success too.

Don't Believe the Deprivation Lie

Deprivation is a feeling stimulated by the survival mechanism the beast uses to get you to pick up your problem foods. It groans and moans about how deprived it is now that (problem food) has been removed.

Don't be gullible.

We don't need problem foods to survive or to be happy.

What we need is Jesus and real food.

We may feel we're missing something. In truth, deprivation is another sign of withdrawal and the tactics your beast uses to get you to engage with your food idols.

Deprivation is a normal feeling as you change highly tasty foods to normal tasting ones.

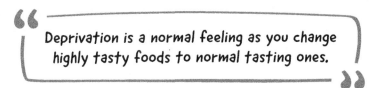

> Deprivation is a normal feeling as you change highly tasty foods to normal tasting ones.

Technically, deprivation is a state of being kept from possessing, enjoying, or using something.[168]

To outsmart feeling deprived, we must firm up our belief that we choose not to have it—that we really don't want it in our systems. You are free to eat whatever you want, whenever you want.

Only you don't want your problem foods. It's not that you "can't" eat them because you can. Only you don't want to eat them because you don't want the cravings, binge episodes, nutrient theft, or mind control.

Make it 100 percent your choice to reject foods that have harmed your life. Don't make yourself a sulking victim but choose victory. I don't is more victorious than I can't.

Plus, can we really be deprived of something we never should've had in the first place? We may feel disadvantaged, but these allergenic, highly palatable foods have taken advantage of our brains, beauty, and desire to be obedient to God's instructions to eat nature's loving foods.

Dive into feelings of deprivation. As we do, the hole in our soul we've filled with problem foods can start to reveal its truth.

As we heal through these feelings and learn to live without the problem foods, we can explore a new world of abundance of foods and fulfillment in life. No food can ever fill that place deep inside that screams for love.

The best thing to do is get on the floor and cry out to God to fill this place, not stuff it. "For He satisfies the longing soul and fills the hungry soul with goodness" (Psalm 107:9).

Decide Your Alternatives

We're super blessed to have many options for alternatives. One of the best ways to shut up the beast is to find alternatives that don't activate Beast Baloney. Over time, we figure out what works and what doesn't.

Marsha found that dark maple syrup didn't drive her out of control like sugar did. She set a guideline and only had up to two tablespoons when desired. She could keep this guideline because maple syrup didn't cause an addictive response for her, but other sugars like agave or coconut sugar were triggers.

Lisa chose a low sugar protein bar instead of the chocolate bar offering only high sugar and high fat. And, as a tasty alternative to wheat-based crackers, Kelly chose rice or flax crackers without added preservatives when she wanted some crunch.

Instead of ordering out, you can make the same thing in, without the added salts, oils, and sugars. Instead of fried fries, make homemade baked ones.

These days, entire meals like lasagna can be made from fresh vegetables, nuts, and seeds. Check out raw foods recipes to get more nutrition.

Research alternatives that won't give you the food crazies or sabotage your health efforts. It may take some experimentation and time, but you can learn to enjoy your food and live without problem foods.

You can do this!

Know Your White Stuff Threshold

The addictive ingredients in the Standard American Diet work kind of like an action movie.

If you were being chased by one ninja (salt), perhaps you'll slide through a window and get away. But if you were combated by a gang of ninjas (sugar, milk, flour, salt, and caffeine), you may not be so enthusiastic about your escape skills.

Most of us can get pretty beat up because we don't have Bruce Lee skills to combat the multiple addictive ingredients without craving more and more.

If you're Bruce Lee, well, praise the Lord for the dead has risen!

When cravings happen, you've gone over your *white stuff threshold* or the amount you can tolerate without initiating the Addictive Game— cravings, binges, and the need for withdrawal.

If it's difficult or you tend to have to strive to let problem foods go, that just means something sneaked into your mouth that shouldn't have, causing urges or cravings to eat the wrong stuff. Perhaps you didn't read the ingredient label or there were added sugars in the restaurant meal you ate the night before.

Any *white stuff* in the blood makes us crave more of it.

The goal is to get these substances out in order to make it easier to keep the beast quiet. But no matter what, a break from problem foods is necessary to gain strength.

Frankly, I don't make a stink when some sugar slips into a meal. I just make sure that it's a miniscule amount that won't cause me to go over my *white stuff threshold* because my tolerance for sugar is low and wheat-flour almost nonexistent. And at this point, I choose none of them because the benefits of none have far outweighed the costs of a little.

We all have a *white stuff threshold.* Monitor your food cravings to get to know yours. And if your beast gets especially loud, you've gone over it.

Get Support

A food addiction recovery group of your choice may support you on the journey. It's great to connect with others who get it.

Personally, I've enjoyed these groups when I needed the support to connect with others who understand and keep me on track. But I've seen some cohorts get more obese because they weren't willing to let go of the addictive foods.

Some participants still search for the root cause without removing the actual cause of food addiction—addictive foods! We need to remove the addictive foods from our lives and do our part to gain full confidence in that decision.

If you need support, reread Chapter 5 for some ideas. It's also preferred to connect with groups that validate your healthiest self, like hiking, fitness, personal growth, or healthy eating groups to stay on track. We'll touch on this point again in future chapters.

I'm Not Ready!

Despite the pain of food addiction, some still prefer a reduction strategy versus elimination to fit in with culture or societal norms. God's grace is sufficient.

And I realize it can all feel very overwhelming, especially if your current way of eating is mostly processed or Standard American Diet fare.

I understand.

Start with replacing one or two problem foods for now as you transition.

Reduction or moderation is possible but not as effective to win for good. If you introduce problem foods back into your system, you'll need strong boundaries and correct frequencies (how often you consume) around these ingredients as well as not living in any food fear (the fear of food dominating and making you binge). We'll discuss more in Chapter 29.

And still pray for a miracle of changing overnight and act accordingly. Remember faith without works is dead (James 2:20).

You've Got This

When it comes to food addiction, we don't have peace with problem foods and ingredients in our lives.

And when we know to do better and don't do it, it's sin (James 4:17). When we let go, we gain. Whenever we let go of sin, God is faithful to reward obedient behavior.

All unrighteousness is sin (1 John 5:7). But he who sows righteousness *will have* a sure reward (Proverbs 11:18). Amen.

What is it that you've been waiting to come through that hasn't yet? How long have you been praying about your health? Or body weight? Or food freedom?

Perhaps, it's the constant regret from these problem foods that God may want you to lay down so that He can provide you that reward.

God's intention is certainly for us not to be a slave to food.

In response to questions around continuing to sin, Paul said, "Certainly not! How shall we who died to sin live any longer in it?" (Romans 6:2). "Therefore, do not let sin reign in your mortal body, that you should obey its lusts. And do not present your members as instruments of unrighteousness to sin but present yourselves to God as being alive from the dead, and your members as instruments of righteousness to God" (Romans 6:12–13).

Funny, how he says that sin reigns inside the body. Nothing gets inside our bodies more than food!

A part of you will get very excited about all the possibilities you can create by letting problem foods go from your life once and for all.

Jack Trimpey calls this excitement the Abstinence Commitment Effect, which is the sustained, uplifted feelings that arise from your food plan, restoring your human spirit, family values, and joy![169]

I hope you feel ecstatic that you'll release weight and get your energy and life back.

Keep your reasons for change in front of you.

"Let us lay aside every weight, and the sin which so easily ensnares us, and let us run with endurance the race that is set before us" (Hebrews 12:1).

In other words, you've got this!

REFLECT & SHARE

1. Why do I want to let go of my problem foods and ingredients?
2. Where will I end up if I don't change my food choices?
3. What does my beast say to get me to eat poorly?
4. What benefits will I gain as I let my food addiction go?
5. What support do I need to let my food addiction go?

PRAYER

Heavenly Father,

Thank you so much for helping me to understand that my cravings aren't my fault! You've opened my eyes to walk the narrow way and restore my sanity around food. I pray for a miracle to take hold of my taste buds. Help me to love the abundance of the food you've provided to heal my body, soul, and spirit.

I give you all my food idols. I repent for replacing my need for you with food. I repent for eating harmful things to my body. Please help me to walk in freedom. Increase my wisdom, knowledge, and understanding to reject the Standard American Diet and Satan's Agenda of Death for my life and ministry.

I rebuke the Sugar Demon and all her Cheesy Cousins right now. I choose to stand for truth over the Satanic Addictive Deception. Thank you for going before me to win the weight and eating war to help others get free as well!

In Jesus's mighty name we pray, amen.

CHAPTER 23

PERFORM A GLUTTONECTOMY, STAT

Battle #2 – Overeating

"Do not mix with winebibbers or gluttonous eaters of meat. For the drunkard and the glutton will come to poverty, and drowsiness will clothe a man with rags"

–PROVERBS 23:20-21

*"I felt it kick," I said, touching my belly.
"Oh, that was the jalapeno in my salsa, baby; I'm not pregnant."*

Part One: Understanding Overeating

An exciting baking contest was on television. The gourmet bakery chef teams were to construct a candylike, floury monument of each of the seven deadly sins. The crowd cheered as cakes of lust, greed, and sloth rounded up for the judges.

To represent gluttony, the bakers created a snarling pig with a bulging belly, sitting upright in piles of sauced up spaghetti noodles and surrounded by pastries.

Its mouth was stuffed with a dripping, nasty-looking bite while its hooves were ready with the next oversized food stuffing.

Who could bear to eat that explicit cake?

This gruesome cake depicts our cultural subconscious about

gluttony—an exposé of a sin masked as obesity, eating disorders, diets, and a plethora of diseases.

Gluttony in this chapter's context, isn't only our sweet, innocent inner child screaming for help as in Book 1. In Book 2 we're looking at the other side of overeating as an act of our blatant rebellion, puffed egos, and comfy culture, muting conviction and quenching the Spirit.

I'm warning that this chapter—who am I kidding, this whole book—is convicting for me as well as for you. But conviction creates the deepest change.

Trust the plans are good and defeating this doozey of a giant requires your openness.

Any ouch is the Holy Spirit doing surgery on our hearts since this issue is as tender as much as it's a pinch.

It's not my goal to offend.

It's my goal to set the captives free.

And we need to be real to be free.

So, keep reading. No matter how upset with me you get, remember that He chose me, a recovered glutton, to deliver the message! I cannot throw any stones. And my readers mean the world to me. Trust that the Holy Spirit is doing a mighty fine work!

By fine, I mean—fine, as in improved good looks.

A Little of This, a Little of That

What does overeating look like? Well, it doesn't have to be a formal, feast-like occasion, although it may be. It's the times you get repeated food ideas, a little of this, a little of that, and next thing you know—it's several calories later.

My brain may get the idea to eat some peanut butter an hour after I've eaten. Do I really need the peanut butter?

No, I just ate.

But mentally, the brain compels me to rumble through the cabinet to get a jar of peanut butter to stick my finger into.

I eat the peanut butter and then wonder how it would taste with nuts and cheese to go with it. Then it turns into tea with half a jar of honey and crackers to go with this random after-dinner party for one.

A healthy snack turned into 1,000 excess fat calories. Compulsive eating episodes are just that; you stop at the store and get one thing that leads to another and before you know it, the food is in your mouth, which ends up with an unamusing free ride on your thighs.

There are four types of overeaters:

- **The Binger** – A binger eats an objectively large amount in a short period of time.[1]

- **The Grazer** – A grazer eats all day and desires to eat all the time.

- **The Piler** – A piler eats normal meals with abnormal portion sizes; they pile it on.

- **The Driver** – A driver eats the wrong stuff; when they do eat, it's fast and packaged foods, although it may not be too much.

Which overeater type(s) do you resonate with most? Each overeater consumes more energy (calories) than their body functioning (organs, tissues, systems, and activity level) needs.

Each overeater demands much from their body's digestive resources. And each overeater may be a combination or flow in and out of types. Studies show that we consume more than we think we do, especially when we're overweight.[2]

All overeating stresses the body significantly. Overeating depletes gastric juices causing many of us to have low stomach acid and low counts of digestive enzymes causing malabsorption (see Chapter 7). Because we're more and more depleted over time in our digestive power, overeating is the primary reason we can't get away with the problem foods and ingredients we used to when we were younger.

Overeating also spikes insulin levels which causes continued weight gain and difficulty releasing weight despite our best efforts.

In a study by the University of Pennsylvania, binge eaters lost 1.9 percent of body weight over four years whereas the non-binge eaters lost 4.6 percent.[3] That's almost 250 percent more weight reduction for the non-bingers. We already know that one bad episode can hinder our health efforts.

So, healing overeating is vital to *Win the Weight & Eating War for Good.*

And overeating doesn't just stress the stomach, it stresses every single organ in the body—your heart, brain, intestines, liver, gallbladder, spleen, and kidneys.

We're designed to take heed to the voice of leptin, telling us to stop eating. If we keep eating ingredients that put duct tape on leptin's mouth and hide it in the closet, we're not going to yield the fruit of temperance in our lives.

What No Diet Book Told Us

Compulsive overeating is a primary behavioral, physiological, and spiritual component of weight and eating bondage that's most certainly missing in the average diet book.

No diet book says, "Hey Glutton, stop eating so much! Let yourself be hungry for once. Give the choppers a break for goodness sake!"

No, they give all sorts of meal plans and tell us, the gluttons, to eat in moderation. Like it's so easy to just not eat so much.

The victory for this battle is a commitment to move from periodic binge episodes, poor food choices, and overeating to recovered.

We're performing a gluttonectomy.

Once you have a gluttonectomy, all of life is better.

So, what's a glutton, let alone a gluttonectomy?

By definition:

Glutton
(glut·ton)
one given habitually to greedy and voracious eating and drinking[4]

Gluttonectomy

(glut·ton·nek·to·mi)

a commitment of removal of the behavior of compulsive overeating
(bingeing) and health demoting food choices in one's life

Gluttony is a compulsion to eat without discretion or control. Not
to be mistaken for the occasional gustatory fun or special occasion, but
what's become the common lifestyle of obsession with excessive, non-
health promoting food and drinks. In truth it's much bigger than foods
and has to do with our drive for more or excess.

Compulsive overeating or bingeing is the pull toward foods, typically those fun foods that aren't really food ... the highly palatable ones
we talked about that do nothing except jazz taste buds in a two second
sublime experience of the tongue.

With all those television food commercials oozing sexy cheese over
a burger or chocolate sauce over vanilla ice cream, of course we're falling
prey to temptation. As discussed, the nature of these highly palatable
foods causes us to eat more than we need.

Lately it seems as though our nation is taking glory in what should
be our shame. What if the shame of gluttony with our shameless supersized, extra-large portions of greasy indulgence was as socially acceptable
as people having orgies in the grocery store?

Nowadays, gluttony is just as socially acceptable as murder and sex
on television, even in ministry.

A pastor went to a weekend retreat with ministry leaders and was
disgusted.

"Jendayi, they ate so much it was blatant gluttony. The amount of
food and constant eating was beyond normal, and they were unashamed.
It made me sick to see it. I had to leave the table," the pastor confessed.

To witness gluttony can derive a feeling of disgust in others because
we know something is out of order. Just like we'd be disgusted if we
actually saw an orgie in the grocery store.

Watching folks who openly struggle with pre-diabetes, diabetes, pre-hypertension, hypertension, heart disease, cancer, and/or obesity have a food orgie around a long table can warrant nausea.

A mother confessed, "My daughter looks at me with disgust whenever I eat my cupcakes, so I eat them while hiding in my bedroom."

And a wife said, "My husband is so turned off by my eating that he doesn't eat with me anymore, and we don't go out to dinner." A man was divorced for his eating behaviors and the consequence of his binge eating on his relationship's emotional and sexual intimacy.

For some couples, gluttony eats away marriages because it affects all levels of intimacy. It can be a challenge for a spouse to be aroused by a partner whose gained significant weight over the years. And men especially have a need (not a want) for an attractive spouse to thrive in their marriages. But we've accepted the cultural norms of gluttony and the consequences.

What if we've been deceived that this sin reflected on our health and bodies is sin, leading not only to natural death and disease but spiritual death and disease?

An estimated 1 percent of those who struggle with weight and eating have a legitimate medical condition.[5] Most are challenged with binge eating and eating the wrong stuff.

The Global Burden of Disease 2017 study reports poor diet as the primary cause of death, above tobacco.[6]

Mike Atnip drove this point home. In his article titled *The Sin of Gluttony* he said, "We've convinced ourselves that our sin is an eating disorder or a medical problem and not a sin ... Because obesity is a leading preventable cause of death worldwide, and is preventable through temperance, then are we not called as Christians to prevent it?"[7]

Convicting or convicting?

> **The Global Burden of Disease 2017 study reports poor diet as the primary cause of death, above tobacco.**

Early Church Views of Gluttony

Back in the day, gluttony was looked at as a sin in that's not just overeating but food worship that directs our appetite away from Christ, dulls the mind, and causes sloth.

We've been quiet about our disorderly conduct around food choices in recent decades. *Christianity Today* published an article in 1995, "To Hell on a Cream Puff," saying, "Gluttonous impulse is a sign of disharmony with God's provision and creation, and it can disrupt the spiritual lives of people of every size."[8]

In 1840, *The Oberlin Evangelist* reported, "Excessive eating is the most common form of intemperance that prevails among mankind."[9]

And later in the nineteenth century, Russian Bishop Ignatius Brianchaninov said, "Wise temperance of the stomach is a door to all the virtues. Restrain the stomach, and you will enter Paradise. But if you please and pamper your stomach, you will hurl yourself over the precipice of bodily impurity, into the fire of wrath and fury, you will coarsen and darken your mind, and in this way you will ruin your powers of attention and self-control, your sobriety and vigilance."[10]

Ouch.

I told you this chapter hurts.

What are we doing?

The early church thought that the abundance of their food produced bodily ailments and, thus, damaged their bodies. Meanwhile, other people are damaging their bodies because they don't have enough nourishment and their bodies waste away.

Atnip said the two evils of gluttony are that we both harm our bodies (health) and don't give enough to those in need, which is a sign of greed.[11]

As of 2018, the World Health Organization reports 872 million people worldwide that are obese to 672 million that are starving.[12] In 2017, two billion people were overweight or obese, which is more than double the amount starving.[13] And more people die from obesity and obesity-related causes than those who are starving.

Both are forms of malnourishment.

The seven deadly sins were also the "fruits of a self-centered life or the "me-first" syndrome. They are lust, greed, wrath, envy, pride, sloth, and gluttony. In the same way, dieting can make us ignite vanity. Gluttony was eating for indulgence over nourishment, a reflection of the carnal versus spiritual Christian (see Chapter 4).

Alfonso Maria de Liguori, an 1835 author, said, "It's a defect to eat like beasts through the sole motive of sensual gratification ..."[14]

In summary, Gregory "The Great" called eating intemperance the following:[15]

- Eating to satisfy the tastes buds, not at appropriate mealtimes (snacking)
- Seeking delicacies and the best quality of food
- Seeking after sauces and seasonings for taste pleasure
- Exceeding the necessary amount of food
- Taking food with too much eagerness (overzealous to eat)

Gluttony also involved the "matter of timing, quality of food, use of stimulants, quantity, and undue eagerness in eating."[16]

The Anabaptists, an early Christian group, had very holy conduct that denounced "covetousness, pride, profanity, drinking, and gluttony."[17]

Perhaps they knew certain activities, including excess nibbling, could make God feel distant and also mute hearing the Holy Spirit.

Carnality is to do things only for self-indulgence and pleasure. Ascetism disapproves of doing anything for pleasure at all.

God has called us to the balance of holiness.

Holiness is to do what is right and joyfully accepts either the pleasure or the pain that accompanies the act.

It's seeking God's will in all things. Being intentionally unhealthy is unholy. It's necessary then for us to overcome overeating and dramatically improve our food quality.

Gluttony is:

- Idolatry – Seeking an end/deliverance/relief from excess food instead of God
- A hindrance in our relationship with God
- Greed and takes more than our fair share of food
- Consistent indulgence
- A lack of discretion

Gluttony isn't:

- Eating cardboard to satisfy only nutrition needs all the time
- Enjoying dessert
- Overeating or feasting on occasion
- Only about food
- Only a problem for heavy people

Gluttony can't be reduced to how much we weigh, although a heavy weight is a sign, but gluttony is a heart matter that affects every size.

A compulsive pull toward unhealthful foods is an issue for a normal weight or thin person just as much as a heavy person. It gives our heart to molten creations of our hands.

 A compulsive pull toward unhealthful foods is an issue for a normal weight or thin person just as much as a heavy person. It gives our heart to molten creations of our hands.

We love God when we obey Him. If we obey our stomach or the call for rich foods often, isn't that food and belly worship?

I'm guilty. How about you?

We reap what we sow.

Eating isn't just a nice meal, it's sowing.

It's an investment or a withdrawal into our bodies, souls, and spirits.

Like a bank, if we sow into our body excess food deposits, we create withdrawals that show up in medical bills, lethargy, depression, emotional and spiritual disconnect, and rather snug clothing.

God's View on Gluttony – A Bible Study

We've heard what the early church had to say. Let's hear what the Word of God says on the matter.

Gluttony first appeared in Genesis 2.

Eve was tempted by the serpent, who knew if she was truly hungry, but she surely ate the wrong stuff. She saw it was good for food, like our processed foods, and it was edible.

She ate, rebelling against God's instructions.

Then gluttony appears in Numbers. The children of Israel became frustrated with their provision, the manna, and whined about it to God.

"We want quail," they said to God.

And God said, "I'll give you quail."

Therefore, the Lord will give you meat, and you shall eat. You shall eat, not one day, nor two days, nor five days, nor ten days, nor twenty days, but for a whole month, until it comes out of your nostrils and becomes loathsome to you, because you have despised the Lord who is among you, and have wept before Him, saying, "Why did we ever come up out of Egypt?" (Numbers 11:18b–20).

Longing for the food they had when in bondage wasn't good. So later ...

And the people stayed up all that day, all night, and all the next day, and gathered the quail (he who gathered least gathered ten homers); and they spread them out for themselves all around the camp. But while the meat was still between their teeth, before it was chewed, the wrath of the Lord was aroused against the people, and the Lord struck the people with a very great plague. So he called the name of that place Kibroth Hattaavah, because there they buried the people who had yielded to craving (Numbers 11:32–34).

Don't we crave every day?

To yield to our cravings wasn't on His happy list.

See, these cravings were the pining for more than what was provided due to discontent and contempt with God.

It was a heart issue.

Let's look at Deuteronomy again. This one broke my heart.

And they shall say to the elders of his city, 'This son of ours is stubborn and rebellious; he will not obey our voice; he is a glutton and a drunkard.' Then all the men of his city shall stone him to death with stones; so you shall put away the evil from among you, and all Israel shall hear and fear (Deuteronomy 21:20–21).

Don't you want to thank God, yet again, for Jesus Christ who has reconciled us to the Father and saved us from the former law of sin and death?

Gluttony was a problem for God because He dwells in us.

Do you not know that you are the temple of God and that the Spirit of God dwells in you? If anyone defiles the temple of God, God will destroy him. For the temple of God is holy, which temple you are (1 Corinthians 3:16–17).

We don't defile with occasional feasting.

We defile by bringing poor health intentionally into our bodies.

We defile by stuffing ourselves with food as a means to fill our souls.

The Spirit of God want to fill our souls.

Think of it like this: have you ever driven by a beautiful church and thought, *Wow, that looks beautiful?*

The lawn was manicured, the building was well kept, and the freshly painted walls pose the most picturesque image of God's place. I love when I see a well-kept church. It feels like it represents God so well and His people.

But what would you do if you drove up to your church and found someone had vandalized it? Someone had shamelessly driven over the bushes, battered the glass windows, trashed the grounds, and stole its precious art and furniture—even the coffee bar.

Can you feel your heart sink?

If you were sad about the coffee bar alone, revisit the last chapter.

If someone did that to our church, I'd weep for that person who just didn't understand what they had done.

When we habitually indulge on certain foods, we're robbing our bodies of key nutrients, promoting disease.

God's Spirit dwells in us, evidenced by the act that moves of God are often performed through people. Our Builder values our temples to a higher degree than food giants lead us to believe.

We think it's okay to eat however we want and how much we want.

We break the biological laws of the holy temple, also known as our bodies, when we overeat physically, and we destroy our character when we have no temperance or discretion in our food and beverage choices or amounts.

To habitually choose to be a glutton is to love food, satisfying your flesh, more than God. To be carnally minded is death and against God (Romans 8:6–10). It's being governed by another master; therefore, it's idolatry.

Solomon said it this way:

> *When you sit down to eat with a ruler,*
> *Consider carefully what is before you;*
> *And put a knife to your throat*
> *If you are a man given to appetite.*
> *Do not desire his delicacies,*
> *For they are deceptive food*
> *(Proverbs 23:1–3).*

To be given to appetite or craving was a poor character trait that could put someone in a vulnerable position in life and cause them to sell their souls to evil practices.

When we're under the rulership of food, we gain a host of problems, especially deceit.

To be given to appetite meant that if we have no temperance with food, we could deceive ourselves of the motives of others.

In Proverbs 23:1–3, the ruler represents Satan who is luring the victim to his table or agenda instead of God's best agenda. The ruler can also be our own kingdom of self or what Pastor Paul Tripp calls our flesh pleasing nature.[18]

Deceptive food is bait to lure one from the right agenda to agree to a wicked one.

As Proverbs 23 warns, we need to carefully consider what we're consuming because it could place us in an agreement with an evil ruler's plans.

For we do not wrestle against flesh and blood, but against principalities, against powers, against the rulers of the darkness of this age, against spiritual hosts of wickedness in the heavenly places (Ephesians 6:12).

Addictive ingredients and processed foods are a part of that wicked agenda, Satan's Agenda for Death.

Let's sharpen our discernment to see our fuel as important to our impact in the kingdom. The ruler of this world wants to derail you by any means necessary to get you off track from God's agenda.

The best way to get you off track from God's best plans for your life is to make you sick from an addictive, deceiving diet. If he succeeds,

> The best way to get you off track from God's best plans for your life is to make you sick from an addictive, deceiving diet.

your time, energy, and money will go to pay for your illness via doctors' visits, prescriptions, and more addictive food than to nurture the good works God has called you to do to build the kingdom. Or they will cut your current ministry short.

See how the Satanic Addictive Deception all works in Victory Morsels.

Another example is when Esau wanted Jacob's red stew, so he irrationally sold his birthright to Jacob to get a taste of it (Genesis 25:29–34).

As Paul put it, "For a morsel of food" (Hebrews 12:16).

Esau regretted this choice; he was deceived on what he was giving up for the food he wanted in the moment.

Remember food that promises a good time now robs you of your healthiest you later.

We're deceived every time we yield to cravings or overeating. We're deceived that, "It's okay." But overeating isn't okay. Consistent poor choices need God's conviction because these poor choices can also make one poor.

> *Do not mix with winebibbers,*
> *Or with gluttonous eaters of meat;*
> *For the drunkard and the glutton will come to poverty,*
> *And drowsiness will clothe a man with rags (Proverbs 23:20–21).*

Overeating makes us drowsy and hurts our pockets. In a survey of 212 *Never Binge Again* readers, the average amount spent on binges per month was $360; that's $4,320 per year.[19] About 13 percent spent $11,520 per year on their binge foods.[20]

How much do you spend on yours?

America isn't only dealing with chronic health issues due to poor diet, but our favorite pastimes are eating and spending.

We're not only overweight, but we're in debt.

Northwestern Mutual research reported that the average American has $38,000 of non-mortgage related debt in 2018.[21] Ironic that thirty-eight is the scriptural number for bondage.

This Scripture sums up everything:

Look, this was the iniquity of your sister Sodom: She and her daughter had pride, fullness of food, and abundance of idleness; neither did she strengthen the hand of the poor and needy (Ezekiel 16:49).

In the fullness of food, it's implied that overeating takes away from others because we're too idle to help others, which validates what Jesus said, "The harvest truly is plentiful, but the laborers are few" (Matthew 9:37).

Ezekiel 16:49 also implies that those who are okay with overeating have taken more than their fair share of food, leaving someone somewhere with less.

And to complete our study:

For many walk, of whom I have told you often, and now tell you even weeping, that they are the enemies of the cross of Christ: whose end is destruction, whose god is their belly, and whose glory is in their shame—who set their mind on earthly things (Philippians 3:18–19).

We want to love God with everything, not our food or bellies. We reject every idol.

As we review the Scriptures, we can see where the early church came from as they looked at gluttony. However, overeating is more prevalent today because it's also a widely accepted part of the Satanic Addictive Deception.

Don't our restaurants serve portions fit for a gladiator?

So, even though there are psychological (see Chapter 14–16) and spiritual aspects (see Chapter 19), there's also practical matters that create and cause overeating.

The Satanic Addictive Deception Strikes Again

Overeating is a tremendous giant to overcome for those in weight and eating bondage. I do believe it is another symptom of the Satanic Addictive Deception, which again is synonymous with the Standard American Diet (S.A.D.).

One hundred years ago overeating was a rare, non-issue. People naturally ate when hungry and stopped because they didn't have access to exploiting foods. They had whole food nutrition and simpler lifestyles.

Since then it seems that our stomachs have stretched and that our foods are a hundred times more addictive causing us to overeat as well as calorically dense.

We also eat more calories overall.

In 1970, we ate 2,016 calories and in 2014, we ate 2,390.[22] Also, notice in the illustration below the types of foods eaten. There's been significant increases in added fats and oils, mostly refined grains and added sugars.

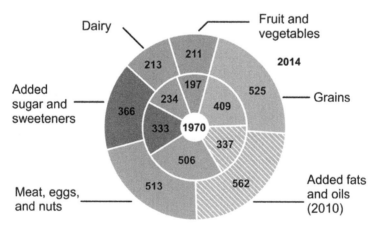

Note: Loss-Adjusted Food Availability data serve as a proxy for food consumption. Data on added fats and oils and rice were unavailable after 2010. Added fats and oils and added sugars are added to foods during processing or preparation. They do not include naturally occurring fats and sugars in food (e.g., fats in meat or sugars in fruits).
Source: USDA, Economic Research Service, Loss-Adjusted Food Availability data.

Illustration 23.1   USDA 1970 to 2014 Calories by Food Group[23]

The average restaurant meal today is more than four times larger than in the 1950s

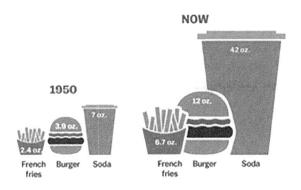

Image 23.2 Fast food meals 1950 – 2016, CDC[24]

We've created gluttony with portion sizes. For example, the portion size of fries grew 279 percent, burgers by 307 percent, and sweet drinks by 600 percent.[25] Even the McDonald's quarter pounder is a quarter pound bigger than a quarter pound.[26]

On average, restaurant meals are half our daily calories, and we eat at least 20 percent more calories when we eat out versus at home.[27]

In restaurants and at home, we have portion distortion. We have an abundance of food available to us at any given time.

In *Times* article, "One Big Fat Truth," Tamar Haspel writes, "Large size portions are normal. High calorie foods are normal. To fix obesity we need to fix normal ... Normal—not carbs, not fat, not insulin, not bacteria—is the problem."[28]

Is our normal a blessing or curse?

We've also covered up the gluttony issue with clothing size deception. Size inflation is also real. What used to be a female size 8 in 1958 was a size 14 or 16 in 2008.[29]

There's no doubt that slim folks or skinny fat people are affected in large numbers as well by gluttony, but our most obvious indicator of excess is the fast-growing 73.6 percent of Americans over 20 years old that are overweight and obese.[30]

Our bodies aren't supposed to be fed the way we feed them with the Standard American Diet's giant-sized candy bars and supersized fast-food meals.

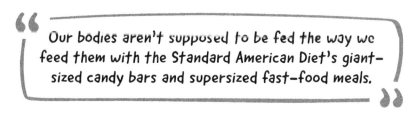

> Our bodies aren't supposed to be fed the way we feed them with the Standard American Diet's giant-sized candy bars and supersized fast-food meals.

To further emphasize how our disordered eating affects us, look at the trends in the images. By 2030, the number of overweight and obese individuals in the USA is expected to be 86.3 percent.[31]

Sin multiplies.

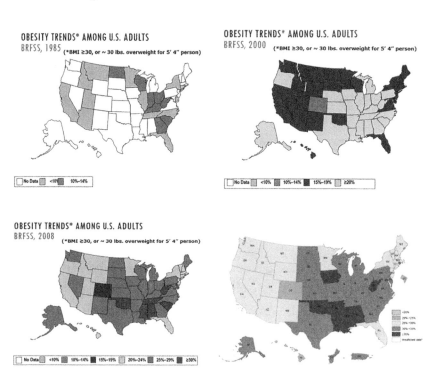

Illustration 23.3 Obesity Epidemic[32] *Last image is 2019

America is both blessed and plagued with an abundance of choice when it comes to foods that offer taste but insufficient health benefits. Temptation is everywhere, and our eyes and taste buds certainly lust.

A study of 102 mentally ill obese individuals concluded that they ate very little fruits and vegetables and mostly fatty cuts of meats in their diets.[33] This and more research suggests that our diet is also a part of the reason for mental health problems including eating disorders.

Abnormal Eating

The Standard American Diet is the biggest eating disorder because its plate lacks actual food and its motive is greed. However, Hosea 4:6 tells us that God's people perish for lack of knowledge. I didn't know I was dealing with an eating disorder for years after I started healing.

In the United States, 20 million women and 10 million men suffer from a clinically significant eating disorder at some time in their lives.[34]

It's common for eating disorder patients to also have depression, seasonal affective disorder, obsessive compulsive disorder, social phobias, alcohol abuse, PTSD, and body dysmorphic disorder.[35]

It's my hope to give you psychological ammunition. Knowledge makes you more equipped to help yourself and others who struggle with abnormal eating.

The four classified psychological eating disorders are anorexia (AN), bulimia (BN), binge eating disorder (BED), and other specified feeding/eating disorder not otherwise specified (OSFED)—as in, not the first three exactly but something else funky!

Eating Disorder Quick Reference Chart

EATING DISORDER	MANTRA	WEIGHT PROFILE	KEY MARKER
Anoerxia (AN or "ANA")	"Starve"	Very Thin Weight	Intense Fear of Fatness
Bulimia (BN or "MIA")	"Purge"	Normal Weight	Binge Episodes with Compensatory Behaviors to Minimize effects on Weight Appearance
Binge Eating Disorder (BED)	"Stuff"	Over Weight/Obese	Binge Episodes
Other Specified Feeding Eating Disorder (OSFED)	"Strange"	Various Weight	Varies

Chart 23.4 Eating Disorders Quick Reference Chart

I want to help you understand bulimia and binge eating disorder because they both involve overeating behaviors. We'll discuss anorexia in Chapter 25.

An Introduction to Bulimia Nervosa (BN)

Bulimia (BN) is an eating disorder of bingeing then purging to rid of the effects of the binge. For example, one may binge eat and then work out excessively to reduce the binge effects on weight.

Others vomit and take laxatives or diuretics to rid the body of excess to maintain a normal weight. In other words, bulimics compensate for poor eating with exercise, laxatives, vomiting, or fasting. Most bulimics are normal weight, but a growing sect is also overweight.

Bulimia is one of the top killers for young females.

Eating disorders are the leading cause of premature death for young women.[36] Of that, 3.9 percent report bulimia as the cause of death; however, sudden cardiac arrest is frequent amongst sufferers which isn't reported as bulimia.[37]

In America, about 1.5 percent of women and 0.5 percent of men have bulimia.[38] That's approximately 4.7 million females and 1.5 million males.

Bulimia Illustrated – Roger's Story

After work Roger was quick to hit the gym. He'd go for three hours at time, religiously. His colleague Dan never heard the end of Roger's comments about his cardio and lifting routines.

Whenever Dan would see him in the bathroom at work, it seemed like Roger was always checking himself out in the mirror. During lunch time Dan was always baffled by Roger's lack of discretion in his eating. *How could someone workout yet have no discretion in their intake?* Dan thought.

They'd frequent burger joints and Roger spared no impulse. Roger often raided the snack machine or got ice cream after a rather large lunch.

Roger seemed to work out so much to compensate for his poor diet.

This belief was validated when Roger said openly that he had worked out to maintain his weight and work off what he had eaten.

He looked good but treated his body poorly.

Roger also complained about feeling too skinny and not muscular enough.

Dan was confused about the matter and just thought something seemed off. So, he asked his girlfriend about it, and she mentioned that it could be an eating disorder. Dan looked up eating disorders and realized that Roger may have bulimia. He binges then exercises for hours to get rid of the binge effects on his weight.

Bulimia Eating Disorder Check[39]

YES (X)	BULIMIA NERVOSA CRITERION
	Do you binge eat more than once per week?
	Have you binge ate weekly for at least three months?
	Do you suffer with negative thoughts and feelings about your body?
	After a binge, do you try to reduce the weight effects by compensating with behaviors such as fasting, excessive exercise, medications, diuretics, enemas, laxatives, or vomiting?

Important: This check is not a diagnosis. Please see a professional for help if you believe you have bulimia nervosa for a full evaluation and treatment plan.

YES (X)	BINGE SEVERITY CRITERION
	A binge episode is a large caloric intake within a discreet period of time with feelings of loss of control over food
	Mild: 1-2 binge eating episodes per week
	Moderate: 4-7 binge eating episodes per week
	Severe: 8-13 binge eating episodes per week
	Extreme: 14 or more binge eating episodes per week

Bulimia Nervosa Medical Complications

- Erosion of tooth enamel because of repeated exposure to acidic gastric contents
- Dental cavities, sensitivity to hot or cold food
- Swelling and soreness in the salivary glands (from repeated vomiting)
- Stomach ulcers
- Ruptures of the stomach and esophagus
- Abnormal buildup of fluid in the intestines
- Disruption in the normal bowel release function
- Electrolyte imbalance
- Dehydration
- Irregular heartbeat and in severe cases heart attack
- A greater risk for suicidal behavior
- Decrease in libido

Bulimia Nervosa Signs and Symptoms

- Eating uncontrollably followed by strict dieting/ fasting
- Vigorous exercise
- Vomiting or abusing laxatives or diuretics to attempt to lose weight
- Using the bathroom frequently after meals
- Preoccupation with body weight and or food
- Depression or mood swings
- Feeling out of control
- Swollen glands in neck and face
- Bloating, indigestion, constipation, and heartburn
- Irregular periods
- Dental problems
- Sore throat
- Weakness and exhaustion

An Introduction to Binge Eating Disorder (BED)

Binge eating disorder (BED) involves bingeing but does not make efforts to get rid of its effects like bulimics. One may binge and sit on the couch instead of going to the gym or vomiting.

BED affects 3.5 percent of women and 2.0 percent of American men.[40] It's the fastest growing eating disorder, and although validated as early as 1987, it just attained recognition in the *Diagnostic and Statistical Manual of Mental Disorders* in 2013.[41]

BED affects 65 percent of obese persons and even more of us who are overweight.[42] Those with binge eating disorder can be any weight but are typically overweight or obese.[43]

An estimated 30 percent of people who are in weight control programs such as Weight Watchers, Jenny Craig, or Nutrisystem have binge eating disorder.[44]

BED keeps you in the bed. More than 45 percent of those with BED also are plagued with depression.[45] They're also plagued with anxiety disorders, alcoholism, panic attacks, and a variety of other ailments.[46]

Binge Eating Disorder Illustrated – Tanya's Story

Tanya, a single, attractive worship leader in her thirties, lived with her roommate Jan. Jan noticed Tanya's struggle with weight. Tanya worked out regularly at the local gym and ate healthy, but Tanya's weight never seemed to change after over a year of living together.

In fact, her weight was rapidly increasing.

Jan was afraid to bring up the topic of weight to Tanya as not to offend her.

Tanya shared about her recent struggle with her role as a worship leader, and she was conflicted about the demands the role had on her over the past year.

Jan thought Tanya may have been stress eating but wasn't sure.

Then, it came to a head.

When Tanya was sick with the flu, Jan helped her by taking out her trash and cleaning her room while Tanya was asleep on the living room sofa.

Jan was alarmed to find pizza boxes, large bottles of soda, family sized bags of chips, and several other snack food packages completely empty. She found a stash of unopened junk food in her closet.

Shocked, Jan realized that Tanya had a problem.

After praying for guidance on how to talk to Tanya, Jan asked her about the hidden food. Tanya cried and confessed her out of control eating binges to Jan. Jan was able to support Tanya to get help from the local Christian counseling center.

Binge Eating Disorder Check[47]

YES (X)	BULIMIA NERVOSA CRITERION
	Do you binge eat at least once per week?
	Have you binge ate weekly for at least three months?
	Do you suffer with negative thoughts and feelings about your body?
	Do you eat rapidly, when not hungry, or under duress?
	Do you avoid doing things that get rid of the damage such as working out excessively or taking laxatives?

Important: This check is not a diagnosis. Please see a professional for help if you believe
you have binge eating disorder for a full evaluation and treatment plan.

YES (X)	BINGE SEVERITY CRITERION
	A binge episode is a large caloric intake within a discreet period with feelings of loss of control over food
	Mild: 1-2 binge eating episodes per week
	Moderate: 4-7 binge eating episodes per week
	Severe: 8-13 binge eating episodes per week
	Extreme: 14 or more binge eating episodes per week

Binge Eating Disorder Medical Complications [48]

- Diabetes
- Cardiovascular diseases
- Obesity
- Gallbladder diseases
- Depression
- Insomnia/sleep apnea
- Muscle/joint pain

- Enzyme deficiencies
- Dental abnormalities
- Hypoglycemia
- High cholesterol
- High blood pressure

Binge Eating Disorder Signs & Symptoms[49]

- Continually eating even when full
- Inability to stop eating or control what is eaten
- Stockpiling food to consume secretly at a later time
- Eating normally in the presence of others but gorging when isolated
- Experiencing feelings of stress or anxiety that can only be relieved by eating
- Feelings of numbness or lack of sensation while bingeing
- Never experiencing satiation: the state of being satisfied, no matter the amount of food consumed

Other Specified Feeding and Eating Disorder

Other Specified Feeding and Eating Disorders (OSFED) make up 44 percent of all eating disorders.[50] If there's atypical situations such as purging but no bingeing, strange activity with food such as repeatedly chewing and spitting out food, not swallowing, or hiding food, it fits here. Many of the same symptoms and signs exist as other disorders presented.

Eating disorders are difficult to read about, aren't they? It's so important for believers to have this insight to support those in need. While it can take a decade or more to heal from eating disorders, keep your hope in Christ and do the work. Our God is a healer.

Get the Right Help

We may need professional therapeutic help due to trauma experienced earlier in life that promotes eating disorder pathology.

A therapist can support you to rebuild your relationship skills, self-worth, and your place in the world beyond food.

The most significant results are from therapeutic modalities: cognitive behavioral therapy (CBT) and/or dialectical behavioral therapy (DBT). Work with someone who specializes in these modes for eating disorders.

There are powerful stigmas about getting help for psychological health that lie to us and say that if you seek help, you're crazy. I assure you; the opposite is true. If you keep doing the same thing over and over and don't get help or make change, that's more evidence of mental health problems.

You are a worthy investment.

Did you want to schedule that gluttonectomy?

Part Two: Win the Overeating Battle

How to Perform a Gluttonectomy, Stat! and Win the Battle of Overeating for Good!

Since the giants of overeating are so large, we have much to cover to gain the victory, so brace yourself. You can try mastering one or two battle strategies at a time if it's overwhelming.

However, the following battle strategies will support you to surrender, balance your body, and ultimately let go of overeating so that you can finally see results from your health pursuits.

Let's jump in.

Battle Strategy #1 – Commit to Stop

The best thing we can do is become resolute in our decision to stop overeating. We do this when we eliminate and prevent all excuses—emotional, physiological, mental, chubbological, spiritual—to overeat.

To stop being addicted to food we need to stop the addictive foods and ingredients. To stop overeating we need to, you guessed it, stop overeating. It's simple, yet we need strategies to help us with our commitment. As we work on our commitment to stop, we have fewer and fewer episodes of binges.

As believers we're accustomed to letting go of worldly behaviors.

We stop swearing, telling people off, wearing offensive T-shirts, being inconsiderate, having sex outside of marriage, neglecting sex if in marriage, and stealing office supplies, I hope. What behavior(s) did you change when you came to Christ?

Are you willing to stop your beast who drives your compulsion to overeat, too?

One way to support your decision, besides singing "Who let the beast out?!" is to include behavioral aspects to your eating plan we discussed in the last chapter.

What does your beast get you to do or not to do that leads to overeating?

Perhaps, you overeat at night because your beast makes you feel like you don't have time for breakfast or can reduce calories by skipping breakfast. Your new guideline would be, "I always eat breakfast" or, "I plan and eat balanced meals every day."

What behavioral eating aspects do you need to add to your eating plan?

Your beast will go to any lengths necessary to get you to binge and often sets up pre-binge scenarios all day to get you to overeat. It's a war strategy to weaken you, its opponent. You can weaken your beast as you master your addictive overeating voice.

Dr. Glenn Livingston, PhD, struggled with severe binge eating for much of his life. Some nights he would visit up to seven different food places. Many days he struggled to win the battle of the binge. Until, he caged his Pig for good.[51]

As author of *Never Binge Again*, Dr. Livingston has helped overeaters to master their food related addictive voice and stop bingeing.

Checkout his *Never Binge Again* podcast, webinars, coaching programs, and many books to target specific issues around overeating like *An End to Nighttime Eating, The Food Demon Interviews,* and *45 Binge Busters.*

I highly recommend his programs to help you defeat this lifelong issue by working to cage your pig, Sugar Demon, or Cheesy Chucky, so much so, that you can download a free copy of his book here: *www. theovereatingsolution.com.*

Battle Strategy #2 – Heed the Call to Heal

Mastering the addictive voice in your head is great, but we also must look at the heart. More than likely overeating has been the reliable companion we've had trouble saying goodbye to since a young age.

Over 40 percent of overeaters started overeating before eleven years old.[52]

The food choices may have been wrong, but the act of eating itself has felt so right. If we're willing to continue to binge and overeat, we will remain bound in the Weight & Eating War for life. We must surrender our desire to overeat.

No matter what we eat the act of eating soothes anxiety and helps us to process emotions. And it has done so since we were babies.

> No matter what we eat the act of eating soothes anxiety and helps us to process emotions.

We're scared to let go of our companion for good reason. Overeating is a heart issue. It's an anxious heart, lonely heart, neglected heart, resentful heart, fearful heart, hurting heart, hungry heart issue.

Whenever I notice my intake is higher, it's almost always an emotion asking to be processed. A fear. A grief. A worry. Or a commitment I can't keep because there's too much on my proverbial plate, which manifested on the dinner plate.

Overeating is an act of anxiety. Our anxiety seeks comfort in the act of eating itself. We may have been deprived in emotional support and comfort. But at this point, that old security blankie of eating needs to be donated to the local shelter.

In Book 1, I said, "My addiction to the food obsession was an attempt to control and manipulate my out-of-control identity crisis, like a child seeking love and protection from a hamburger mistaken as mom and dad."

Overeating truly was my mother replacement in times I needed comfort or to help me cope with fears as I advanced to new levels of being.

I told you my dad story. But I didn't tell you my mom story yet. One day, after a few days of senseless overeating for no reason, of all healthy foods nonetheless, I knew it came time to surrender overeating itself.

God knew that this behavior was a deep deprivation in my soul. He knew it was a way I coped when I needed some love and comfort due to not having a safe mother relationship.

I ran to food because I couldn't run to my mother. See, she was addicted to pain pills for most of my life. So not only did I not have my dad around, but my mom was also emotionally absent and left me feeling like a neglected orphan.

It was just me and my food.

It's always been just me and my food.

A mother's love is so needed, even when she's not there or can't love. Food has faithfully partnered with me to cope with the lack of relationship with her. And praise the Lord, God was faithful to do a miracle to restore her and our relationship.

Perhaps He wants to heal you in a deep way that a parent should've been there for you. Or a sibling or a romantic partner.

If relational bonds were spotty with primary caregivers—if they were tuned out, absent or self-absorbed, inconsistent, or terrifying (abusive) instead of secure—it makes us very insecure in human relationships and makes us prone to rocky food relationships.[53]

Karol Truman in *Feelings Buried Alive Never Die*, says overeating represents emotions, a material-emotional lack, craving closeness, anger and resentment energy, and a symbol of power and desire to throw one's weight around.[54]

> **If relational bonds were spotty with primary caregivers—if they were tuned out, absent or self-absorbed, inconsistent, or terrifying (abusive) instead of secure—it makes us very insecure in human relationships and makes us prone to rocky food relationships.**

Can you relate to these feelings?

Overeating as a means of dealing with difficult emotions only postpones your best life. Instead process your emotions.

Do Emotional Fitness Workouts™ (see Chapter 18) and emotionally clear so you won't eat over them.

Lisa Morrone, physical therapist and author of *Overcoming Overeating,* created the chart below to escape overeating and food addiction emotionally by exploring the pain or spiritually by repenting and forgiveness.

I recommend that at any point you can stop the shame-guilt cycle perpetuated by overeating with an Emotional Fitness Workout™ to process fully as well.

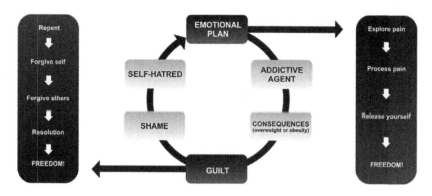

Illustration 23.5   Cycle of Food Addiction & Overeating Escape[55]

To remind you of The Emotional Fitness Workout™ to process triggers and pain:

Chart 23.6   The Emotional Fitness Workout™ [56]

THE EMOTIONAL FITNESS WORKOUT™	
Step #1: Stop	How can I disengage in self-harming pursuits?
Step #2: Pinpoint	What triggered me and what emotions am I feeling exactly?
Step #3: Evaluate	Why am I feeling this way?
Step #4: Experience	How can I best process my feelings right now?
Step #5: Release	What or who do I need to let go of?

> **When you're overeating, it's also the Holy Spirit asking for you to come to Him.**

When you're overeating, it's also the Holy Spirit asking for you to come to Him. Anytime you overeat be open to healing—healing emotions per Chapter 18 and healing by the Holy Spirit.

Take a moment and reflect on the behavior of overeating in your life.

How has the act of overeating served you all these years?

What's it been like for you?

What or who has it replaced?

Sit with the answers.

Then pray, "Father I give you my companion and all emotional bonds with overeating. Please heal what's underneath. Where my heart longs for a close mother, heal me. Where my heart longs for my father's love, heal me. Where my heart longs for close companionship, heal me. Where I am in fear or grief, heal me. Where I fear changing, heal me. I give you the wounds of my heart and ask for healing to never binge and overeat again. Please help me eat the right portions. Transform my heart. And I ask to receive the fullest manifestation of my healing in my physical body."

Ahh.

Feels good to surrender, doesn't it? But we're not done yet.

Speak to your old companion out loud.

Say, "Overeating, thank you for helping me cope when things were tough. Thank you for being a faithful friend. But now the time has come to say goodbye so that I can cope in healthier ways. I will miss you, but I need to stand on my own and enter into the promises God has for me. Goodbye."

I hope grieving tears came to you as you released your good friend of overeating. I surely cried as I had to say goodbye.

And I've had to pray these types of prayers more than once. So, it's okay if you do, too. Just remain committed to ending the overeating behavior in your life and you will.

Battle Strategy #3 – Eat Greens Daily

More than emotional upsets, nutrient deficiencies drive binge eating behavior. Addictive foods increase appetite hormone ghrelin and decrease appetite suppressant hormone leptin which causes overeating.[57]

Processed foods also cause us to overeat because they deplete nutrients at lightning speed. Zinc, Vitamin D, Iron, B vitamins, and chromium deficiencies as well as others lead to binge eating behaviors.[58]

Recall from Chapter 7, overweight and obesity are signs of mal-nourishment. Our cells are ravenously hungry for real food. Cells look at collard greens like we salivate at a sizzling steak.

Cells don't want to taste the counterfeit rainbow that Skittles® can offer. They want the real rainbow of fruits and vegetables that nourish abundantly. Your taste buds may not be overly excited, but your insides and organs get giddy when they see real nutrient dense food coming their way.

And to reduce overeating and cravings we may need to not only eat vegetables with dinner but do what Chef AJ suggests and eat vegetables for breakfast (VFB).[59]

Yes, start early with at least three cups of green vegetables with your breakfast most days. Green vegetables contain thylakoids in the green chloropropyl cells of the plant.

Eating thylakoid containing green plants, including spinach, kale, collards, seaweed, chard and others, you can reduce your urges to overeat by 95 percent and stop cravings.[60]

> **The more greens you eat, the more your body heals.**

The more greens you eat, the more your body heals. And the easier it is to eat three meals per day with less snaccidents between or after meals.[61]

The other good news is that you can eat as much greens as you want because the minerals, fiber, and water content make it nearly impossible to overeat them. This is the divine genius that is in God-based foods. They come with zero guilt, shame, or regret, quite contrary to packaged counterparts.

I love a good craving-squashing smoothie most days blended up with a few cups of greens and a cup or two of fruit or a huge salad with thinly chopped collards, mustard greens, and cabbage. The recipes are endless.

So, go ahead and have loads of fun with an eat-all-your-produce-before-it-goes-bad game! And enjoy overeating spinach, broccoli, green beans, celery, kale, romaine, green lettuce, collards, chard, mustard greens, cabbage, and any other green vegetables you'd like. For more motivation, check out *By Any Greens Necessary* by Tracye Lynn McQuirter.

Battle Strategy #4 – Practice Normal Eating

We've heard what abnormal looks like. Let's talk about normal eating.

Karen Koenig, author of *The Rules of "Normal" Eating* says, "You will achieve your goals when you're ready and not a moment before. And you won't be ready to receive the gift of "normal" eating until you have cleaned out the mental and emotional space that's been occupied by compulsive, emotional, and restrictive eating ... If you work hard to become a "normal" eater, it's highly likely that you will be creating an abundance of every one of these qualities: curiosity, compassion for self, care of self ..."[62]

A few ways to practice normal eating are:

Get In Tune With Hunger

Due to the Standard American Diet (S.A.D.), those of us who've struggled with food tend to be disconnected from our body's natural signals. If we've had abuse, that disconnect can feel worse.

We know when we need to pee or go to sleep, but hunger has been short-circuited. Thankfully, hunger signaling can be re-learned.

Normal eaters eat when they're hungry or have a specific (non-addictive ingredient related) craving. And they stop when they're satisfied, not stuffed.

Can you gauge your hunger or fullness?

Whenever you eat, check in with your hunger by using a scale from 1 to 10 to measure your fullness.

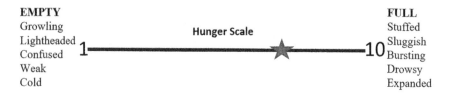

Illustration 23.7   Hunger Scale

A one (1) on the hunger scale may cause hunger signs such as a sense of hollowness in chest, stomach grumblings, brain fatigue, weakness, cold shivers, confusion, or irritability. Typically, if you haven't eaten in four or more hours, you're hungry.

And, if you don't have ready healthy meal options, you'll be vulnerable to overeat junk.

A ten (10) on the hunger scale feels stuffed, bloated, full, and gain less pleasure from food. We don't want to go to a ten anymore.

Since it takes twenty minutes for feelings of fullness to occur, when you eat, aim for the star or sweet spot between 6 or 7 on the scale.

A simple check in with your hunger can prevent overeating as can regular mealtimes.

Remember grade school lunches? Didn't your hunger meet you at lunchtime? It's highly recommended to eat at regularly scheduled mealtimes to avoid eating late or choosing poorly.

I have found, when overeaters attempt to be guided solely by hunger it leads to poor choices and poor meal timing that affects health negatively such as eating late at night. And sadly, they don't experience long term results.

So please eat at regular mealtimes to avoid eating at ridiculous times. You can also aim to eat meals two to three hours apart or four to five hours apart to balance blood sugar and reduce ravenous eating. A balanced meal sustains you for hours. If you're hungry after an hour, that meal failed.

> "
> **Eat at regular mealtimes to avoid eating at ridiculous times.**
> "

Also, don't skip meals. Binge eaters are notorious for skipping meals which only sets us up to binge.

As you listen to your body and learn your hunger signals, you get better at discerning if you're physically or emotionally hungry. Physical hunger can only be solved by food, and emotional hunger can be solved by clearing your emotions.

> **Physical hunger can only be solved by food, and emotional hunger can be solved by clearing your emotions.**

Embracing hunger between meals also makes everything tastier. Tastes buds seem to be more open to savor a meal when the body isn't overloaded with food. They say absence makes the heart grow fonder. Well, hunger makes the taste buds more excited to eat vegetables.

And if we're not willing to eat vegetables, are we really that hungry anyway?

Eat With Gusto and Mindfulness

Have you ever felt like your beast clubbed you to voraciously stuff food in the piehole? Like you've gone somewhere else? From now on when you eat, eat.

Get present with your food.

Mindfulness is the art of focused attention to be where you are with all your senses. Jesus modeled a strong present sense of awareness in that no matter what was going on around Him, He was there, in the moment.

Allow eating to be the same way. Know what's happening. Slow down the eagerness that turns into fast eating. I'll breathe before I take bites. I like to prepare everything and then sit down and eat it.

These habits are a complete shift from my former days of holding the cell phone in one hand, burger in the other, fries in the lap, and knees driving the car. I was comically, and dangerously, not present with my food.

Won't He do it?

Concentrate on eating and being present. Be grounded. Sit and eat at the table. Take the time to chew and taste.

Use all your senses.

Enjoy every bite.

Savor the flavors.

Slow down and learn how to sit and eat without distractions of cell phone, television, driving, or rushing. And make the time to eat. It's the most nourishing, health promoting thing we do to support our lives.

Accept That You're Not A Normal Eater

One thing we abnormal eaters want is to eat normally. But you must realize that the only way you become a normal eater is by understanding you're not a normal eater.

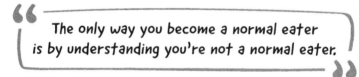

> The only way you become a normal eater is by understanding you're not a normal eater.

Problem ingredients affect our brains and mood causing us to be abnormal eaters.

Therefore, we'll take precautions with foods, ideally eliminate them or use alternatives to stay free and normal. Because we all eat an abnormal Standard American Diet (S.A.D.), doing the opposite will help you easily become a normal eater.

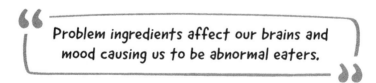

> Problem ingredients affect our brains and mood causing us to be abnormal eaters.

You'll sense hunger signals, leave food on the plate when satisfied, won't overeat or binge at all or much, and you'll have the energy to do other things besides dwell on food. It's really a radical shift in your relationship with food when you let go of problem foods and ingredients. But you've got to let go to receive the benefits of an amazing food relationship and an energetic body.

It's a paradox. The more we accept that we're not normal eaters, we'll normally eat. As problem foods and ingredients are removed, they have a direct positive impact on eliminating binge eating behaviors.

Battle Strategy #5 – Eat Enough

Countless health advocates have proven that the eat less, move more hypothesis has been grossly misleading. And we should know because we've been there and done that to no avail. Calorie restriction leaves us hangry (hungry and angry), and when we're hangry, we binge.

Overweight and obesity are hormonal disorders, a result of the types of calories (energy) we eat and the imbalance of our intake—a piece of chicken here and a candy there, instead of a meal that covers nutritional needs in a balanced way.

To refrain from lop-sided daily intake with binge episodes, we'll balance those calories over meals. We also need to eat the right types of calories for our best overall health.

Remember it's not God's intention for us to ever diet or count calories. But we've been derailed, so to get back on track we'll need data.

Weight loss is not based on calories as much as it is the types of calories.

And the types of calories and amount of them does impact our fat loss more than the exercise more, eat less lie.

How do we know we've overeaten and how much we've overeaten?

Don't we need to know the number of calories we need?

Only makes sense, doesn't it?

Nutrition labels are misleading because they base those labels on an active person who maintains weight at 2,000 calories. However, 2,000 calories may not be what feeds your best health and body.

Most women need less than that. The American standard 2,000 calories per day recommendation is for maintaining current weight and doesn't consider gender, height, and lifestyle factors such as breast feeding, a physically demanding job, health needs, or activity level.[63]

Tips to be sure you eat enough:

Find Your Bio-Individual Calorie Needs

A BMI of 20–21 is the range for the best health and energy outcomes. But, it's important to consider your ancestry and body shape. For example, African American females, like me, are naturally very curvy, and we have more natural fat deposits in shapely areas compared to our Asian friends.

In the same way a seal is a cute and super fat animal. Does it need to lose weight? Not at all, they're made to be nice and fat and don't get chronic diseases. So, what if they're nude and hang out in their birthday suits all day, they're not complaining nor worried about joining Jenny Craig.

People too can carry sturdy fat cells in some areas as divine design. So, maybe a 22–23 BMI range provides the curves that naturally suit you, or a 19–20 BMI range is more fitting for your ancestral body type. If within the healthy ranges, you're still better off from a disease perspective.

The basal metabolic rate (BMR) is the minimum number of calories you need to sustain your body's needs for life and functioning—organs, muscles, tissues, systems, cellular health, etc. We're going to do a little math. So that you don't get lost, I'm outlining the steps.

Step One

On the chart find your healthy BMI weight range. I prefer to stick within a range so it's not overly rigid feeling. A BMI of 20–22 (see top of the chart) for someone 5'6" has a target healthy weight range between 124–141 lbs.

Body Mass Index (BMI) Table
(Adult Men & Women)

	UNDERWEIGHT			NORMAL				OVERWEIGHT									OBESE			
BMI	16	17	18	19	20	21	22	23	24	25	26	27	28	29	30	31	32	33	34	35
Height										**Body Weight (pounds)**										
4'10"	77	82	86	91	96	100	105	110	115	119	124	129	134	138	143	148	153	158	162	167
4*11"	79	84	S9	94	99	104	109	114	112	124	128	133	13X	142	148	153	158	162	168	173
5'	82	82	92	97	102	107	112	118	123	128	133	138	143	148	153	158	163	168	114	179
$1"	85	90	96	100	106	111	116	122	127	132	137	143	148	122	158	164	169	124	180	185
5'2"	88	93	99	104	109	115	120	126	121	136	142	147	153	158	164	169	115	180	186	191
5'3"	91	26	102	107	112	118	124	130	135	141	146	152	158	163	169	175	180	186	191	197
5'4"	91	99	105	110	116	122	128	134	140	145	151	157	163	169	174	180	186	192	192	204
5'5"	96	102	108	114	120	126	132	128	144	150	156	162	168	174	180	186	192	198	204	210
56"	99	106	112	118	124	130	136	142	148	155	161	167	173	129	186	192	198	204	210	216
5'7"	102	109	115	121	127	134	140	146	153	159	166	172	178	185	191	198	204	211	217	223
5'8"	105	112	119	125	131	138	144	151	158	164	111	177	184	190	197	203	210	216	223	230
5'9"	109	UL5	122	128	135	142	149	155	162	169	176	182	189	196	203	209	216	223	230	236
5'10"	112	119	126	132	139	146	153	160	162	124	181	188	195	202	202	216	222	229	236	243
511"	115	122	129	136	143	150	157	165	172	179	186	193	200	208	215	222	229	236	243	250
6'	118	125	133	140	147	154	162	169	122	184	191	199	206	213	221	228	235	242	250	258
6'1"	121	129	137	144	151	159	166	124	182	189	192	204	212	219	222	235	242	250	252	265
6'2"	121	133	140	148	155	163	171	122	186	194	202	210	218	225	233	241	249	256	264	222
6'3"	128	136	144	152	160	168	176	184	192	200	208	216	224	232	240	248	256	264	272	229

Table 23.5   Healthy Weight Range Body Mass Index Chart[64]

Step Two

Calculate your BMR based on the healthy weight you want to be within your range. Be realistic.

Go to *https://www.active.com/fitness/calculators/bmr* and put your healthy desired weight goal into the calculator to find the number of calories you need per day. I've found the BMR target much more helpful to aim for than the caloric needs, which even if sedentary is still too high.

Add half the calories you burn to see results over time. If you've worked out and burned 300 calories, eat another 150 calories.

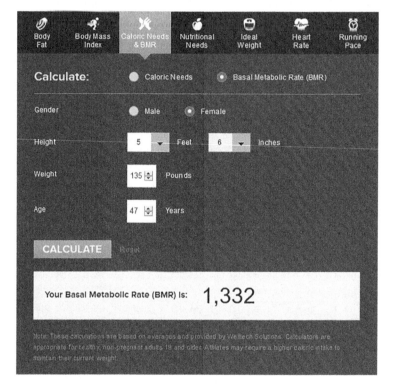

Illustration 23.8   BMI Calculator

Track for Protection and Insight

To train yourself not to over or under-eat, I strongly recommend handling the learning curve scientifically with real data from tracking all you consume in an app for at least six months, but ideally for life if vulnerable to overeating.

The best way to manage money is to look at it and know how much we're working with. Each day we have a caloric budget as well, and now you know what it is. Fifty years ago, we didn't have to monitor calories because there was no need. With processed food temptation and out of whack hormonal levels, now we do.

The conveniences of grocery stores, the abundance of restaurants, desk jobs, and let's be real, our elastic pants, make it that much more of a necessity to protect ourselves from gluttony.

Using a scientific approach, we'll finally see results. We can finally master eating the appropriate amount and types of foods.

In a study of 1,685 mostly obese women with hypertension and other ailments, those who kept a food diary lost twice as much weight than those who didn't.[65] Many other studies show the exact same thing: those who track will have better results than those who don't. I prefer to track on an app like *www.MyFitnessPal.com* or *www.Cronometer.com*.

Invest ten to twenty minutes per day to track your intake because it pays you back with less binges, less Beast Baloney, more clarity, and rich data on what foods work for you and what foods don't.

It's awesome.

Data matters.

Your beast hates the accountability because self-accountability to what you're eating sets you free. If it's emotionally harmful for you to track calories because you've done this in the past in an unhealthy way, please keep a food diary on paper.

Track for Consistency and Balance

Undereating has always promoted overeating, hasn't it? Instead of swings from a low-appetite day to a ravenous day, track for consistency and balance. Aim to eat all your calorie needs to reduce over and under-eating.

Tracking apps, like MyFitnessPal, show you how much you ate, burned, as well as your macro (total proteins, carbohydrates, and fats) and micronutrient (vitamins and minerals) intake. It's encouraging to see progress.

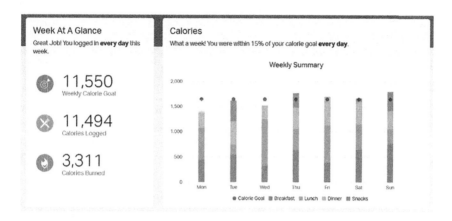

Image 23.9 My Fitness Pal Report Example

A focus on eating enough and three balanced meals is the primary way to prevent over-eating.

Dr. Susan Pierce, PhD, also a recovered food addict, supports men and women to get free in her successful online *Bright Line Eating Program* based on recommended Food Addicts Anonymous eating plan.

This online program is highly recommended to support eating in a balanced way to remove the bondage of weight and eating from your life.

Balanced meals do wonders for emotional, mental, and physical health. It's also fun to get your calories from God foods because you'll always feel like you have plenty to eat, which we'll discuss in the next chapter.

Do you see how these strategies will set you up for success?

In the past you may have avoided knowing your caloric intake. You may have tried to cut calories and only focused on weight. This time we're focusing on health and learning to eat in a way that balances us nutritionally and prevents us from overeating.

This time is different.

This time you win.

FAA Basic Food Plan

BREAKFAST	LUNCH (4 HOURS AFTER BREAKFAST)	DINNER (5 HOURS AFTER LUNCH)	METABOLIC ADJUSTMENT (MA) (4 HOURS AFTER DINNER)
1 Protein	1 Protein	1 Protein	1 Dairy or 2 oz. Protein
1 Dairy	1 Cooked Vegetable	1 Cooked Vegetable	1 Fruit
1 Fruit	1 Fresh vegetable	1 Fresh Vegetable	
1 Grain or Starchy Vegetable	1/2 Daily Oil	1 grain or starchy vegetable	
	Men: Add 1 fruit or 1 grain, or 1 starchy vegetable	1/2 Daily Oil	

The daily requirement for oil is one serving for women and two servings for men, to be divided among two or three meals.

NOTE: Men need to add two ounces of fish or poultry or one ounce of red meat at each meal to the amounts shown on the list. At lunch, men also add a serving of one of the following: a fruit, a grain, or a starchy vegetable.

Chart 23.10 Food Addicts Anonymous recommended food guidelines.[66]

Strategy # 6 – Meal Plan and Prep

When we better prepare, we protect ourselves from overeating more effectively. Driver overeater types zoom through drive-throughs because there's nothing tasty on hand. When you've chopped the onions, have a can of beans handy, or eggs boiled, you'll be more equipped to reduce binges.

The "I'm too tired" excuse goes away when we remove problem foods and ingredients which makes meal planning and preparation near effortless because of the natural energy boost that comes from removing problem foods.

The habit of meal planning and preparation is foundational for success we must learn it. So here's some keys to get this habit down.

Keys to Meal Plan and Prep effectively

Pick meal prep days and times

You can decide if you want to meal prep once a week, once a month, once every few days, or the night before.

If you're running a household with children, you may need a weekly time. If you're single, you may want to prepare every few days. It needs to work with your lifestyle. What day and time works best for you?

Recipe Shop

Spend some time shopping for recipes from cookbooks or going online to search so that you know what you want to prepare. I keep a list of easy meal ideas on my cell phone.

Nowadays there's amazing meal planning apps you can download on your phone. Browse your phone's app store to see which apps appeal to you. Many apps work with various dietary preferences. Meal planning apps make it easy to grocery shop and know what to eat so there's no excuse.

Online there's tons of options for recipes: raw foods, vegan, plant-based meals, vegetable dishes, and the list goes on to getting more vegetables into your diet. You don't have to be a vegan or vegetarian to find great new vegetable dishes.

Check out Tabitha Brown, Forks over Knives, Food Revolution Network, and Chef AJ on apps or YouTube.

Keep Supplies Handy

One of the most magical things we can do is have quality food choices on hand. You'll need ingredients for easy prep and grab and go.

God created bananas, apples, oranges, grapes, nuts, and carrots already packaged and ready to munch on. Always have fruit and quick greens like baby kale, baby spinach, or arugula handy. If pre-prepared healthy options work for you and your family, try them.

You can find prepackaged items that support healthier eating, such as hummus, guacamole, salsa, or cucumber dip or full meals like salads or healthy food delivery or pick-up options. When you don't have the highly palatable taste bud competition, you'll be surprised how delicious simple foods taste.

Schedule Time

It takes time to shop and prepare food. But when you schedule the two to four hours a week it takes, you'll protect yourself from Beast Baloney, food crazies, overeating, and weight and eating stress the rest of the week.

Groceries can be ordered online and then dropped off. Ideally, pick the same time each week. If short on time, it's more important to plan the time for meals than for workouts, as food predicts over 90 percent of our weight and health outcomes.

Use Batch Methods

See the chart below on how to use your meal preparation time effectively.

Batch Cook	Make several servings of foods that hold easy in the refrigerator such as baked sweet potatoes, brown rice, beans, fish, or meat, hard boiled eggs, collard greens. Whenever you prepare a meal, make 2-3 at the same time to store for later.
Batch Chop	When you chop, chop a lot. Foods such as: salad greens (or buy already chopped), fruit, and toppings/ingredients such as tomatoes, red peppers, red onions, or olives.
Batch Bag	Make several servings of foods that hold easily in the freezer and in bags such as soups, fruit salads, and smoothies.
Batch Mix	Use sandwich bags that have 3-5 ingredients for simple dishes or toppings ready to go such as omelet fillings, tofu scrambles, soup ingredients, or salad toppings. For example, in one bag would be your onions, tomatoes, and parsley.
	Batch Mix Ingredient Ideas – olives, red onions, peppers, pumpkin seeds, sunflower seeds, walnuts, green onions, leeks, artichoke hearts, garbanzo beans, chopped avocadoes, shaved carrots, sliced red peppers, or sundried tomatoes.

Meal planning and preparation is a learning curve, so treat it like a great new job. It's nonnegotiable to make time for the learning curve of recipes, foods, meal preparation, and grocery shopping. These habits must be learned to master weight and eating for the rest of your life. In a survey of over 40,000 people, those who meal planned had the healthiest weights and the best variety of food.[67]

Don't put meal planning off any longer. We've avoided the learning curve because it's difficult, but it's only temporary.

When you start a new job, you learn policies, procedures, culture, politics, people, and systems. You're drinking from a fire hose for a few months. But after a while, things click, and you're acclimated to the job.

So, consider yourself hired!

Take on the job of finding your best foods, eating, and lifestyle. Embrace the learning.

For the next several months try new meals and dishes. When you get a new job, other things in your life may be put on hold, and the same holds true here.

What can you move off your plate to give time to meal planning and preparation? If you make time for this season and it will pay you back every day of the rest of your life.

Strategy #7 – Lean on Support

Twelve-step groups are rarely ever mentioned in diet books because self-help diet books don't address the sin-help we really need to defeat the spirit of gluttony.

I have read many books on nutrition, health, and diets, and I've always wondered why none of these books recommend a twelve-step group.

Gluttony Anonymous won't sell T-shirts, that's for sure.

Other names are more politically correct, I guess.

Or maybe because it's anonymous, free, or requires a higher power.

When I first went to a meeting, it was difficult for the words, "Hi, I'm J, and I am a compulsive eater" to come out of my mouth.

For a while, I thought my prideful ego constantly blocked my healing and success.

But it wasn't my ego. It was my Whole & Free self that knew there was more to the story.

I just needed to be willing to quit my problem foods and ingredients, commit to stop eating compulsively, and stand in my God-given wholeness and freedom.

However, I found the support to be very healing. I noticed that the weeks I went I had more progress than weeks I didn't attend. The ability to share with people who understood overeating comforted me. I saw how the behavioral addiction to overeating doesn't discriminate. It affected everyone—all races, sizes, religions, and economic statuses. I wasn't alone.

The scriptural principle enacted for this sin-help group was confession. We're called to confess our sins one to another to be healed (James 5:16).

With confession, sin can't cause destruction.

With conviction, sin dies altogether.

Hidden things bound in darkness die when put into the light. Sharing in a group that understands puts our shame into the light. Confession is a way for us to be humble with one another and before God.

The power of confession is validated by the 90 percent who feel improvements in their mental and emotional health, spiritual relationship, and daily functioning by participating.[68]

And 80 percent who attend regularly have improvements in their weight.[69] Over 54 percent maintained a healthy weight for over six years.[70] (See Victory Morsels.)

As we lean into support, we're strongest in every area and get results.

We're healed when we confess.

Any twelve-step group is a tool.

A support system is necessary in any form of recovery from anything. It felt good for that one hour a week to share with people who really did understand what it's like to go from place to place to get a hit of your food high and have to deal with the shame aftermath.

They were with me. They knew the pain. God knew the possibility.

Go After It and Do Not Quit

So many of God's people succumb to the enemy's plans to keep them broken and bound. He does everything to keep us hopeless in food addiction and a slave to compulsive overeating. His victim's think, "It's too much to change, so I'll be fat and happy."

But it's false happiness based on a false exchange of the truth for lies. And the very essence of who you are, your beauty, and what you're truly designed to do is to give God glory and be the brightest light you can be.

You are not meant to be low in energy, minimal in joy, emotionally up and down, stuck in a chubby suit or surviving but barely getting by.

As we'll learn in Chapter 26, nothing says identity more than your face and how you look. Poor heath and continued eating dysfunction is an attack on your identity—who you really are, how you really look, and how Whole & Free you can be!

It's a direct attack in the area of life that brings the most life, power, and joy—health! Health and holiness go hand in hand.

Benaiah is described as a valiant warrior in the Scriptures. He killed two of Moab's mightiest warriors. (We'll call them problem foods and overeating.) Later he chased a lion down into a pit, and despite the snow and slippery ground, he caught the lion and killed it. And another time he was armed with a modest club and killed a great Egyptian warrior who was armed with a lethal spear (2 Samuel 23:20–23).

Now that's a warrior.

What if you had the type of warrior faith inside of you that instead of getting beat up by the beast, you decided to take charge, hunt down the thoughts, emotions, lies, habits, and triggers taking you down and destroy them?

What if you decided the obstacles couldn't and wouldn't make you back down?

That no matter what you'd win.

See overeating is an issue that requires spiritual, mental, emotional, nutritional, and physical weapons. It's a stronghold.

But because we're called to overcome every single lie of the enemy according to Revelation 12:11, we will.

Let me bring this home in a situational success verse, "And I overcame Satan's lies by the blood of the Lamb, and by the belief and truth in Jesus Christ and didn't love my hoagies (or your preferred problem foods) and overeating unto death (Revelation 12:11).

Go after your victory. David said, "I have pursued my enemies and destroyed them; Neither did I turn back again till they were destroyed. And I have destroyed them and wounded them, so that they could not rise; they have fallen under my feet" (2 Samuel 22:38–39).

And I promise there is a reward for you beyond your wildest dreams!

As you lay down the sin and do whatever it takes to keep it far from you, you will be promoted in your life and family. David said, "I was also blameless before God, And I kept myself from my iniquity. Therefore, the Lord has recompensed me according to my righteousness, according to my cleanness in His eyes" (2 Samuel 22:24–25).

Benaiah was promoted to commander of the bodyguards. David got the blessing of His family line forever; Jesus was birthed out of that line. Jesus conquered sin and death, and we received eternal life.

Be the warrior of God that you are and destroy every kryptonite.

REFLECT & SHARE

1. Why do you want to let go of overeating in your life?
2. Which Battle Strategy do you want to execute right away?
3. What obstacles do you need to remove to succeed?
4. What information on eating disorders surprised you?
5. What support do you need to take down the giant of overeating?

PRAYER

Heavenly Father,

You are great! Wise beyond measure. Thank You for breaking every stronghold of overeating in my life! Thank you for the freedom to let go of eating as my only joy.

I pray for deep conviction over the behaviors that aren't pleasing to You.

Give me conviction and strength to get all forms of gluttony out of my life for good. I cast out every demon of gluttony, pride, arrogance, rebellion, and destruction!

And I tell the enemy right now that I've already won. Back off! I'm a child of God, and I've been given the power to overcome.

Thank you, Great Physician, You are faithful to perform a gluttonectomy, stat!

In the mighty name of Jesus, amen.

CHAPTER 24

EWW, SPIT IT OUT, THAT WASN'T FOOD

Battle #3 – Unclean Eating

"Therefore, whether you eat or drink or whatever you do, do all to the glory of God"

−1 CORINTHIANS 10:31

"'Eat bacon,' said no pig ever." —Anonymous

Part One: Understanding Unclean Eating

B acon lovers, hold on to your skillets. I may shock you right out of that B.L.T.

In 2004, I realized something wasn't quite right with pork. As I cooked up porkchops for my grandparents, I noticed weird squiggly things. I reasoned, *the squigglies were from the oil and vinegar sauce.* A second later, I shoved the image out of my consciousness and served the dish.

The next year I went to school for nutrition and learned about the grossness of pork and rats of the sea otherwise known as shellfish.

As a former, all-you-can eat barbeque ribs girl, who ate bacon with, well, everything, and as one who cooked up shrimp and broccoli on a regular basis, this new nutritional insight was an unwelcomed surprise.

My favorite dish my mother made for me was porkchops smothered in cheddar cheese!

By the power of the Holy Spirit, before I knew where God's food plan was in Scripture and before I understood why some Jews and Christians didn't eat pork, I learned through nutritional wisdom.

In Part One: Understanding Unclean Eating, we'll take a bite into biblically clean and unclean eating, further evaluating problem foods and practices of the Standard American Diet. Then in Part Two: Win the Unclean Eating Battle, I'll provide battle strategies to adopt the Life Abundantly Standard.

The Master Dietician

While you've heard the terms clean eating, paleo, whole foods, or organic, it's God who was the originator of the term clean for foods and God who thought of food and our dependency on it in the first place. This makes God the Master Dietician.

And without getting into a debate around Jewish and Gentile dietary issues, I'm going to keep this profoundly simple: God was, is, and will always be way smarter than me, you, and every other human on the planet—combined.

> God was, is, and will always be way smarter than me, you, and every other human on the planet—combined.

He is infinite intelligence. He gave us His teaching and instruction in our beloved Bibles. To know His ways, which are higher than ours, leads to the abundant life Christ promised.

He says, "I, the Lord, am the one who brought you up from the land of Egypt to be your God. You must therefore be holy because I am holy" (Leviticus 11:45).

"This is the law of the animals and the birds and every living creature that moves in the waters, and of every creature that moves in the waters, and of every creature that creeps on the earth, to distinguish between the unclean and the clean, and between the animals that may eaten and the animals that may not be eaten" (Leviticus 11:46).

Since He is the Creator of all things, it's important for us to take His advice.

It's no different than if we instructed a guest in our home not to eat food from the fridge if it's spoiled. God instructed us not to eat what's already spoiled from His intimate and infinite knowledge on the manufacturing of His products: the pig, snake, or hare.

In God's grocery store, pork sausage nor lobster bisque would be for sale.

We eat clean foods as willful obedience to God's instructions for what to eat to the best of our ability and to counteract diseases that denatured foods perpetuate.

God's Idea of Clean Eating

Unclean eating is when we consume what's considered unclean as outlined in Deuteronomy 14 and Leviticus 11.

God labeled certain meats as clean or unclean. Foods we may think are foods are not good for food at all. Like Eve, we think all that we want to eat is good, it's edible, and it could make us wiser, but God instructed otherwise.

God didn't see foods that we call foods, as food. When we think, *What's for dinner?* cockroaches don't cross our minds. We don't think of cockroaches in the scope of what we consider food in the United States. And can you imagine if a new friend made you *Snake served Al Dente* for lunch? That new friend would, no doubt, fade into a memory.

In the same way, foods such as catfish, shrimp, lobster, crab, scallops, ham, bacon, chitterlings, and genetically modified meats treated inhumanly, pumped with hormones to grow faster, and raised in depressed factory farms are not considered a part of His recommended meal plan.

If we love food more than we love God, we will always have a problem with food since we can't serve two masters (Matthew 6:24). We're to shun evil to bring health to our bodies and nourishment to our bones (Proverbs 3:7–8).

> If we love food more than we love God, we will always have a problem with food since we can't serve two masters (Matthew 6:24).

It's only like a loving God to inform us what's best to eat and drink. And it's our mission to know the difference between holy and unholy and discern the difference between the unclean and the clean (Ezekiel 44:23; Leviticus 11:47).

When we accept the Bible as a love offering from God to mankind, we see everything in it as instruction for our good. This perspective opens your heart to letting go of foods and agricultural practices prohibited from the mouth of God.

> It's only like a loving God to inform us what's best to eat and drink.

The Word of God is the same yesterday, today, and always. The biblically based food plan was an identification marker as a follower of our Hebrew God. God's ways involved how we ate and was the case with Daniel, Jesus, John, and Peter.

This is not out of any form of religiosity or condemnation but because we know Papa knows best. Neither can we be yoked under the law to earn salvation or make God love us any more than He already does. But we can continuously grow in Him to become like Him and do as He did.

And I highly doubt that when Christ returns, He'd say, "Fry up some of that bacon, would, ya?" It would go against scriptural accuracy; Jesus only did what the Father instructed. And the Father clearly instructed kosher.

What's Kosher Anyway?

The foundation of kosher is written in Leviticus 11 and Deuteronomy 14. It's God's meat plan also known as the Jewish dietary laws or laws of Kashrut. Kosher means *fit for consumption.*

A kosher summary:

- All seafood is to have both scales and fins and be from fresh or salt waters. Eel or catfish don't meet those standards, but trout, halibut, tuna, salmon, flounder, Mahi Mahi, and anchovies are fine.
- Any meat should only be from animals that both chew the cud and have split hooves. If the animal doesn't have both, it's considered unclean.

    If the animal has paws, crawls, or scurries on the ground, it's unclean. Cats, raccoons, mice, horses, rabbits, and pigs aren't mentioned in God's cookbook.

    Lamb, bison, elk, beef, venison (deer), or veal is alright, assuming they are treated and handled properly.

- Insects that jump on hind legs like crickets, bald locust, and grasshoppers can be eaten. Insects that crawl or walk on the ground are unclean. Spiders or ants are terrible appetizers. Chew on crickets or grasshoppers for something different.
- For the most part, poultry is fine but no vultures, bats, or other birds of prey. Chicken and turkey are good to go.
- And in case you were wondering, it's not okay to eat roadkill (Leviticus 11:40; Leviticus 22:8; Acts 15:29).
- Don't eat the blood of an animal (Deuteronomy 12:23).
- Don't eat the fat of cattle, sheep, or goats (Leviticus 7:23).
- Don't eat food sacrificed to idols (Acts 15:29).

Kosher meat is also raised and killed in a humane way. This means the animal, if used for food, should be treated healthfully and humanely and should have the least pain and shock to it at death.

In addition, animals are valued by God as His creations, and while we have dominion over them, we are to treat them right.

Proverbs 12:10 says a righteous man has regard for the life of his animal, but even the compassion of the wicked is cruel. Animals belong to God and are to be stewarded with care (Psalm 50:10–11, Isaiah 40:11, Matthew 6:26, Proverbs 27:23, Matthew 10:29, and Genesis 2:15).

In the United States, animals earmarked for food aren't treated right. Modern agriculture is another aspect of the Standard American Diet and lends itself to one of the unequivocal immoral issues we face. Most meat, kosher or not, is quite unkosher (unfit for consumption).

See, we're not only misaligned with our waistlines; we're misaligned with how we care for living beings.

We treat animals in such a horrific way that lends to many problems for the earth, animals, and our health. So, even if you're eating clean from a biblical perspective, the meat and the meat industries are rather dirty.

Let me explain.

The Standard American Diet's #1 Offender – Factory Farmed Meat

The USDA reports that 98.75 percent of the meat we eat in United States is from a factory.[1] If you eat at any restaurant, any fast-food place, or buy meat from the grocery store or kosher deli, you partake in factory meat.

Our meat is a millennia of grocery stores away from where it used to be. The meat industry in the United States shifted from normal agricultural practices to downright abominable factory farming practices in the 1960s.[2]

> Our meat is a millennia of grocery stores away from where it used to be.

The government incentivizes these practices to support animal product demand for a growing population.

Namely, with Animal Feeding Operations (AFOs) and Confined Animal Feeding Operations (CAFOs).

As the facility names imply, they're not traditional family farms where kids can feed the chickens. These feeding operations deprive animals of their God-given nature to use the land to roam, graze on grass, warm beneath their mothers, cool themselves in pond water, or lay leisurely throughout the day in the sun.

In factory farms, animals don't roam, enjoy their mothers, or see the light of day. Factory farmed animals are treated as though in a prison, only they didn't do the crime. Chickens get beaks cut off and walk around with broken wings.[3]

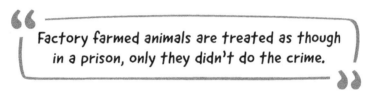

> **Factory farmed animals are treated as though in a prison, only they didn't do the crime.**

The difference between AFOs and CAFOs is the number of animals confined. CAFOs are typically in the tens of thousands, and some are in the hundreds of thousands. They're packed in like the sausages they turn into. There's more than 19,000 CAFOs in the United States.

Total U.S. CAFOs, 2011-2017

In seven years, CAFOs in the United states grew 7.66 percent, adding 1,421 operations.

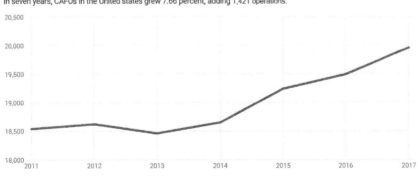

Chart: Christopher Walljasper / Midwest Center for Investigative Reporting • Source: EPA • Get the data • Created with Datawrapper

Graph 24.1 Number of CAFOs in the United States of America [4]

They're described as "infernos of nauseous smells, pools of blood, and screams of terrified animals."[5] Just because an animal is deemed for food versus pet care, should they be treated with such disrespect?

The recommended amount of meat is no more than 5 ounces per day, but Americans eat double that amount.[6] Since the meat and dairy industries spread the marketing campaigns on thick, we're conditioned to believe we need meat and dairy for iron, calcium, and protein to be considered normal and healthy, but this couldn't be further from food truth.

In fact, factory and processed meat is making us quite sick. Regarding your meat consumption, like Dr. Phil, I'll ask, "How's that working for you?"[7]

In 1910 we ate 120 pounds of meat per capita, and it's increased to 220 pounds in 2018, doubling in the past century.[8] And dairy consumption has increased from 294 pounds per capita in 1908 to 653 pounds in 2019.[9,10]

These facts should raise an eyebrow because it's no coincidence that we've also had astronomical increases in chronic diseases during the same timeframe. Chronic diseases have increased due to the unhealthful amount of saturated fat, sodium, and cholesterol, which are root causes for chronic diseases that diets high in meat, dairy, and fish intake promote.

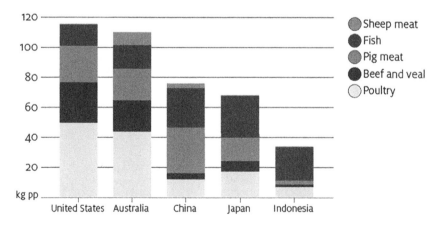

Graph 24.2 Global Meat Consumption [11]

As wealth (the middle class) and population grows, our meat habits will reap greater havoc on animals, the earth, and our health.

See, the only diet proven to reverse health conditions is no meat at all.

Due to the billions of animal products produced in factory farming, we're brainwashed by commercials that promote for us to eat more. So, we bow our mouths down to the sacrificed idol on our plates. You have a right to be empowered to make the best choices for your health.

> " See, the only diet proven to reverse health conditions is no meat at all. "

How Meat-Eating Drives Public Health Concerns

The costs to mitigate the effects of this toxic lifestyle will far outlive our sixth generation if not longer. If we continue to feed ourselves by overconsuming factory farmed meat, we will continue to propel our world into a disastrous future.

Avarice may be the root of all evil, but a lust for food or as the Bible says in gluttonous eaters of meat may surely follow (Proverbs 23:20–21).

Dr. Yuval Noah Harari, PhD, lecturer at The Hebrew University of Jerusalem, historian, philosopher, and bestselling author of *Sapiens*, is quoted regarding modern agriculture as one of the "worst crimes in history."[12,13]

This sentiment is due to several factors. Let's discuss them.

Killing Practices

The United States puts one hundred million animals to rest in abattoirs (slaughterhouses). Many die before they get there due to slum conditions. These animals are flung around one rear leg, breaking the hip, and they hang upside for a few minutes on a rack until it's their time, making their killing worse.[14]

Chain saws are used to cut up the carcasses and pick apart pieces to then send to meat packers. As to be expected, most deaths, mental health issues, amputations, and injuries on the job happen on factory farms because these animals fight back.[15]

Factory farms are the animal version of the Nazi Germany holocaust, and it's been happening to animals since the 60s.

Deception always calls for hiding.

> " Factory farms are the animal version of the Nazi Germany holocaust, and it's been happening to animals since the 60s. "

Industry has pushed legislature to block whistleblowers, in Ag-Gag laws, which are pending in several states.[16] These laws prohibit the use of cameras or photographs in these places to protect the public from seeing what happens.

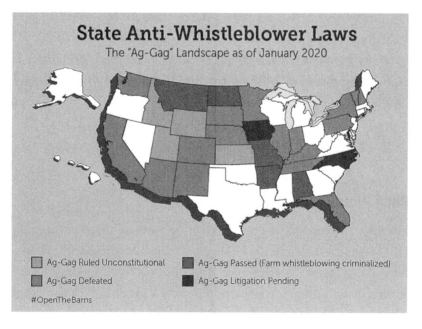

Illustration 24.3   State Anti-Whistleblower Laws[17]

As the name implies, industry wants to gag the throats of those who speak out against the shameful treatment of animals earmarked for food.

Anyone who catches a glimpse of a factory farm video is turned off from eating meat that comes from them. If these animals were dogs the American public would make sure candidates don't approve CAFOs in their cities.

Astronomical Waste Pollutants

Another reason for how meat-eating drives public health concerns is animal waste. There are three times as many animals as there are humans. Animal waste produced in CAFOs is over 1 billion tons per year from the U.S. alone.[18]

A single cow produces as much as sixteen humans.[19] Just one large CAFO can produce up to 1.6 million tons of waste per year, which is one and half times the waste of Philadelphia.[20]

Human waste has a sophisticated sewage system supported by tax dollars.

Animal waste does not.

Because there is no system for the pee-infused manure, we can't imagine the number of infestations, pollutions, and such this can cause to water, land, and air. And the flies? Enough to coat a windshield in these places.

Due to tight living quarters, animals live in their excretions. These excretions are stored in fields, lagoons (man-made manure pools), and ditches causing toxic gases, bacteria, parasites, and microscopic poop compounds to fill the air, water, and grounds in the cities they affect.[21]

The Environmental Protection Agency (EPA) is responsible for public health concerns for CAFOs, which are managed under the Clean Water Act.[22]

However, toxins to land and air are not at all regulated or under-regulated. Toxic stenches can reach up to six to twelve miles in communities affected.[23,24]

Our water comes from ground water (deep in earth, wells) and surface (fresh water sources, rivers). The pollutants from factory farm animal waste contribute to more than ten times as much water pollution from the entire human population.[25] Animal waste contributes to both nitrates and ammonia in the water supply.[26]

If you recall from Chapter 8 on cleansing, Dr. Hulda Clark said that all disease is a product of pollutants and parasites.[27] Diabetes or cancer needs ammonia and other pollutants to survive in the body.

> " The pollutants from factory farm animal waste contribute to more than ten times as much water pollution from the entire human population. "

Toxic gases from CAFOs as well as manure sites impact lung health and function and promote respiratory problems including asthma.[28] All manure produces methane, an odorless, flammable gas that contributes to global warming.[29,30]

CAFO EMISSIONS	SOURCE	TRAITS	HEALTH RISKS
Ammonia	Formed when microbes decompose undigested organic nitrogen compounds in manure	Colorless, sharp pungent odor	Respiratory irritant, chemical burns to the respiratory tract, skin, and eyes, severe cough, chronic lung disease
Hydrogen Sulfide	Anaerobic bacterial decomposition of protein and other sulfur containing organic matter	Odor of rotten eggs	Inflammation of the moist membranes of eye and respiratory tract, olfactor\T neuron loss, death
Methane	Microbial degradation of organic matter under anaerobic conditions	Colorless, odorless, highly flammable	No health risks. Is a greenhouse gas and contributes to climate change.

CAFO EMISSIONS	SOURCE	TRAITS	HEALTH RISKS
Particulate Matter	Feed, bedding materials, dry* manure, unpaved soil surfaces, animal dander, poultry feathers	Comprised of fecal matter, feed materials, pollen, bacteria, fungi, skin cells, silicates	Chronic bronchitis, chronic respiratory symptoms, declines in lung function, organic dust toxic syndrome

Table 24.4 Toxic Pollutants from CAFOs.[31]

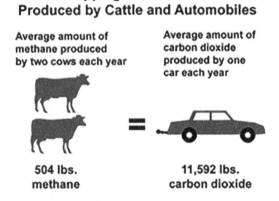

Heat Trapping Greenhouse Gases Produced by Cattle and Automobiles

Average amount of methane produced by two cows each year

Average amount of carbon dioxide produced by one car each year

504 lbs. methane

11,592 lbs. carbon dioxide

Each year, 2 cows produce as much heat trapping greenhouse gas as 1 car driven 10,000 miles.

NWFarmsandFood.com

Illustration 24.5 Cows to Cars[32]

The amount of waste requires constant water irrigation to dilute. This is where things get scary. Each day of meat eating requires 4,000 gallons of water to reduce the effects of waste.[33]

Humans are dependent on aquifers for fresh water.

For example, the High Plains or Ogallala Aquifer provides water to 82 percent of people living within its eight states, including Colorado and Texas.[34] Modern animal agriculture for grain fed cows depletes it by 13 trillion gallons per year.[35] Its once vast resources are now estimated to last until 2028.[36] Should this happen, it would make the land uninhabitable.[37] And it will take thousands of years to replenish this natural resource.[38]

The Worldwatch Institute reported, "Raising livestock accounts for roughly 23 percent of all global water use in agriculture."[39] In the U.S., all of this water is subsidized by the government; otherwise, that fast food burger meat would cost you at least $35.[40]

However, the cost to states is just too much to bear.

As far as global warming concerns, besides cars, electricity is our second largest contributor. Irrigation systems require much electricity to get water to land areas—some require as much as it takes to light the entire nation for a month and a half.[41]

Animal blood is waste too. Over 4 billion liters of cattle blood alone is produced in the United States of America. Imagine all the animals that are slaughtered.[42] Where does the blood go?

I'm sorry to say that 30 percent goes into the food supply in uses such as imitation crab meat, baked goods, and even products for red coloring.[43] The rest goes into pet food products and pharmaceuticals such as wound care.[44] Years ago, it was solely discarded, which has become illegal due to harsh environmental effects.

A Loaded Bite

Ever drive by a cattle ranch? If so, you know half a cow's day is spent chewing. A healthy cow is grass fed and takes a full day or so to digest its intake, ensuring toxins exit its system, which is why God labels cattle as clean.

Cows eating pesticide grains are like people eating processed foods.

They're supposed to eat real, whole foods grass. But 36 percent of all wheat and corn crops as well as soy goes to feed animals to fatten them quickly.[45] The meat of the animals is loaded. Not loaded like a chicken cordon bleu, but they're loaded with pesticides, pharmaceuticals, parasites, and bacteria.

Factory farm raised animals are injected with antibiotics every single day. After decades of these practices, some animal bacteria we consume are immune to antibiotics.[46]

See, factory farms use over 70 percent of all manufactured pharmaceuticals.[47] That's $2 billion worth of pharmaceutical revenues per year for antibiotics and hormone stimulation drugs for these animals.[48]

This means that when we eat these meats, our human gut microbiome is agitated, which makes us prone to a weakened immunity for fighting off infectious diseases.[49]

PATHOGEN	DISEASE	SYMPTOMS
Bacillus anthracis	Anthrax	Skin sores, headache, fever, chills, nausea, vomiting
Escherichia coli	Colibacilosis, Coliforin mastitis-metris	Diarrhea, abdominal gas
Leptospira pomona	Leptospirosis	Abdominal pain, muscle pain, vomiting, fever
Listeria monocytogenes	Listerosis	Fever, fatigue, nausea, vomiting, diarrhea
Salmonella species	Salmonellosis	Abdominal pain, diarrhea, nausea, chills, fever, headache
Clostirdum tetani	Tetanus	Violent muscle spasms, lockjaw, difficulty breathing
Histoplasma capsulatum	Histoplasmosis	Fever, chills, muscle ache, cough rash, joint pain and stiffness
Microsporum and Trichophyton	Ringworm	Itching, rash
Giardia lamhlia	Giardiasis	Diarrhea, abdominal pain, abdominal gas, nausea, vomiting, fever
Cryptosporidium species	Cryptosporidosis	Diarrhea, dehydration, weakness, abdominal cramping

Table 24.6   Common Harmful Bacteria in CAFO Meat[50]

Food inspectors will tell you that you can't see bacteria and other harmful microorganisms just by looking at the meat.[51]

In 300 packages of ground beef tested, all had bacteria. Eighty percent had harmful bacteria, and 20 percent super harmful bacteria.[52] All of these added strands as well as other factors in red meat, such as

TMAO, causes irritated bowels and inflammation, which is why red meat is strongly correlated to colon cancer.[53,54]

And if not for that, consider the saturated fat, sodium, and cholesterol heart disease causing content itself. All CAFO and AFO raised livestock, including chicken and pork, carry more harmful bacteria than sustainably raised meat.[55]

As reported, "In 1950, there were 5.6 million farms raising 100 million farm animals. In 2017, there were 2 million farms raising 9.32 billion farm animals."[56]

To feed us, these cows, pigs, and chickens are given reproductive hormones to be pregnant without breaks between, which would weaken and deplete any mother. Reproduction demands a ton of nutrients from the mother's body, and these animals aren't getting them.

> We're not just eating the meat.

We're not just eating the meat.

We're eating added fattening hormones, antibiotics, bacteria, fecal matter, and parasites.

A Breeding Ground for Disease

Ultimately all these factors and more create a breeding ground for disease. For example, in 2019 we had an outbreak of e-coli on romaine lettuce. And a while back the same thing happened with spinach.

In both outbreaks the lettuce was produced in areas where CAFOs were only 400 feet or less apart.[57] Since the outbreaks, buffers of 1,200 feet were established to prevent the waste irrigation systems and effects from the vegetation.[58]

But is that enough?

Mark my words: if we don't take care of animals, they will not take care of us. Dr. Michael Greger's recent book *How To Survive a Pandemic* validates evidence for other

> We're eating added fattening hormones, antibiotics, bacteria, fecal matter, and parasites.

coronaviruses and zoonotic diseases (diseases that transfer from animals to humans) are expected to increase. According to the National Institutes of Health, 75 percent of emerging infectious diseases are from animals.[59]

Per Greger, these strands can infect livestock such as pigs quickly and 'jump' on humans. The recent coronavirus was predicted, which was caused by China's trading of exotic, unclean meats to please the palate for delicacies. As of January 2020, wild exotic meats were banned for food in China.[60]

Unsustainable Effects on Global Warming

Soon we'll reach 9 billion people on the planet. Billions of humans eating animal foods regularly is unsustainable because it depletes natural resources and contributes to greenhouse gases warming the planet and raising sea levels.

We need to question our consumption—at what cost? The efficiency gained from packing animals in isn't efficient whatsoever according to researchers of *CAFOs Uncovered: The Untold Costs of Confined Animal Feeding Operations*, a free public health report that outlines exactly why factory farming is inefficient.

Global warming is a proven and growing concern as shown by evidence of a hotter planet and ice melting like wax over the last decade.[61] Global warming puts island countries and coastal cities like New Orleans and Florida at risk of drowning.[62]

The primary source of global warming is burning fossil fuels, and the second is use of electricity.

What we eat has an impact.

Emissions from different food types vary across farms and countries

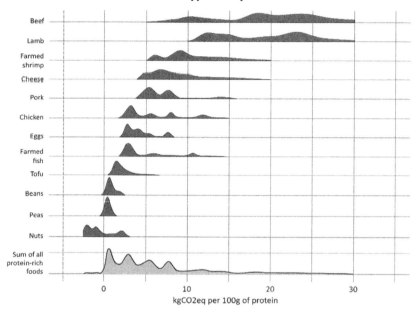

The spread of greenhouse gas emissions (per 100g of protein) created by the production of different food types from 38,000 farms. Adapted from Dr Hannah Ritchie/Our Woad in Data (2020) Data source: Poore & Nemecek (2018)

Chart 24.7 Emissions from Various Protein Sources [63]

Factory farming contributes an estimated 18 percent to global warming, which is more than trains and planes.[64] Studies show that if we reduce meat to one day a week, we can all impact efforts to slow global warming.

With all this insight on how meat-eating drives public health concerns, you may still wonder, *What does one do with bacon?*

The Bacon Dilemma

Like a 90's love song, you're singing to your memories of bacon: *It's So Hard To Say Goodbye.* You're not alone. The average American eats at least fifty pounds of pork a year.[65] Let me give you a love nudge. I'll provide you with a few reasons to trim the pork belly.

See, those squigglies I mistakenly fed my grandparents were a form of parasite carried in pork called Trichinella, which can be seen with vinegar while cooking.

Seriously, search the internet. I did, and here's what I found:

Trichinosis is a disease of man and other animals caused by a tiny parasitic worm, Trichinella spiralis. Humans may be infected by eating the meat of infected domestic pigs, wild bears, wild pigs, or walruses ... An estimated 10 to 15 million people in the United States have been infected with trichinosis. An estimated 1.5 million Americans carry the parasite, and between 150,000 and 300,000 new infections occur each year.[66]

Yuck.

Pigs excessively overeat, nibble, and tail bite other pigs, which can turn into cannibalism where they start eating the pig. They have zero discretion on what they eat. And because they have a four-hour digestive cycle, whatever they ate isn't adequately cleansed from toxins in their system, so pig meat is loaded with bacteria and parasites.

Swine has also been unfavorable in scriptural occurrences, such as in the following:

- "Do not give what is holy to the dogs; nor cast your pearls before swine, lest they trample them under their feet, and turn and tear you in pieces" (Matthew 7:6).
- The Prodigal Son hit rock bottom when he was surrounded by pigs and wanted to eat what they were eating (Luke 15:11–32).
- Jesus cast demons out and put them in swine. Over the cliff the swine went with the unclean spirits that matched the unclean pigs (Matthew 8:28–34).

Several health concerns are either indirectly or directly related to pork consumption, such as the following:[67]

- Hepatitis E

- Trichinosis
- A number of parasitic infections (Taenia solium tapeworm, genotype 3, Nipah virus, menangle virus, Paramyxoviridae viruses)
- Multiple Sclerosis
- Liver Cirrhosis
- Hepatocellular Carcinoma (liver cancer)
- High nitrosamines – in processed pork products
- Yersiniosis (bacterial infection causing deaths and food poisoning each year from undercooked pork)[68]

Mouth Excellency

Daniel wasn't willing to eat just anything. He and his cohorts were sure they weren't eating like the Babylonians. Daniel is known as a man of excellence, and part of that excellence was what he put in his mouth (Daniel 1:9–16).

- When Peter was impressed by God to "kill and eat" after seeing unclean animals, Peter responded, "Surely not, Lord!" Peter replied. "I have never eaten anything impure or unclean" (Acts 11:8). God was using unclean food to represent an unclean people whom God made clean for Peter to disciple, not for unclean foods for Peter to eat (Acts 11:1–18).
- And Job said, "I have not departed from the commands of His lips; I have treasured the words of His mouth more than my daily food" (Job 23:12).

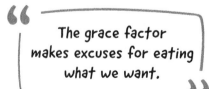

The grace factor makes excuses for eating what we want.

I don't believe these faith runners honored God with food out of a religious spirit. I believe they wholeheartedly trusted God enough to follow His advice.

The grace factor makes excuses for eating what we want.

But if God had His perfect way with us, we wouldn't choose to eat what He doesn't consider food. However, His abundant grace doesn't place a burden on believers in this way. It's not the priority when one is saved, but as we mature, we're to become more like Christ in all our ways. And eating food fit for consumption is a part of maturing.

To eat solely based on tastiness at the expense of health is spiritually immature.

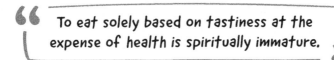

> **To eat solely based on tastiness at the expense of health is spiritually immature.**

Your beast doesn't care what God's thoughts are about food or about the health of the body. Food may be edible and all things God created are good, but this doesn't mean we should eat it. To summarize what Paul said in 1 Corinthians 6:12, just because we can doesn't mean we should.

With all of this said, what we do with bacon is transition your pig bacon to an organic, uncured, nitrates-free, turkey version or skip it altogether.

Factory fish farming also has severe effects to the environment and human health. Over 150 million pounds of fish are also produced in an unsustainable way.

Except for direct revenues, there is no logical reason morally, financially, or environmentally that supports factory farming—from the mentally ill institutions participating. The only logical reason is the Father of Lies driving the agricultural bus (John 8:44).

We don't need to eat meat every day. Despite the meat industry's promotion of iron or protein, we're still anemic and unhealthy. There are better ways.

Once again, our best bet is to take responsibility for ourselves and align with God.

The Standard American Diet's #2 Offender – Chemicalized Ingredients

The other side of clean eating has to do with processed foods. Not only do we eat unclean foods from a biblical perspective, but we also eat impure foods dramatically denatured with chemical engineering to support preservation, softness, and taste in fast and processed foods.

Clean eating from the world's perspective is eating foods that haven't gone through severe manufacturing processes and don't have added chemicals or ingredients to pump up the flavor and get you hooked.

While the authors of *It Starts with Food*, *Think and Eat Yourself Smart*, and *The Micronutrient Miracle* are pushing forward positive messages on whole food eating, God said it first in Genesis 1:29–30, which we'll discuss in Part Two.

Do your most frequently eaten foods resemble the ingredient list of this popular doughnut?

Popular Doughnut Chain Glazed Doughnut[69]

*Ingredients: **Doughnut** (Enriched Wheat Flour (Wheat Flour, Niacin, Reduced Iron, Thiamine Mononitrate, Riboflavin, Folic Acid), Water, Palm Oil, Soybean Oil, Sugar. Contains 2% or Less of Each of the Following: Yeast, Soy Lecithin, Hydrogenated Soybean Oil, Salt, Mono and Diglycerides, Wheat Gluten, Calcium Sulfate, Monocalcium Phosphate, BHT, Dried Milk Powder, Egg Yolks, Cellulose Gum, Calcium Propionate (to maintain freshness), Ammonium Sulfate, Ascorbic Acid, Dicalcium Phosphate, Sorbitan Monostearate, Tocopherols, Tricalcium Phosphate, Diammonium Phosphate)*

***Glaze** (Sugar, Water, Corn Starch, Palm Oil, Calcium Sulfate and/or Calcium Carbonate, Agar, Dextrose, Natural and Artificial Flavors, Salt, Disodium Phosphate, Locust Bean Gum and/or Mono and Diglycerides).*

Homemade Doughnut

Ingredients for doughnut and glaze: active dry yeast, sugar, salt, eggs, shortening, flour, vegetable oil, butter, confectioners' sugar, vanilla, water (hot and lukewarm)

You're probably thinking, *I cannot pronounce some of the ingredients in the first list.* And your liver is thinking, *I can't either! I know what to do: I'll store them in weird places in your body since they'll probably live in here longer than you!*

Your beast is thinking, *Come on, let's make some donuts!*

Shut-up, beast.

Some of these ingredients are banned in other countries because of possible ill effects. When you look up the ingredients, you'll find a variety of health issues that go with them.

For fun, let's do it again. Check out a very popular chicken sandwich.

Fast Food Chain Chicken Sandwich[70]

Ingredients: Chicken (boneless, skinless chicken breast filet, seasoning [salt, monosodium glutamate, sugar, spices, paprika], seasoned coater [enriched bleached wheat flour {with malted barley flour, niacin, iron, thiamine mononitrate, riboflavin, folic acid}, sugar, salt, monosodium glutamate (MSG), nonfat milk, leavening {baking soda, sodium aluminum phosphate, monocalcium phosphate}, spice, soybean oil, color {paprika}], milk wash [water, nonfat milk, egg], peanut oil [fully refined peanut oil, with Dimethylpolysiloxane, an anti-foam agent added])

And if that wasn't a mouthful, now for the bun of that chicken sandwich:[71]

(enriched wheat flour [wheat flour, malted barley flour, niacin, reduced iron, thiamin mononitrate, riboflavin, folic acid], water, sugar, yeast, soybean oil, wheat gluten, contains 2% or less of salt,

*cultured wheat flour, vinegar, calcium sulfate, monoglycerides,
DATEM, calcium propionate, ascorbic/citric acid, enzymes, soy
lecithin, potassium iodate), bun oil (soybean oil, palm kernel oil,
soy lecithin, natural flavor, beta carotene), pickle (cucumbers,
water, vinegar, salt, calcium chloride, alum, potassium sorbate
[preservatives], natural flavors, polysorbate 80, yellow 5, blue 1)*

Interesting finds, huh? Each chemicalized ingredient has severe consequences even with a tiny amount. Dyes, for example, can cause mood problems including violence.[72] DATEM (Diacetyl Tartaric Acid Esters of Monoglycerides) can cause headaches, nausea, leaky gut, and adrenal growth.[73]

You may wonder if the food is so good, why do you need Monosodium Glutamate (MSG), twice? Because without it, the food isn't going to sell by the multimillions.

Again, food addicts are the best, frequent shoppers.

MSG is made from an isolated sodium salt from the naturally occurring amino acid Glutamate. However, it's proven to create addiction in the brain as well as to raise insulin levels. These are two problems that cause obesity.

> "Food addicts are the best, frequent shoppers."

These are just a few chemicalized ingredients, but the others follow suit to health problems from asthma, high blood pressure, diabetes type 2, and heart disease.

And I must say, by nature of the fast-food business, this chicken sandwich is one of the best on the market as far as ingredients are concerned. Most companies don't even list the ingredients because their ingredients are far worse health bombs.

Just note that it's not God who causes disease and sickness, it's addictive, man-made, chemically engineered foods that lead to death of energy, organs, vitality, effort, and accomplishment. It's also our willingness to partake in the Satanic Addictive Deception that causes disease, early death, and lethargy.

It's not God who causes disease and sickness, it's addictive, man-made, chemically engineered foods that lead to death of energy, organs, vitality, effort, and accomplishment.

What Are Processed Foods Anyway?

Processed foods are foods that are denatured from their original intention by way of the manufacturing process. They include:

- Processed meats: ham, lunch meats, sausage, bacon, cured meats like salami, and hot dogs. Note: The World Health Organization has directly linked these meats as causal to cancer in the body due to high levels of nitrosamines.[74]

- Anything on the market from food giants

- Anything that must advertise what's no longer in it such "no arsenic" or "no trans-fat"

- Any item that has a laundry list of ingredients and any you can't pronounce

- Most food that comes in a bag, container, can, or box

- And Spam or Scrapple. (That's for our friends in a more distinguished generation.)

Overall, we need to eat more nutrient dense, higher quality meats, vegetables, fruits, and grains. Not every one's budget can afford to eat the highest quality meats or products. But can we afford not to?

With medical costs skyrocketing, perhaps we could consider our health as both an investment and a protection from costs later on.

And the good news is that the healthiest way to eat is very inexpensive.

As Paul Nison, author of *Health According to the Scriptures* says, use *common sense* Kosher; that is to not to be obsessive about Kosher approvals but to do what you *can* do to stop eating what isn't food.

Are You an Unclean Eater?

We're way off from God's intention with food; therefore, we're way off from His intention from vibrant health, energy, and wellbeing. Despite the prayer lines, we need to make change to reduce processed foods toward elimination to whole, real, honest food.

However, don't limit God. It's possible to have a miracle deliverance from fast food, just don't keep eating it expecting one.

Again, the Standard American Diet (S.A.D.) is 70 percent processed foods. But when I was a fast-food junkie, I ate 100 percent processed food—S.A.D. indeed because this was before McDonald's stopped making their burgers with "pink slime."[75] But God did it for me, and He'll do it for you too.

You can reduce your non-foods too.

Ready to spit out unclean foods? Let's win the unclean eating battle.

Part Two: Win the Unclean Eating Battle
How to Spit It Out because That Wasn't Food for Good!

There's nothing like a chapter poking at die-hard, meat-eating habits for revealing the real food idols of hearts is there?

I get that some of the information presented wasn't exactly your favorite, but wasn't it a needful conversation? God loves you. And real love delivers the truth. The fact that you got to this point proves that you can handle the truth.

Our God loves the pork eating folk just as much as He loves the non-pork eating folk, but I'll still need to drop some food truth.

To win the battle of unclean eating, instead of focusing on what not to eat, we'll focus on what to add to your food selections. In earlier chapters, I said it's not the calories, but it's the nutritional make up of calories we eat. Let's get the type of intake right.

Battle Strategy 1: Focus Eating According to Genesis 1:29–30 [The Life Abundantly Standard]

No matter which way of eating you choose, a certain food truth reigns throughout all of them. Well, maybe not the Breatharian diet, where one lives on air alone for a low fee of $100,000 up to one million.[76] Go figure, the main advocate of that false plan was caught coming out of 7-Eleven with a Slurpee® and Twinkies®.[77]

Clearly, any healthy eating plan requires some level of adherence to God's original order for how human beings were to eat. I call this adherence to Genesis 1:29–30, the Life Abundantly Standard (L.A.S.).

The Life Abundantly Standard sets a minimum daily intake of 50 percent of calories from whole plant-based, fresh, alive foods, and the rest to whole, clean, real, non-plant, or plant foods.

Basically, it's the opposite of the processed, refined, fast, factory-farmed foods of the Standard American Diet. The Life Abundantly Standard works with any diet you choose because it's a guideline for healthy obedience to lead to prosperous health, not a diet.

> The Life Abundantly Standard works with any diet you choose because it's a guideline for healthy obedience to lead to prosperous health, not a diet.

Life Abundantly Standard	Standard American Diet
And God said, "See, I have given you every herb *that* yields seed which *is* on the face of all the earth, and every tree whose fruit yields seed; to you it shall be for food. Also to everything … in which there is life, I have given every green herb for food" [Gen 1:29-30]	Consuming foods and ingredients that create and cause addictive nature in brain, altar taste buds, inflammatory states in the body, disordered eating, or unbalanced, inadequate nutrition promoting disease of body, soul, and spirit.
Daily Calorie Intake 50-100% - fresh 'alive' whole plant food, uncooked [Gen 1:29] 0-50% - whole plant and non-plant 'clean' food, cooked [Gen. 9:3; Lev. 11; Duet. 14]	**Daily Calorie Intake** 60-100% processed, highly processed foods, refined, 'dirty', 'dead' and animal foods [addictive, dead foods] 0-40% whole plant foods, much cooked

Illustration 24.8 Life Abundantly Standard versus Standard American Diet

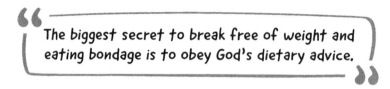

> **The biggest secret to break free of weight and eating bondage is to obey God's dietary advice.**

The biggest secret to break free of weight and eating bondage is to obey God's dietary advice. Therefore, we listen less to the constant confusion of the media on what to do with food and listen to God's instructions in Genesis 1:29–30 and our own bodies.

And God said, "See, I have given you every herb [plant] that yields seed which is on the face of all the earth, and every tree whose fruit yields seed; to you it shall be for food. Also, to every beast of the earth, to every bird of the air, and to everything that creeps on the earth, in which there is life, I have given every green herb for food"; and it was so (Genesis 1:29–30).

Commit this Scripture to memory. I'll make it easy for you. Say this out loud, "No matter my diet, I still eat mostly fresh whole plant foods!"

Ah, good job, you'll grow into it.

The question is how much nutrient dense foods do you eat now?

On a scale of 0 to 100 percent, how much do your foods/beverages adhere to Genesis 1:29–30?

_____ percent of Genesis 1:29–30 (Life Abundant Standard) foods [whole plant foods – fruits, leafy green vegetables, starchy vegetables, nuts, seeds, whole grains, beans, legumes/lentils – in uncooked/baked/ boiled or other natural form – fried foods, fast foods, refined foods, and meats are not included.]

On a scale of 0 to 100 percent, how S.A.D. (Standard American Diet) are your foods now?

_____ percent of non-Genesis 1:29–30 foods [denatured foods, addictive ingredients, chemical ingredients, processed foods, fast food, factory farmed meats and/or fish, regular meats, unclean meats or fish, and/or fish, fried/deep fried]

It's simple and filled with grace. Aim to increase your current percentage of total caloric intake per day to real, clean, mostly whole plant foods.

For the record, I don't advocate any specific diets.

I want us to focus on adherence to our Master Dietician's primary advice because it brings health.

So, note that you are the master of your mouth.

It's totally fine to eat meat, eggs, dairy, and fish if you desire to eat these foods. I'll give you ideas to not do the harmful versions.

You can also work your chosen dietary plan (keto, paleo, vegan, vegetarian, pescatarian, etc.) with the Life Abundantly Standard.

Whole plant-based foods are food truth: fruits, vegetables, beans and legumes, whole grains, nuts, and seeds. The Creator, who is life, created sustainable, life-giving foods for us to enjoy and provide life to the body, soul, and spirit.

They also reduce oxidative stress and free radicals, make blood thinner and easier to flow, improve thinking, balance hormones, hydrate cells, cleanse the intestines, feed healthy bacteria in the gut, and so much more.

If you're interested in more specific food, check out *What the Bible Says about Healthy Living*. In it, Dr. Rex Russell, MD, breaks down details of food benefits and detriments with Scripture. It's so good.

In a world of deception, His truth always remains.

Please let go of confusion against any of His foods, such as not eating this or that vegetable or fruit. Scientific research proves the same obvious truth: we need to eat fruits and vegetables in more abundance.

Here's how:

Eat More Low-Calorie Dense Foods

God is so abundant in all things, especially food. Calorie density is the number of calories per pound of food. The more calorie dense a food is, the more caloric it is with the least amount of food, so eat less. The less calorie dense a food is, the less caloric it is with the most amount of food, so eat more.

Oil, for example is 4,000 calories per pound, yet it barely fills the stomach. For one tablespoon of oil, you can eat twenty-five strawberries. Can you see God's abundance?

Table 24.9 Calorie Density Scale

FOODS	CALORIES/POUND
Vegetables	60-195
Fruit	140-420
Potatoes, Pasta, Rice, Barley, Yams, Corn, Hot Cereals	320-630
Beans, Peas, Lentils (cooked)	310-780
Breads, Bagels, Fat-free Muffins, Dried Fruit	920-1360
Sugars (i.e. sugar, honey, molasses, agave, corn syrup, maple syrup)	1200-1800
Dry Cereals, Baked Chips, Fat-free Crackers, Pretzels, Popcorn	1480-1760
Nuts/Seeds	2400-3200
Oils	4000

Note: Chicken, turkey, pork, and red meat are 820–1,300 per pound.

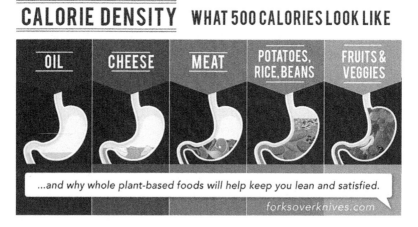

Illustration 24.10 Forks Over Knives Calorie Density[78]

Not only is the volume of low-calorie density foods we can eat huge, but most are nutritionally dense too. With all those strawberries you gain 300 percent of vitamin C, 29 percent fiber, and 9 percent iron. Friends, daily nutrition like this is potent healing power to years of damage from the S.A.D.!

Many non-starchy vegetables are barely 100 calories per pound, which allows us to eat more. Only eating vegetables will make one weak if you don't eat enough calories of them. So, we pair with a variety of vegetables, including starchy ones, as well as fats and proteins to be strong.

Since low calorie dense foods allow for more food abundance, servings sizes may need to change. I think we're designed to be abundant eaters, and we've gotten that confused with overeating because we've been eating the wrong things. We can eat more abundantly if we switch from the dark side of the S.A.D. and come to the light of the Life Abundant Standard.

Here's the deal from Chapter 23. Like the manna given from heaven, we're to eat enough for our needs each day. If your calorie needs are 1,500 per day and you divide that over three meals, at breakfast you'll eat 500 calories. A cream filled donut (370 calories) and coffee (130 calories with cream and sugar) adds up fast and leaves you wanting more because they're empty, worthless calories that don't do anything for the whole body only the tongue.

A mono meal is a meal of a single type of fruit or vegetable.

For example, you'd have to eat five oranges, a whole watermelon, five bananas, or almost three whole cantaloupes to get 500 calories. Or make a big bowl of each fruit up to 500 calories.

It may look bad psychologically to eat a whole watermelon at one sitting in the presence of food under-schooled friends compared to a donut and coffee, but you'll certainly look and feel good physically.

How abundant is God?

An *Abundant Green Salad* recipe could have five cups of thinly chopped collards, chard, and kale greens with sprouts, a chopped baked

sweet potato, 1 tablespoon of pumpkin seeds, and quarter cup of walnuts with a pear balsamic dressing to fill a mixing bowl, yet it is barely
500 calories. That's the power of calorie density. You get to fill your
stomach with foods that are nutritious and delicious, eat more, and
transform.

Dr. Barbara Rolls, PhD, an author and researcher for obesity at
Penn State University, is credited for calorie density understanding in
what she calls volumetrics, eating more lower calorie dense foods for
nutritional abundance.[79]

Be abundant. "And God is able to make all grace abound toward
you, that you, always having all sufficiency in all things, may have an
abundance for every good work" (2 Corinthians 9:8).

Seek Nutrient Density

Nutrient density is about selecting foods that are packed with fiber,
water, vitamins, minerals, antioxidants, and phytonutrients that prevent and reverse disease, inflammation, and free radical advancement
in your system.

A nutrient dense food provides more nutrition per bite. Foods
such as collard greens or broccoli as staples in your diet impact focus,
memory, circulation, and freedom from cravings.[80]

These foods are loaded with vitamin K, magnesium, vitamin A, vitamin C, and many more antioxidants and blood cleansing chlorophyll
richness. Kind of like a spray cleaner for the kitchen, nutrient dense
foods support your body's natural healing process.

See, fiber and water-based foods are like a scrub brush and soap,
and toxins are like stains. The more you eat the right foods, the more
fiber and water you get, and the more fiber and water you get, the more
toxins get out of cells.

Adipose (fat) tissue is filled with toxins.

We want an eating plan that is nutritious and delicious. Be mindful
because we all know there's junk food versions of every eating plan.

Junk food vegans and vegetarians, as they're called, barely touch green vegetables and still gorge on chips and deep-fried, fast-food veggie burgers. True whole foods, plant-based eaters are superior in nutrition over S.A.D. and meat-eating counterparts.

Seek nutrient dense options. Foods that have more life, raised by the energy of the sun, also have more energy for you. Light is sweet and it is pleasing to the eyes to see the sun (Ecclesiastes 11:7).

Increase Raw Food Intake

Be conscious about how much of your food is cooked or uncooked. Fresh, alive, uncooked foods, also called raw, are packed with lifeforce, and have power to heal damage done by the S.A.D.

Temperatures over 117 degrees (F) strip life out of food that is otherwise abundantly blessed with enzymes, minerals, and vitamins that aid in digestion.[81]

Fruits are raw if fresh or frozen and should be eaten ripe.

Dates, dried figs, raisins, dried apricots, or dried pineapple are raw, but eat them sparingly. They're God's candy. And do still brush after eating starches or sweets because teeth aren't exempt from the residues of sugar they leave behind.

Non-starchy vegetables are great raw. They include cucumbers, tomatoes, broccoli, onions, mushrooms, bell peppers, lettuces, parsley, cilantro, kale, spinach, cauliflower, cabbage, any lettuce, carrots, radishes, chard, onions, green beans, jicama, zucchini, beets, daikon radish, watercress, garlic, and artichokes.

Starchy vegetables like green peas, corn, beets, and parsnips can work raw, but sweet potatoes, white potatoes, pumpkin, butternut squash, and acorn squash work best baked, boiled, or steamed.

Check out the list of raw food options:

Karen Knowler's Raw Foods Group [82]

- Fresh fruits (apples, pears, pineapple etc.)
- Vegetables (carrots, turnips, sweet potatoes etc.)
- Salad vegetables (tomatoes, bell peppers, cucumbers etc.)
- Leafy green vegetables (kale, watercress, chard etc.)
- Herbs (basil, mint, parsley etc.)
- Wild greens (dandelion, nettle, purslane etc.)
- Nuts (almonds, pine nuts, macadamia nuts etc.)
- Dried fruits (prunes, raisins, sultanas etc.)
- Sprouted beans, pulses and legumes (aduki, mung, lentil etc.)
- Sprouted grains (wheat, rye, barley etc.)
- Seeds (pumpkin, sesame, sunflower etc.)
- Sprouted seeds (quinoa, buckwheat, chia etc.)
- Indoor greens (wheatgrass, sunflower greens, pea shoots etc.)
- Sprouted vegetable seeds (broccoli, mustard, cress etc.)
- Edible flowers (wild rose petals, honeysuckle, lavender blossoms etc.)
- Mushrooms (oyster, portobello, reishi etc.)
- Sea vegetables (dulse, wakame, kelp etc.)
- Algaes (chlorella, spirulina, Klamath lake blue-green algae etc.)
- Oils (olive oil, sesame oil, hemp oil etc.)
- Stimulants (onion, garlic, cayenne pepper etc.)
- Spices (turmeric, cumin, nutmeg etc.)
- Flavourings and sweeteners (cacao, honey, mesquite meal etc.)
- Superfoods (aloe vera, bee pollen, maca etc.)
- Pre-packaged/prepared raw foods (nut butters, seed butters, flax crackers etc.)

While I am not advocating any diet, some people choose to eat all raw 90 to 100 percent of the time like Dr. Douglas and his wife, Rosalind Graham. Dr. Doug Graham is the author of *80/10/10,* an all-raw eating plan. As a coach to elite athletes and an athlete himself, for optimal performance and energy he advocates calories to come from macronutrients (macros) of 80 percent carbohydrates (mostly fruits), 10 percent fat, and 10 percent protein.

Rosalind admits to having no more disordered eating problems after she adopted a raw lifestyle and divorced the Standard American Diet.[83]

There are many great raw foods teachers out there. My favorites are Drs. Rick and Karen Dina at Raw Food Education and Karen Knowler, who calls herself the Raw Food Coach. They've supported thousands of people in learning how to eat more raw foods.

A sauce of fresh tomatoes, mangos, and basil over zucchini noodles is one example of many delicious all raw food meals. Again, you don't need to be 100 percent raw to learn how to make raw food lunches and dinners.

Aim for 50 percent of your nutrition to be from raw foods. It's okay if it takes time. But if you have dreams of doing cartwheels like in grade school, vacuuming at warp speed, springing out of bed early, or a refund on your gas bill, eat an abundance of raw foods.

Set Simple, Clean Food Goals

One of the fastest ways to get somewhere is to set a goal. To make health changes fun, set targets of what you'd like to achieve. Then have a blast winning your own health game to increase clean food intake.

It may take time, but you know where you're headed. And the weight and eating victory is unmatched when you're all cleaned up from the S.A.D. with its unclean meats and seafood. You can get there by setting specific food goals. Mark examples of daily or weekly food goals that you want to try:

- Make baked fries at home.
- Eat only at fresh foods places instead of fast food.

- Eat one *Abundant Green Salad* per day or three times per week.
- Eat 3–5 cups of vegetables per day or with dinner.
- Drink one green smoothie per day.
- Eat kale chips instead of potato chips.
- Make cacao powder hot chocolate with nut milk with stevia instead of a chocolate bar.
- Drink coffee black.
- Use spaghetti squash, zucchini noodles, or lentil-based pasta instead of wheat pasta.
- Eat Ezekiel or other whole grain bread instead of white bread.
- Reduce meat intake to once or twice per week.
- Substitute cheese with avocados.
- Eat turkey bacon instead of pork bacon.
- Buy grass-fed beef instead of factory farmed.
- Exchange white rice for brown rice.
- Switch from cow milk to nut milk.

Set yourself up for success by making goals simple and achievable. Be sure to read the ingredients on the label to know what's going into your system—after all it could be animal blood disguised as cookies. Just saying.

Eat To Heal

As if God wasn't already smart enough, He shows us how thoughtful He is when we consider the natural remedies of food to heal our bodies. For instance, take the walnut. It's loaded in omega 3's and looks like a brain, doesn't it? And it does, in fact, support brain cell signaling and reduces oxidative stress to it.[84]

How cool is it that? I'm going to eat some right now.

And what body part does celery look like? Right, bones.

170

Celery is loaded in 37 percent of the daily recommended dose of vitamin K, a known factor to support reversing autoimmune conditions, Alzheimer's, and free radical distribution.[85]

The kicker, vitamin K can prevent osteoporosis in bones!

Take a piece of the green, leafy beauty Kale. Doesn't it look like a capillary system? Kale and other green, leafy beauty queens support blood circulation as well as breathing.

From kidney beans that benefit the kidneys to carrots that when broken in half look like two eyes staring back at you, God's divine intelligence for nourishing our organs with life is all around us.

As Hippocrates said, "Let medicine be thy food, and food be thy medicine." And as God said in Genesis 1:29–30, use food to heal.[86]

Battle Strategy #2 – Avoid the Meat Department

Humans have eaten meat, dairy, and fish for a long time, but the quality and amount has changed to be detrimental. Even in the public journal, *Meat Science*, meat industry researchers' question if they should be vegetarian. They opted out due to economic effects, not for alarming and highly researched public health concerns.[87]

In 2017, Global Health Burden researchers found, "Poor diet is responsible for more global deaths than tobacco, high blood pressure, and any other health risk."[88] They strongly advocate avoiding the meat, fish, and dairy departments.

> " In 2017, Global Health Burden researchers found, "Poor diet is responsible for more global deaths than tobacco, high blood pressure, and any other health risk." "

There are hundreds of studies that connect factory farmed products with at least eleven different cancers, heart disease, autoimmune diseases, obesity, and diabetes type 2.[89]

In addition to the unwanted sides these factories farmed meats serve (bacteria, parasites, pollutants, etc.), diets high in these protein sources are by default high in saturated fat, sodium, and cholesterol-proven problem ingredients in leading killers.

And by the way, besides being the single dietary factor in all chronic diseases, meat eating also affects body fat.

The Adventists are a group of Christians that honor biblical eating practices for the most part. In a famous study of over 50,000 participants of these Christians and their diets, those who ate dairy, eggs, and cheese weighed on average twenty-five pounds less than meat eaters.[90]

In the same study, those who ate no animal products had the lowest body mass index, averaging forty pounds less than meat eaters.[91] Most of the meat eaters were overweight or obese with an average BMI (Body Mass Index) of 28.[92] Studies showed those with troublesome visceral fat around the middle eat more meat.

Chicken should get an award as the most utilized food for weight loss attempts, shouldn't it? How often have you tried the ol' chicken and broccoli? A chicken today has 1,000 percent more fat today than it did one hundred years ago due to factory farming.[93] We can't eat factory farmed meat and expect major health gains.

Here's why: all meat and dairy increases both insulin and IGF-1 (insulin growth factor hormone), which grows cancerous cells and is found in all chronic diseases, such as heart disease and type 2 diabetes.[94] A mere 10 percent of calories from meat increases IGF-1.[95]

In men and women tested, those eating meat-free, whole-plant foods have double the IGF-1 binding hormones than those on a meat eating or dairy and eggs only vegetarian diet, which means plant-based eaters can fight cancerous cell growth. And the longer one eats vegan the more IGF-1 reduces.

Insulin itself is another factor. Meats, poultry, cheese, and seafood increase insulin just as much as sugar and more than eating white rice or mashed potatoes alone.[96] And after just three weeks or no meat, insulin levels reduce significantly. Plant-based fats, such as nuts, seeds, and avocados, slow insulin levels.

Meat eaters have 50 percent higher insulin levels than non-meat eaters.[97] Given that insulin is the primary cause of weight gain, it's best to reduce or eliminate meat to have more ease in weight reduction.

One of the biggest worries about reducing meat is protein deficiency. But no worries because we're more protein bamboozled than deficient in America. Excess protein stores as fat, taxes kidneys, and depletes gastric acids.[98]

Males need about 56 grams and women 46 grams of protein. To get your specific protein needs in grams, multiply your body weight by 0.36.

Protein is made from amino acids.

We get amino acids from fruits, grains, vegetables, and legumes and build a better, healthier body. And while seafood and animal products are a whole protein source, a few heaps of beans, collards, or broccoli can easily meet your needs.

Unlike sugar, meat isn't addictive, only habitual.

It's easier than other S.A.D. problem foods and ingredients to let go of. Only cured and processed meats like salami, pepperoni, ham, sausage, bacon, as well as fast food chicken, beef, and fish can be addictive due to bliss point factors like sugar, fat, and salt combinations as well as additives.[99]

Did a tear drop when you read about bacon?

Would you be interested in fried chicken without the crispy flour, salt, and oil? Or a rotisserie without the liberal salt?

Probably not.

Again, the addictive ingredients make these meats irresistible.

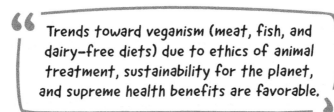

Trends toward veganism (meat, fish, and dairy-free diets) due to ethics of animal treatment, sustainability for the planet, and supreme health benefits are favorable.

Trends toward veganism (meat, fish, and dairy-free diets) due to ethics of animal treatment, sustainability for the planet, and supreme health benefits are favorable.

Tabitha Brown is a wonderful example who felt called by God to veganism and shares her spirit-filled journey and recipes on YouTube. Since letting meat go, she was able to eliminate a two-year long headache, neck problems, depression, and obesity.[100]

Think about this, before quarantining you may have struggled to get the basement cleaned out because you had to focus your attention on getting to work. But because you worked from home, your basement is sparkling.

Without bacteria-laden foods, your body can put its energy into healing the adverse cellular affects caused by years of habitual meat eating.

Here's some ideas to let go or to keep:

Substitute

I want to invite you to do an experiment. I'm a big fan of experimenting because it supports the steep learning curve to find what foods work for healing your body.

For two weeks substitute your usual meat choices with black beans, navy beans, garbanzo beans, lentils, brown rice, quinoa, millet, oatmeal, or starchy vegetables like potatoes or peas. And substitute your dairy with alternative options like nut milk or plant-based cheeses.

Avocados are also a great cheese alternative if mindful of the portion size which is a quarter of the avocado. I usually cut a small avocado in half and cut it up small so that the creamy delicious flavor lasts longer. Plant-based cheeses are widely found on the internet and are still high in saturated fat, but they don't come with the added hormones, bacteria, or other non-goodies.

Some like meatier, plant-based options like portobello mushrooms, non-GMO tofu, or tempeh for more meat-likeness. Some consciously packaged, whole, plant-based food products are available, such as bean or veggie burgers.

Quorn®, despite being a highly processed food, is a plant-based, meat-like alternative that offers more satiation, fullness, and no insulin spikes compared to chicken.[101] My mom makes a dish using Quorn meatballs, and no one can tell the difference.

Most plant-based alternatives have little fat and are good sources of protein. Remember to check your caloric needs to determine how many servings make sense for your body size—maybe 2 to 3 servings (1/2 cup is one serving).

But due to their fiber, water, and satiation levels, most don't need to worry about calories or intake. For ease check out whole-plant-based programs online or with apps such as Forks over Knives, Mastering Diabetes do it yourself food program, or 21-day Vegan Kickstart. You don't have to be vegan to learn how to make more Genesis 1:29–30 recipes.

Shana, a Whole & Free Health course participant didn't think she'd ever be meat free, but after two weeks of letting animal products go, she felt vibrant again, her skin cleared up, and she stopped craving junk foods. And yes, she had random episodes of eating a chicken wing offered to her, but for the most part, she hung in there. And she's been animal product free for over two years.

Dr. Neal Barnard, MD, wrote a quick read called *The Vegan Starter Kit* to help those in transition to whole foods, plant-based eating.

Take a before and after photo of your face as well as measure your waist, hips, and weight.

Log changes such as softer skin, brighter eyes, more energy, joyful mood, less digestive problems, or regular, fuller bowels.

Cutting back helps too. If you prefer to reduce meat, do so after the two weeks, and let's discuss ways to bump up the quality.

Bump Up the Quality

If you prefer meat, make the investment for better quality options. Because they're pricey you'll consume less—a win-win.

Thankfully, there are great options for beef that's humanely raised as 70 percent of beef is factory farmed versus 99.9 percent of chickens.[102] Sustainable products have more nutrients than factory farmed.

Grocers sell well-treated bison or beef, wild fish, and organic eggs (which have a bright orange yolk) and often have sales.

Otherwise, do a search for local, sustainable family farms. Lately there's been a shift of quality farms going direct to consumer. You may even be able to visit and milk the cows. Organic, raw cow's milk dairy products like the old milkman days can be found in most states.

In our tech age, online organic kosher or regular butchers are also available.

Wild game meat and wild caught fish, sardines, or anchovies can be bought at any health food store and wholesale markets like Costco. Watch for sales. As a conscious buyer know where your meat, fish, and dairy come from and remember you don't need meat to live. But we do need nutrients and God! "My soul shall be satisfied as with marrow and fatness, and my mouth shall praise You with joyful lips" (Psalm 63:5).

Conviction to Clean It Up

When I learned about unclean meats like shellfish and pork from a nutritional point of view, it was rather easy to give them up overnight. But chicken and beef were a different story.

After exhaustive research, the evidence kept coming back the exact same: meat consumption is a fundamental cause to all chronic diseases. But I didn't have conviction. I do my best to eat the healthiest meat I can afford. But I ate factory-farmed meat, eggs, dairy, and fish while traveling, and I travel often.

So, I asked God. I wanted to know what He thought of the food

EWW, SPIT IT OUT, THAT WASN'T FOOD

> " After exhaustive research, the evidence kept coming back the exact same: meat consumption is a fundamental cause to all chronic diseases. "

industry, the way animals were treated, and how the earth was being treated. I got on my knees and prayed.

Deep in the night, I had a terrifying dream. It was Jesus in the middle of a deep, dark, vast, fiery, never-ending pit in what seemed like an endless ball of blackness. Then I heard the voice of God—powerful—with the words, "My son took the fall for all evil."

And I had a sense that the wrath of God wasn't just a hot sauce; it was real for those who do not repent.

I got out of bed and fell to the floor on my knees. I cried out to God, shaking.

My deep, soul-wrenching sobs were for the injustices of inhumanity, the pure void of moral consciousness, the money god worship, and the food god worship blinding conviction in our nation and silencing the discernment of His voice.

I was terrified, humbled, and in awe. I cried out for the Earth, the animals, the evil wickedness of industry, and the humans who operate apart from God's teachings and instructions. My soul anguished at its core.

I knew what I saw was hell.

I'm not a hell and brimstone teacher because that doesn't matter. God is an end in Himself. I focus on my Creator.

What matters is that we get to love Him, know Him, obey Him, and walk with Him. As we put our own opinions aside and lean into His ways and truth for the current times, we humble ourselves, and He gives us grace to endure (1 Peter 5:6) and fills us with hope (Romans 15:13).

So, focus on knowing Him and allowing Him to mold and change your heart. He'll align your choices to His.

The real heart of a nation is demonstrated in how we treat those without a voice—children (born and unborn), animals, the sick, elderly, special needs, disabled, and the underdog.

I didn't expect to share all the details about factory farming, but the Holy Spirit had other ideas. Even so, some will get convicted and make changes, and some won't.

It's all okay.

Again, there is no condemnation in Christ Jesus (Romans 8:1).

If you're weight rises and health conditions ensue, you know your prayers (faith) may need some action (changes in your diet).

And the Scriptures are clear: if you don't feel led to eat something (including meat) and your neighbor does, don't criticize them for not eating like you. "Let not the one who eats despise the one who abstains and let not the one who abstains pass judgment on the one who eats, for God has welcomed him" (Romans 14:3 ESV).

It's only to him that knows to do good and doesn't do it—to him it is sin, not the neighbor who doesn't have the same conviction (James 4:17).

We all get to have our own journeys with God.

If you struggle to let go of pork, shellfish, or factory farmed meat eating and want to let go to achieve greater health, ask God directly for conviction. The Holy Spirit will guide you. "And when he comes, he will convict the world concerning sin and righteousness and judgment" (John 16:8 ESV).

Even with everything you've read, you are free to eat unclean foods and shellfish. I am not your judge. See, God's grace is sufficient for you and me (2 Corinthians 12:9), and faith does have a place in all we choose to eat (Romans 14:2).

I consider myself "mostly vegan" to give space and grace to my food choices. And I trust that our loving God isn't going to rebuke you or me if a big wild turkey leg at the annual food festival is licked to the bone. "Therefore, whether you eat drink, or whatever we do, do all to the glory of God" (1 Corinthians 10:31).

REFLECT & SHARE

1. What about factory farming surprised you?
2. How conscious about your food do you feel?
3. Which unclean foods have captured your heart?
4. What chemicals are you ingesting from the processed foods in your diet?

PRAYER

Gracious Father,

I love you! Thank you so much for convicting me around all my food idols. I give you my weakness so that your power will be made strong.

Thank you for increasing my knowledge that I may not perish before my time. Help me to desire to live more abundantly, to be around and influence others for change. Rapidly advance my health and wellbeing for your glory! Help me to choose life in what I consume. By your Spirit, please overhaul all Satanic Addictive Deceptions of the Standard American Diet in my life and help me to adopt your Life Abundantly Standard.

I pray a supernatural miracle pertaining to my decisions around what I choose to consume. I will change. I will stand like Daniel and not defile myself with food and beverages that aren't your best for me. Thank you for purifying my choices and purifying me as your vessel to spit out of my life anything that isn't real food.

In Jesus's mighty name, amen.

CHAPTER 25

FORGO FLESHY FASTING

Battle #4 – Undereating

"However, this kind does not go out except by prayer and fasting"

–MATTHEW 17:21

God are you sure you meant to call me on fast?
I think you have the wrong number.

Part One: Understanding Undereating

Have you ever woken up and thought, *I need to fast today,* motivated by the pizza binge you had the night before? Or after an evening out with friends, you ate all the boxed food in the house, and you think, *I'll fast tomorrow,* and then wake with the intention to fast, only to binge two hours later?

Both scenarios are common in believers who struggle with weight and eating bondage. Fleshy Fasting is calorie restriction under impure motives. We don't want to be spiritually free, only free from the weight gain itself.

> " Fleshy Fasting is calorie restriction under impure motives. We don't want to be spiritually free, only free from the weight gain itself. "

Truth be told, some in the church fast as a guise for an eating disorder. Because fasting is both a spiritual thing and an eating disorder thing, we need to put some guidelines around fasting to address our next giant, Battle #4 Undereating.

Some Chubby Church members may wonder, *Why a chapter on undereating?* Well, the habit of undereating is almost as strong as the habit of overeating.

Basically, to undereat is to set ourselves up to overeat, while to eat enough and appropriately stop eating will allow us to win the battle. In this chapter we'll discuss undereating and fasting for the victory. And like you may suspect, the undereating battle is easier to win than the ones we've discussed.

> "To undereat is to set ourselves up to overeat."

Which type of undereater are you?

Types of Undereaters:

- **The Restrictor** – not enough caloric intake, denies signs of hunger, a traditional dieter
- **The Skipper** – regularly neglects physical needs and skips meals, sparking a physiological reaction to overeat or choose poorly later
- **The Fleshy Faster** – motivated to fast due to binge or overeating previously

Undereaters may be malnourished because caloric deficiency starves cells and undereaters often don't choose healthy foods when they do eat. See, we can self-harm by overindulging or depriving.

We can struggle with both under and overeating because meals are haphazard or unplanned. This leads to skipping meals, which makes us vulnerable to overeat or choose poorly.

Chronic undereaters eat late, binge, obsess with weight, or control food. Those who resonate with undereating have practical concerns, like getting total caloric needs or meal planning, and mental concerns, such as anxiety or eating disorders.

In the past have you restricted caloric intake?

Calorie restriction, dieting, skipping meals, and fasting are all forms of undereating if done with the motive to punish oneself or lose weight fast. Therein lies the destruction.

We talked about the dieter's mindset in Chapter 17. And I pray you've taken heed to the stats around dieting, such as the 95 percent of folks who lose weight will regain it back.[1]

Dieting is the mindset and actions of restricting oneself from food in a legalistic way. Dieters are rigid with food, applying difficult, self-imposed rules to restrict calories to unhealthy levels or fasting extensively.

> " Dieting is the mindset and actions of restricting oneself from food in a legalistic way. "

Dieter's fear fatness, food itself, and food groups (like fat or carbs). Undereaters may also over exercise to restrict overall calories or ignore signs of hunger—thinking about food, poor mental focus, or weakness. While the U.S. Army Handbook says we can survive on 600–1,000 calories per day with little activity, we can't do it for long, nor can we thrive with too little.[2]

Calorie restriction is not supportive to winning the Weight & Eating War. Calorie restriction creates intense craving of problem foods and ingredients and exacerbates health conditions such as hypothyroidism.[3]

Undereaters may feel cold, fatigued, lose hair, have difficulty in reproductive health, depression, low libido, and susceptibility to illness.[4]

Calorie restriction also makes us more prone to fatness. Too little calories will stimulate holding on to body fat.

Faith-based, registered dietician Laura Schoenfield puts it like this, "When you don't eat enough, your body reduces active thyroid hormone, shuts down sex hormone production, and raises adrenal stress hormones like cortisol. Chronically elevated cortisol leads to both leptin and insulin resistance, an unhealthy hormonal state that

> " Too little calories will stimulate holding on to body fat. "

promotes body fat and water retention and causes long-term health issues that go way beyond weight loss resistance."[5]

I do want to acknowledge that undereating isn't always due to weight loss motives. In studies of older adults, a variety of factors such as oral health problems, economic constraints like food insecurity (unsure when you'll have access to food due to financials), functional issues such as needing help eating, as well as medical conditions.[6] For these issues, it may be impractical to solve by planning to eat balanced meals.

Going forward, if you identify with being an undereater, work on eating enough, tracking foods, and possibly eating more. Continue to execute the Battle Strategies outlined in Chapter 23 as the exact same strategies for defeating overeating work for undereating as well.

As Christians, we're called to undereat in a fast, aren't we? As mentioned, there's a difference between undereating and fasting. So, how do we know the difference between a fleshy versus spiritual fast? Well, let's discuss.

Fleshy Versus Spiritual Fasting

What comes to mind when I mention fasting? What has been your experience? To not eat food sounds foreign to many in the church. The early church knew the benefits of fasting and prayer, but the modern church can only go so far as a Daniel fast once a year, if that.

Greek author, Saint Gregory Palamas said, "Fasting and self-control are a double wall of defense, and those who live within them enjoy great peace."[7] And Athanasius, an early Egyptian church father who defended the divinity of Jesus Christ, said, "To fast is to banquet with angels."[8,9]

All faiths institute some level of fasting. Muslims take thirty days a year to abstain from food and worldly things to seek their god in the month of Ramadan.[10]

Buddhists are encouraged to fast frequently. Catholics use Lent as a time to fast. But to abstain from eating isn't very common in the American church, which makes the stronghold of gluttony all the stronger.

Jesus said that we would fast.

> To abstain from eating isn't very common in the American church, which makes the stronghold of gluttony all the stronger.

And Jesus said to them, "Can the friends of the bridegroom fast while the bridegroom is with them? As long as they have the bridegroom with them they cannot fast. But the days will come when the bridegroom will be taken away from them, and then they will fast in those days. No one sews a piece of unshrunk cloth on an old garment; or else the new piece pulls away from the old, and the tear is made worse. And no one puts new wine into old wineskins; or else the new wine bursts the wineskins, the wine is spilled, and the wineskins are ruined. But new wine must be put into new wineskins" (Mark 2:19–22).

Fasting is a spiritual grenade to our strongholds that we're to utilize more in the church. It's not a coincidence that Jesus gave us the analogy of new wineskins after fasting was discussed. The wineskins represent the body, and the wine represents the Spirit.

Our bodies need to be refreshed and renewed so the Spirit can be best handled by its instrument, the body. The purpose of spiritual fasting is to humble ourselves before God and be refreshed in His Spirit. If you recall from Chapter 4, our bodies are a vessel of His Spirit or our flesh. Periodically, we need to humble our flesh by not puffing it up with food.

Spiritual fasting humbles the flesh (soul and body's lusts), fights food addiction, cleanses the body, and cleans out spiritual ear wax to hear from the Lord about our situation.

Fleshy fasting seeks to counteract binge eating episodes more than the pursuit of spiritual breakthrough to stop binge eating behaviors altogether. Fleshy fasting also may be a sign of the eating disorder bulimia nervosa (BN) as you learned in Chapter 23. Because of this, fasting even for believers can go wrong.

Fasting Gone Wrong

In 2006, twenty-nine-year-old Rosaline Gilbert went on a fast to be like Jesus.[11] On her Jesus fasts, she refused to eat anything except for processed hot chocolate and water. She did these fasts periodically, but her last fast killed her that April.

She died of sudden cardio-respiratory failure, her lungs and heart failed at the same time. Professionals wrote it off as an underlying blood issue—namely a sickle cell trait. But sudden cardiac or respiratory arrest and blood disorders are the leading cause of death in eating disorders and often aren't properly diagnosed in autopsy.[12]

I believe this woman was deceived between what's a godly fast and a fleshy fast. Most packaged hot chocolates have hydrogenated vegetable oils also known as trans-fat, like we discussed in Chapter 22.

Even a small amount of hydrogenated oils or trans-fats can cause an increase of premature death by 25 percent.[13] Because she fasted often in this manner, her body was probably starved of quality nutrients and rich in artery clogging oils caused by her hot chocolate diet disguised as a fast for Jesus.

While I don't know this woman's heart, I do know we perish for lack of knowledge (Hosea 4:6). Jesus warned about people about doing things in His name without the right motive (Matthew 7:21).

Jesus also warned us that we will be deceived (Matthew 24). And that He came to give us life and life more abundantly, yet the adversary comes to steal, kill, and destroy (John 10:10). The adversary's weapons are thoughts that show up as lies in our minds. Fasting can be an invisible, spider-web like trap for members of the Chubby Church.

By no means attempt a dry fast, no food or water, like Jesus did. Our current S.A.D. lifestyles aren't healthy enough to do dry fasting. What Moses and Jesus did in their forty-days and forty-night fasts is not for a person in today's toxic culture.

They had the true stillness of the wilderness; we have Netflix®.

Big difference.

Our current health status makes a dry or long water fast a risky pursuit.

South African Pastor Alfred Ndlovu took that risky pursuit in the summer of 2016.[14] Even though he seemed like a healthy, vibrant man at forty-four years of age, he too acted in ignorance for the modern age. He died due to malnourishment in the wilderness and was found by a hunter. It's not wise to fast for that long in modern times.

We underestimate the power of our flesh and dieting stronghold. Some have a compulsion to fast, but it's not out of a pure motive. It's also a sign of poor mental health.

> " We underestimate the power of our flesh and dieting stronghold. "

Since fasting is an honorable spiritual discipline and socially acceptable with practices such as intermittent fasting, church folks can be more vulnerable to eating disorders going unaddressed.

Emotional health matters. We must be mindful as some things we think we're doing for the Lord are filtered through our mental and emotional vulnerabilities. It's important not to over-spiritualize things by underestimating the power of our flesh's motives.

Our souls weigh heavy on the equation of things we think we hear from God, including the hearing of fasting. If weight and eating issues are prevalent, it's common for a Christian to think, *I'll fast today,* after a food frenzy the day before.

Fleshy fasting is impure because the believer doesn't want to be spiritually free but only free from the weight gain itself. The Day of Atonement is a picture of the day of judgment coming to us all. And the word atonement is reparation for wrongdoing. In our faith we know Jesus is our atonement.

Isaiah 58 is a word from God regarding the wrong and right motives and activities for fasting properly on the Day of Atonement but can be applied to all fasting.

Is this not the fast that I have chosen: To loose the bonds of wickedness, To undo the heavy burdens, To let the oppressed go free, And that you break every yoke? Is it not to share your bread with the hungry, and that you bring to your house the poor who are cast out; When you see the naked, that you cover him, and not hide yourself from your own flesh?

Then your light shall break forth like the morning, your healing shall spring forth speedily, and your righteousness shall go before you; the glory of the LORD shall be your rear guard.

Then you shall call, and the LORD will answer; You shall cry, and He will say, 'Here I am.' "If you take away the yoke from your midst, the pointing of the finger, and speaking wickedness, if you extend your soul to the hungry and satisfy the afflicted soul, then your light shall dawn in the darkness, and your darkness shall be as the noonday.

The LORD will guide you continually, and satisfy your soul in drought, and strengthen your bones; you shall be like a watered garden, and like a spring of water, whose waters do not fail" (Isaiah 58:6–11).

The Chubby Church mustn't fleshy fast. But we do need to fast and pray to shift the major stronghold in weight and eating bondage, so let's talk about how to discern when God's calling you versus an eating disorder.

Spiritual Fasting

While the Day of Atonement is a specific fast, fasting is a natural reaction to certain issues in life. When we're sick, under duress, or grieving, the last thing we want to do is eat. You know this from your own life experience, which is consistent in Scripture as well.

Fasting was not in the Ten Commandments. It was a natural part of the human process to humble the burdened body, soul, and/or spirit.

Oftentimes, life's noisy with entertainment and busyness, isn't it? Our bodies are so burdened by toxins and rich foods that we fail to hear the still small voice of our heart's cry to humble our flesh to be with God and fast. Fleshy lusts will always war against the soul (1 Peter 2:11).

Spiritually you may need to fast when:

1. You're honoring the biblical holy Day of Atonement (Leviticus 23:26–32).

2. You're need a big breakthrough, freedom from addiction, or a move of God (Matthew 17:20–21; Joshua 7:6; Isaiah 58:3–7).

3. Your flesh is out of control (Romans 8:13).

4. You're seeking direction and wisdom (Ezra 8:21–23; 1 Kings 19:8).

5. You need to repent and gain courage for the war ahead (Joshua 7:6).

6. You need wisdom and protection (Esther 4).

7. You're mourning (2 Samuel 12:16).

8. You're standing for revival in your church, city, or nation (1 Samuel 7:1–8; 2 Chronicles 20:3–4).

9. You're about to make a major decision on behalf of God or your church (Acts 13:1–3; Acts 14:23).

10. You're standing for a loved one's breakthrough (2 Samuel 12:13–22).

11. You've been spiritually lazy or complacent and need to repent and revive in the Lord (Psalm 69:10; Joel 2:12).

12. You've got a major assignment, task, or event to spiritually prepare for (Matthew 4:1–3; Luke 4:2; Exodus 34:28–29).

There are so many great resources about fasting where you can learn more. Some resources are Jentezen Franklin's books *The Fasting Edge* or *Fasting*, Marilyn Hickey's *The Power of Prayer and Fasting*, as well as John Eckhardt's *Fasting for Breakthrough and Deliverance*. These are great reads to further study fasting from a biblical perspective.

Fasting is a great addition to the life of a believer for spiritual reasons first and then for health reasons next.

Fast as a Part of a Healthy Lifestyle

Fasting is not only a part of a strong spiritual life but also a healthy lifestyle for our physical bodies. Look at a summary of fasting health benefits in the illustration.

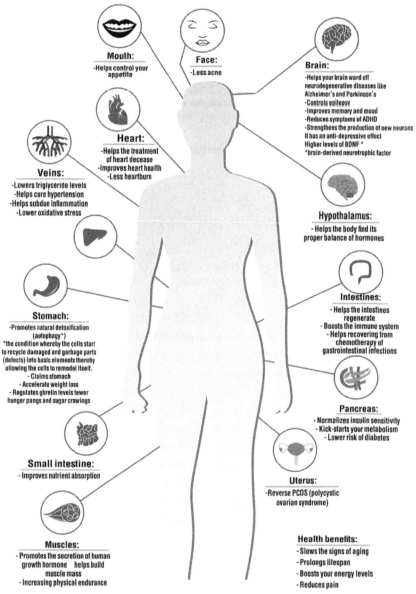

Mouth:
-Helps control your appetite

Face:
-Less acne

Brain:
-Helps your brain ward off neurodegenerative diseases like Alzheimer's and Parkinson's
-Controls epilepsy
-Improves memory and mood
-Reduces symptoms of ADHD
-Strengthens the production of new neurons
It has an anti-depressive effect
Higher levels of BDNF *
*brain-derived neurotrophic factor

Heart:
-Helps the treatment of heart decease
-Improves heart health
-Less heartburn

Veins:
-Lowers triglyceride levels
-Helps cure hypertension
-Helps subdue inflammation
-Lower oxidative stress

Hypothalamus:
- Helps the body find its proper balance of hormones

Intestines:
- Helps the intestines regenerate
- Boosts the immune system
- Helps recovering from chemotherapy of gastrointestinal infections

Stomach:
-Promotes natural detoxification (autophagy*)
*the condition whereby the cells start to recycle damaged and garbage parts (defects) into basic elements thereby allowing the cells to remodel itself.
- Claims stomach
- Accelerate weight loss
- Regulates ghrelin levels fewer hunger pangs and sugar cravings

Pancreas:
- Normalizes insulin sensitivity
- Kick-starts your metabolism
- Lower risk of diabetes

Small intestine:
- Improves nutrient absorption

Uterus:
-Reverse PCOS (polycystic ovarian syndrome)

Muscles:
- Promotes the secretion of human growth hormone   helps build muscle mass
- Increasing physical endurance

Health benefits:
- Slows the signs of aging
- Prolongs lifespan
- Boosts your energy levels
- Reduces pain

"Everyone has a physician inside him or her; we just have to help it in its work. The natural healing force within each one of us is the greatest force in getting well. Our food should be our medicine. Our medicine should be our food. But to eat when you are sick is to feed your sickness." - Hippocrates

Illustration 25.1   Benefits of Fasting [15]

Adding fasting to our lives helps us physically in many ways. As we know, the S.A.D. causes the body to be inflamed with toxins and fat, salt, and sugar overload. The overload keeps the body in a constant overdrive state of cleansing itself.

Think of yourself as a babysitter who was given one child to care for, then the neighbor dropped off a few more kids, and another a few more, and so on until there were hundreds of children. Fasting is like parents picking up their dagone kids. It's getting the toxins out. Not that kids are toxic—they're wonderful, but that many are an absolute burden.

Paul Bragg, health crusader and co-author of *The Miracle of Fasting* said, "Fasting provides the magic formula for retaining youthfulness, natural beauty, and a streamlined body."[16]

> " Because your body is built from the fabric of love, it's always seeking your highest good. "

I've also heard it said that man doesn't die from old age but from toxins over time. Your body is the most amazing machine you will ever get to own. And it's in a constant state of cleansing by nature. It is a profoundly engineered machine, built with the highest regard of care and intelligence that a human could never make on her own.

Because your body is built from the fabric of love, it's always seeking your highest good. When we overload the body with toxins, we stress it like a teenager going to prom.

So, fasting done properly brings forth great benefits, including weight loss, because of the body's natural healing process that happens with fasting as well as from taking a break from addictive allergenic foods we shouldn't be eating regularly anyway.

Jason Fung's book, *The Complete Guide to Fasting,* helps us to understand the benefits of fasting throughout the day or week, which we'll discuss more in Part Two.

Several health benefits take place from fasting.

In one study that compared fasting to bariatric surgery, fasting proved to reduce blood sugar and body weight more effectively.[17] Fasting reduces insulin levels and increases insulin sensitivity, helping glucose work more efficiently and helping us release sticky weight.[18]

In a study of 4,629 participants, fasting reduced risk of heart disease and diabetes.[19]

Three weeks of supervised fasting reduced blood pressure and cholesterol levels.[20] Samantha reported that her blood pressure decreased from 142/92 to 128/83 in one month and 101/75 after four months using fasting protocols.[21]

Inflammation markers like c-reactive protein (should be <1) and others decreased with fasting.[22] This makes sense because we're not contributing to inflammation markers when we take out addictive or allergenic foods like sugar, dairy, salt, meat, and excess saturated fat.

Fasting heals skin concerns like eczema and psoriasis as well as reduces acne.[23]

Fasting can reverse aging affects in animal studies. Rats put on a fast lived 83 percent longer than those that didn't.[24]

When we fast, we increase human growth hormone (HGH), which is supportive in metabolism, youthful looks, weight reduction, and strength.[25] In a small study, after a twenty-four-hour fast, levels of HGH showed an increase and after two days a five-fold increase.[26]

In animal studies, fasting reduced tumor growth.[27] Fasting has many benefits to the human body, soul, and spirit. And the body, soul, and spirit speak to us about when to fast.

Your body is telling you to fast when:

- You have no appetite
- You don't see anything appealing to eat.
- You sense you need to.
- You haven't in a long time.
- You have strong body odors.
- You're not feeling well.

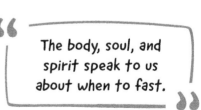

The body, soul, and spirit speak to us about when to fast.

Your soul is telling you to fast when:

- You need to come out of bondage.
- You have a decision to make.
- You're grieving.
- You need change.

Your spirit is telling you to fast when:

- You need breakthrough.
- You need to break free of sin.
- You want spiritual growth.
- You want to hear from God on a matter.

We'll talk about types and strategies for fasting when we win this battle by learning how to undereat (fast) in the right way. But this chapter wouldn't be complete without sharing with you the worst type of fast of all. It's the death fast.

An Introduction to Anorexia Nervosa (AN)

Anorexia nervosa (AN) is starvation by choice. I call it a death fast. Researchers estimate that 0.3–4.3 percent of women and 0.2–0.3 percent of men in America are anorexic.[28]

A study by the National Association of Anorexia Nervosa and Associated Disorders reported that 5 percent of anorexics die within ten years after contracting the disease.[29] And 18 to 20 percent of anorexics die after twenty years.[30]

There's a twelve times higher mortality rate for this disease than all causes of death for females fifteen to twenty-four years old.[31] An estimated 10.5 percent will die prematurely from it or complications that arise like Rosaline's blood or heart problems or by fasting to death or suicide.[32]

Sadly, it's the toughest mental illness to treat with a 21 percent full recovery rate.[33]

Anorexics have an intense fear of gaining weight, a low body weight, and a rejection of eating food. Despite what the scale says, or the obvious skin and bones reality, an anorexic may look in the mirror and see someone who is bigger than in real life. This is called Body Dysmorphic Disorder (BDD), and we'll discuss it and body image next in Chapter 26.

Anorexia Illustrated – Nancy and Steve's Story

Nancy and Steve were a young, career oriented, and God-fearing couple. Steve noticed Nancy's weight loss over the past six months.

He knew something was wrong when he cooked dinner for the two of them and she refused to eat more than a bite or two. She said, "I can't eat all this; I'll get fat!"

When she cooked for him, she would clean the kitchen while he ate. What perplexed him was that every few days she insisted she was fat and asked him about it. His heart sank, "Honey, you're too thin. Please eat more."

It dawned on him that he hadn't seen her eat in long time, so he started asking about her daytime meals. She grew defensive. And they'd started to argue daily about food and her ridiculous speculation that she was fat when she looked sickly to him.

Finally, he Googled anorexia and was sickened by what he discovered.

Deflated, Steve knew Nancy needed professional help.

Anorexia Eating Disorder Check[34]

If an individual meets all four criteria, then they would be considered an anorexic; however, it is best to go to an eating disorders clinic to verify and get the right help.

YES (X)	ANOREXIA NERVOSA CRITERION
	Do you refuse to maintain body weight at or above a minimally normal weight for your age and height and a body weight less than 85 percent?
	Do you have an intense fear of gaining weight or becoming fat, despite evidence of needing to gain weight?
	Do you suffer with negative thoughts and feelings about your body?
	Do others insist you're too thin, but you think you're too fat?
	In females, amenorrhea (absence of three consecutive menstrual cycles)?

Important: This check is not a diagnosis. Please see a professional for help if you believe you have anorexia nervosa for a full evaluation and treatment plan.

Anorexia Nervosa Medical Complications:[35]

- Brain and nervous system problems, bad memory, fainting, changes in brain chemistry, moodiness, irritability, can't think right
- Hair thinning, hair and nails are brittle
- Slow heart rate, fluttering of the heart (palpitations), heart failure, low blood pressure
- Anemia and other blood problems
- Weak muscles, swollen joints, fractures, osteoporosis
- Kidney stones or kidney failure
- Low potassium, magnesium, and sodium levels
- Constipation and bloating
- Hormone imbalance such as ceased periods
- Difficulty getting pregnant, and higher risk for miscarriage, C-sections, and babies with low birthweight
- Skin bruises easily, dry skin, get cold easily, yellow skin

Anorexic Nervosa Signs and Symptoms [36]

- Dieting despite being thin
- Obsession with calories, fat grams, and nutrition
- Pretending to eat or lying about eating
- Preoccupation with food
- Strange or secretive food rituals
- Dramatic weight loss
- Feeling fat, despite being underweight
- Fixation on body image
- Harshly critical of appearance
- Denies being too thin

Sometimes You May Need To Say Something

Once I saw a woman, who was skin and bones, in a workout class working out with light hand weights. I was so disturbed that I was angry. This woman needed to be banned from gyms and given an all-you-can-eat pass to Kentucky Fried Chicken®! Her skin was aged, her body looked breakable, and she was barely seventy pounds on her 5'6" frame.

After class, I caught up to her in the parking lot. I put my judgments, upset, and fear aside to introduce myself. And with Holy Spirit prompting I said, "I notice that you're underweight, and I felt concerned. Is everything okay?"

She shared with me that she struggled with anorexia and claimed she was under treatment with approval to attend the course and do it at her pace. She assured me that she was doing what she was supposed to do. She said how thankful she was that I asked and that most never said anything.

Even if I did believe her, which I didn't, I sent a detailed letter to the workout studio, so they were aware of the great risks they take on without approval from her treatment providers, not to mention allowing patrons to think it's okay to not eat enough and workout. It's not.

Like Steve had to do for Nancy and I had to do for a stranger, if you suspect someone is anorexic, help them get help from the local eating disorders clinic. Do not delay! Their future depends on someone caring enough to help them get professional treatment.

It's easy to see Satan at work when a person doesn't want to eat at all because in their mind, they think they're unworthy or too fat to enjoy food.

When we as the body of Christ are aware, eating disorders can't infiltrate the church so easily under the guise of fasting. Are you ready to win the battle with undereating and learn how to fast properly? Great, let's do it.

Part Two: Win the Undereating Battle

How to Forgo Fleshing Fasting for Good!

For *Chubby Church* members fasting is a potent weapon to break down spiritual and physical strongholds of obesity; however, we need fasting guidelines so that fasting doesn't become a diet or disorder.

Battle Strategy #1 – Follow Battle Strategies from Chapter 23.

Good news, you solve undereating the same way you solve overeating. Revisit the Battle Strategies in Chapter 23 to see what you can implement to prevent under and overeating.

Battle Strategy #2 – Be Led of the Spirit and Guidelines

Something was very wrong. I didn't know what. But I knew something. It was December 2004; I was sick and having panic attacks where my oxygen supply felt cut off and I couldn't breathe.

What was going on? Why did I feel so sick? Why couldn't I breathe? Why was I so tired? And how would I ever get out of the inner turmoil I was in? How would I ever be who I was supposed to be?

My soul cried out for Jesus Christ before I knew to cry out to Jesus. My soul cried to be healed and made worthy by Him. Each body ache and pain was a manifestation of my soul's cry.

I felt it very clear in my spirit, *Fast 41 days from the generational curses.*

His voice riveted me.

I knew the Holy Spirit was leading because, Lord knows, I was not giving up food for forty-one days by choice. I thought I'd die. I had never gone without food—ever.

You ever get a call from God and wonder if he had the wrong number? *Lord, maybe you meant to call my neighbor. Cindy down the street is holy; she's available. Surely, you're not asking me to do this.*

That's how I felt. Yet it was unshakable. I had to obey.

Fast? I thought, *What's a fast? How do I fast? What's a curse?*

It seemed everyone in my family struggled financially, physically with poor health, broken relationships, emotionally with depression, and spiritual disconnection. I questioned our family issues, *Were these curses?*

Sacrifice was necessary to humble the great strongholds of my flesh. Strongholds I did not understand. Strongholds I had not yet learned about. All I knew was something wasn't right, and I needed to be obedient.

I was sick in every way—emotionally, mentally, spiritually, financially, and relationally. Back then, I had struggled to fill my deep soul holes with food, sex, and occasional binge drinking.

My faith in God and my love for God was all I had to work with, which was all I needed. I said, "Father, I could do three days, but I need you to do the rest." And it was so.

The Holy Spirit helped me to fast for forty-one days with fresh water and vegetable and fruit juices. I bought a Jack Lalanne juicer and organic juices and didn't tell anyone.

> " My faith in God and my love for God was all
> I had to work with, which was all I needed. "

Before I started, I researched fasting on an online website called *Freedom You*. I knew how long, I knew when it would start, and I knew what I was supposed to do.

All this to say, I'm still reaping!

The Holy Spirit walked me through amazing healing, broke the bondages of anger, grief, doubt, rejection, fear, lust, guilt, and fifteen pounds of excess weight, which came back some years later per Chapter 3, but you get my point.

My healing journey started before that experience and continues today, but I believe He used that experience to accelerate my alignment with my destiny and to clean up my past and generational sin.

Fasting is a tool to help us walk out our salvation, healing, and freedom. It's used to support our divine alignment to His will by humbling the flesh.

Jesus didn't arbitrarily decide to fast. He only did what the Father told Him to do (John 5:19). Jesus was instructed to fast and pray for the call of salvation. He prepared

> " Fasting is a tool to help us
> walk out our salvation,
> healing, and freedom. "

His spirit, soul, and body to be obedient to the call. He didn't wake up and think, *Boy, that supper made me feel so bloated; I ought to fast for forty days.*

A spiritual fast doesn't have anything to do with weight loss. But breaking the stronghold of the S.A.D. in your life very well may be the reason to spiritually fast.

Ask a few questions to support a successful spiritual fast:

Should I fast?

Pray, "Lord are you calling me on a fast?"

Why would I fast?

Pray, "What's the purpose of the fast?" Clarify and purify your motives for fasting and know your reasons. Strong reasons provide the momentum and completion of the fast.

I knew why: to break of generational curses from my life and family lineage that have affected my life. I heard this confirmed in my spirit before I started. I also researched the meaning of generational curses because it was so hard for me to believe that God, knowing I was a foody, wanted me to fast.

Whether your fast is to humble yourself before God, purify a wrong motive, remove a desire, or to receive a breakthrough for yourself or someone else, know what it is so that you can pray about it and get clarification before you begin.

If your reason is to reduce damages from a binge, stop and get back on track with a nutritious meal.

How long do I fast?

Pray, "How long do I fast?" A specific number of days should feel very clear in your spirit.

What type of fast?

Pray, "How should I fast?" You can fast healthfully with fresh, homemade vegetable and fruit juices by eating 100 percent fruits and vegetables, broths, pureed soups, and/or short fasts of clean water.

The Bible explains the laws of Niddah, which was for a husband and wife to fast from sexual relations due to her menstrual cycle (Leviticus 15:25–30; 1 Corinthians 7:5).

Daniel also abstained from rich foods like desserts for a time (Daniel 10:3). We too can do a behavioral fast from hobbies, screens, dining out, talking on the phone, or spending money. But ideally habits such as criticalness, selfishness, or complaining should be fasted for life.

Ideally you use the fasting time to seek revelation of the Father and His will for your life and enjoy time in the Bible and prayer.

When will I fast?

Pray, "When should I fast?" Get a clear timeframe on when your fast begins. Here's a hint: it's not today or tomorrow. Our minds and refrigerators need time to prepare to successfully complete a fast, which can take at least two weeks.

What confirmations did I receive to fast?

After you pray the above questions and wait for clear answers, look for confirmations of God's calling. One reader felt led to fast, and then read this chapter. It served as confirmation.

Fasting is an act of surrendered obedience. We humble our body, soul, and spirit before God. If He's called you on a fast, it's not haphazard based on what you ate the day before. His reasons are richer. You'll have some measure of strong inclination, the ability to prepare, and confirmation.

You'll gain confirmation through messages that speak to you, sermons, research, dreams, and mentors. Start after you've taken at least a couple weeks to pray about it.

Battle Strategy #3 – Start with Mini Fasts

A mini fast is fasting for short bursts of time. Mini fasts help you to build toward a monthly weekend fast or a bi-annual weeklong fast. A mini-fast could also be a fast between meals. As simple as breakfast, fast, then lunch, fast, then dinner, fast until breakfast again, avoiding snaccidents.

In Book 1, I said, "In 1977, we ate three meals a day. At that time meals were four and a half hours apart. Now we eat five to six times per day, with three and a half hours between meals or less.[37] Because we eat all day and night, insulin is always elevated. This makes our weight set point stay set on high. And although tasty snacks aren't necessary, they're usually highly processed snaccidents waiting to happen anyway. Perhaps we balance by eating enough of the right stuff at meals to sustain not eating processed snacks between meals."[38]

As mentioned in previous chapters, to balance blood sugar and reduce cravings, we can fast between meals. Still, focus on eating enough at meals.

Battle Strategy #4 – Fast for Freedom

Feel free to choose to do a fast to demonstrate your growing power over food. I fasted once a week for a full day for about six months to break free from weight and eating bondage.

Save longer fasts for when you feel you've had traction with more food control by letting go of the aspects of the Standard American Diet that caused problems.

Consider a one day a week fast to break free from weight and eating bondage. A breakthrough weekly fast helps us to overcome food idols. Pick the same day each week, ideally from 5 p.m. to 8 a.m. or 5 p.m. to 5 p.m. A biblical day starts in the evening (Genesis 1).

A few more guidelines:

Be Mindful About Intermittent Fasting

Dr. Jason Fung, co-author of *The Complete Guide to Fasting,* recommends intermittent fasting—the practice of giving your blood fasting insulin and glucose levels time to heal to reduce risks and poor outcomes from chronic diseases.

Ann started intermittent fasting in July. By February of the next year, she had released eighteen pounds. Two nights a week, she stopped eating at seven o'clock and wouldn't eat again until eleven o'clock in the morning. This gave her hormones sixteen hours to get their balancing act together. She also overcame her processed food and sugar addiction.

Intermittent fasting is a fancy term for what used to be normal, not eating after dinner. However, the recommendation is to go twelve, sixteen, eighteen, or twenty-four hours without eating, which includes when you're asleep, and then to eat during the feeding window.

Ann did a sixteen-hour fast with an eight-hour eating window, which Dr. Fung calls a 16:8 protocol. Ben stopped eating at 7 p.m. and ate again at 9 a.m. during his work week and regained his health.

Like a restaurant that gives patrons the opportunity to eat during operating hours, intermittent fasting has open feeding hours. When the feeding hours are over, the kitchen's closed.

These long periods without food at night help to heal elevated insulin levels and reduce inflammation. In the chart, ketones represent fat burn, and glucose represents sugar burn. The arrows indicate mealtimes.

M.P. Mattson et al. / Ageing Research Reviews 39 (2017) 46–58

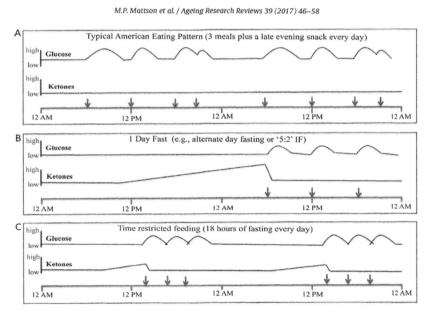

Figure 25.2 Fasting Glucose and Ketones[39]

As you can see on the chart, fat burning is easier with fasting period. I personally just do my best to eat dinner early and not eat anything until the morning because intermittent fasting, although effective, is fad-like and can become an on again-off again fad diet because the sole motive must be bigger than weight loss for long-term success in health.

I don't recommend any Chubby Church member to do more than sixteen hours as an intermittent fasting practice. While there are minor benefits for longer periods, we teeter on eating disorders mental, emotional, and spiritual health that outweigh them.

It's much easier to focus on eating enough at mealtimes, rejecting the Satanic Addictive Deception, and increasing overall nutrients.

Any extreme approach to weight reduction causes weight gain recidivism. Only if you're Spirit led as well as educated around this practice, give it a try.

Intermittent fasting can exacerbate an eating disorder. So, for us, I recommend keeping it simple, work on not eating after dinner, and focus on the Life Abundantly Standard.

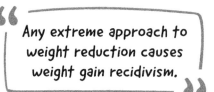

> Any extreme approach to weight reduction causes weight gain recidivism.

Break Your Fast Well

Since your body needs to recover from damages caused by the S.A.D., break fasts with lighter fare such as fruit, broth, green smoothies, vegetable soup, or other soft foods that aren't gastronomic bombs like meat, heavy creams, or processed foods. And do so during normal hours.

If you do a twenty-four-hour fast, start at a mealtime and end at the same meal the next day. A Chubby Church member fasted faithfully once a week in dedication to God, but she damaged her health by breaking her fast with thanksgiving-like feasts at midnight. Heart health, body weight, and sleep is compromised when we eat heavy meals late at night. And to stay up until midnight to eat smells like a food idol. Go to bed.

Don't Tell Everyone

Fasting is between you and God. But it's wise to inform a close confidant or two, especially for fasts exceeding two or three days if you have health challenges. Exercise wisdom by using vegetable and fruit juices. Please don't do a dry (no food or liquid) fast or water only.

Jesus said, "Moreover, when you fast, do not be like the hypocrites, with a sad countenance. For they disfigure their faces that they may appear to men to be fasting. Assuredly, I say to you, they have their reward. But you, when you fast, anoint your head and wash your face" (Matthew 6:16–17). He doesn't want us to fast to look pious to others. We fast to humble ourselves before God.

Seek Supervision

Should you want to fast for spiritual and health reasons, there are many options to do so with medical supervision. Clinics like True North in California and others supervise water and juice fasting. Look up fasting retreats in your area.

Be Encouraged

> Fasting gives us power over our body, soul, and spirit if done with the right intentions.

In Matthew 4:4, Jesus finished His forty-day fast with no food or water, only to be tested by Satan. But Jesus refused to eat anything from the enemy's hand. Fasting gives us power over our body, soul, and spirit if done with the right intentions.

Jesus's fast prepared Him for the ransom He was to pay for our souls.

It's only by God's grace that I am still reaping the incredible benefits of that fast from generational curses; now I can love freely. My default emotions are joy and peace, where in the past they were sadness and anger.

Work with God so that you, too, can be free of the bondages in your soul from your family lineage and your past. Let 1 Thessalonians

5:23–24 be a guide. It says, "May God himself, the God of peace, sanctify you through and through. May your whole spirit, soul and body be kept blameless at the coming of our Lord Jesus Christ. The one who calls you is faithful, and he will do it."

Don't doubt because as you work toward freedom, He will give it you. God is God, and there is none like Him. He is all powerful, and He can change your brain and habits if you work with Him.

Will you fast and pray?

Will you allow the Lord to get rid of every stronghold in your life? Not just food but pride, bitterness, control, anger, grief, fear, stubbornness, and poverty?

Will you let Him do breakthrough after breakthrough in your life?

You can do all things through Christ who strengthens you. God can heal your soul and your past—so much so that you thank Him for all that you have gone through.

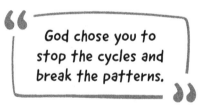

God chose you to stop the cycles and break the patterns.

God chose you to stop the cycles and break the patterns. The generational changes start with you, and the old ways stop with you. Like Esther, God chose you for such a time as this!

REFLECT & SHARE

1. What has your experience with undereating or skipping meals been like?

2. How has undereating set you up to fail?

3. When have you fasted for spiritual reasons, not weight loss?

PRAYER

Dear Lord,

Please speak to me about fasting and when to implement it in my life for my maturing in faith and my weight and eating victory. Give me the ability to discern the difference between a fleshy fast, spiritual fast, or healthful fast. Help me to use fasting and prayer to break the bonds of wickedness in my life and family.

I break every desire to diet or get slim quick!

I can make healthy eating my normal lifestyle. I can stop eating between and after meals. I welcome each day to learn and grow and make better choices. I trust that you're transforming me. Purify my motives in all things that I may have clean hands and a pure heart to worship you. Thank you for allowing me to walk humbly with you.

In Jesus's name, amen.

· CHAPTER 26 ·

JUMP OFF THE BODY SHAME TRAIN

Battle #5 — Body Shame

"I will praise You, for I am fearfully and wonderfully made;
Marvelous are Your works, and that my soul knows very well"

–PSALM 139:14

"The Lord gave me my body. I just added to it,
enhanced it if you will." —Chubby Church member

Part One: Understanding Body Shame

I carried a giant stack of textbooks like a football into my seventh grade English class. My crush, Richard, walked into the class with me when we heard, "You jolly green giant," shouted from the hallway. "Is that Nikki B.?" I asked as I felt the heat in my face.

Earlier that day, I heard that Nikki was the one who spread horrible rumors about me, causing conflict with my friends. She said I had said derogatory things, which I didn't say. I know because I'm not one to gossip or talk about people like that. I just never liked it. So, all that had been said was indeed a lie. I was ready for her. I just wasn't ready for her attack on my height.

I was about 5'9" by the time I was in seventh grade, and although I didn't wear green, the Jolly Green Giant — canned vegetable mascot — triggered my body shame.

Richard came to my defense. "She's just jealous," he said.

I was tickled by his quick defense, but jealous or not, my rage swung me full force into the hallway where I wacked her upside the forehead and grabbed the top of her big hair into a ponytail. Then with Hulk Hogan strength I picked her up by her hair and dangled her there against the wall for a few seconds.

"I'm sorry. I'm sorry!" she said between sobs. I dropped her onto the floor and then gave her a good kick or five before a teacher stopped the madness and broke up the crowd.

All of this happened one handed because the stack of books had my right hand securing it. We were sent to detention where we made up and were cordial for the rest of our school years.

I didn't get into fights often. I was a sweet girl and minded my own business. But she underestimated a fatherless daughter with a chaotic, deprived homelife. At the time I felt justified because I was triggered by her attack on my height in front of my crush, nonetheless.

In hindsight body shame, not Nikki, deserved a good whack upside the head.

Let me tell you another story about body shame that's not riddled in teenage girl drama and is much more spiritually mature.

My aunt and I snapped photos at the *Route 1* scenic area in Key West, Florida, and came across a man and his wife in their late forties. I overheard his wife's complaints about her looks as she prepared to take photos of him alone.

"Hey, I'm happy to take your photo together," I said as I sensed something more.

"I don't take photos," she said. I could see the shame in her eyes.

"She doesn't take photos," her husband reiterated. I could see the sadness in his.

"I'm so ashamed of my weight. I can't stand taking photos," she confessed.

"How long has she been like this about photos," I asked her husband.

"Since I've known her, maybe thirteen years," he said, "It's been a

210

real struggle. I have hundreds of photos by myself or with the kids. See," he showed us his cell phone.

My aunt and I leaned in as he swiped through dozens of photos of only himself. His beautiful wife felt she wasn't picture worthy because she didn't weigh the same as she did in high school.

I felt the warmth of the Holy Spirit come upon me as I turned toward her and said, "Do you have any idea how beautiful you are? When you're ninety, you'll wish you had the youth you do now and a photo to prove it, right?" we chuckled. "More importantly, your children and great grandchildren will long for the photos of their beloved matriarch."

My soap box didn't end there. I am the author of *The Chubby Church* after all. I continued, "Weight will go when you stop obeying its shame. You've been shaming your body and hating how you look, but has it helped? Love God. Love yourself. Love your body. And the weight will follow."

With wet eyes she admitted, "I see my daughter struggle too, yet she's so beautiful."

Gently I responded, "Yes, beautiful like her mother. Where do you think she got this struggle from? Body shame has plagued your family long enough, hasn't it? Don't you want to make memories? And seriously, have you seen some of the folks on the beach?" I said with a funny face to make her smile. We chuckled as we glanced in the direction of glaring suspects who shamelessly let it all, and I mean all, hang out.

"I wish I were one of them," she giggled as she wiped her tears.

"You can be. You can be free. Jesus already did it," I said.

"I believe Him. He spoke to me about my body shame issues just this morning! I can't believe you're saying this to me," she admitted.

"Well, that explains why I'm able to speak freely to you," my hands gestured her over to the *Route 1* sign as I said, "I'm taking your photo."

I took a photo of her and her husband together for the first time in a long time. A memory they'd never forget.

"Thank you," they both said at the same time as all of our eye ducts swelled. He put his arm around his beautiful wife tightly and prepared for the photo that broke the bondage of body shame.

"Smile!" I said with a big grin. *Click. Click. Click.*

Is Your Body Relationship Adversarial?

Do you resonate with this woman? Do you beat up your body with harsh punches of criticism? Does how you feel about your body affect how you live your life?

I deeply empathize.

Before I could ever speak with that lady, I had to recognize and heal the distorted image of my own body. And despite weight reduction, my mind's body glasses needed new lenses.

The fifth battle in the Weight & Eating War is body shame.

We must win this battle because negative body evaluation, the technical term for not liking your body, is not only the common thread in all eating disorders but a strong causal factor to developing one.[1]

Any dysfunctional, adversarial relationship with food reflects a dysfunctional, adversarial relationship with our bodies. How we feel about our bodies predicts and influences our weight and eating behaviors.[2]

Body shame is to hold our bodies and looks in contempt because we think we should look better or different. Our harsh judgments cause our self-esteem to crumble under the pressure placed on our looks, weight, and other physical attributes.

This battle is as fierce as food addiction and overeating.

In Part One: Understanding Body Shame of this chapter, we'll gain understanding about body shame, and in Part Two: Win the Body Shame Battle.

Let's take a quiz to see exactly where you stand in the battle of body shame.

> Any dysfunctional, adversarial relationship with food reflects a dysfunctional, adversarial relationship with our bodies.

> Body shame is to hold our bodies and looks in contempt because we think we should look better or different.

BODY SHAME STRONGHOLD QUIZ

Put a check next to the answer that describes your body relationship and add the total points below. The higher the score the more body shame is present.

1. How often do you need validation around your looks or appearance?
    ☐ (5) ALWAYS ☐ (4) OFTEN ☐ (3) SOMETIMES ☐ (2) RARELY ☐ (1) NEVER

2. How often do you avoid looking in the mirror?
    ☐ (5) ALWAYS ☐ (4) OFTEN ☐ (3) SOMETIMES ☐ (2) RARELY ☐ (1) NEVER

3. How often do you grab, pick, pinch, tug, or pull at your body parts in disgust?
    ☐ (5) ALWAYS ☐ (4) OFTEN ☐ (3) SOMETIMES ☐ (2) RARELY ☐ (1) NEVER

4. How often do you excessively check your perceived flaws in mirrors?
    ☐ (5) ALWAYS ☐ (4) OFTEN ☐ (3) SOMETIMES ☐ (2) RARELY ☐ (1) NEVER

5. How often do you use makeup or clothing (all black, revealing, or over-sized) to hide your feelings of ugliness, inadequacy, discomfort, or shame around your face or body?
    ☐ (5) ALWAYS ☐ (4) OFTEN ☐ (3) SOMETIMES ☐ (2) RARELY ☐ (1) NEVER

6. How often do you get plastic surgery or treatments to improve your looks?
    ☐ (5) ALWAYS ☐ (4) OFTEN ☐ (3) SOMETIMES ☐ (2) RARELY ☐ (1) NEVER

7. How often do you avoid going out because of feeling fat/or overwhelmed by insecurities?
    ☐ (5) ALWAYS ☐ (4) OFTEN ☐ (3) SOMETIMES ☐ (2) RARELY ☐ (1) NEVER

8. How often do you scrutinize or comment on the weight, shape, or body parts of others?
    ☐ (5) ALWAYS ☐ (4) OFTEN ☐ (3) SOMETIMES ☐ (2) RARELY ☐ (1) NEVER

9. How often do you assume others talk about your perceived physical flaws?
    ☐ (5) ALWAYS ☐ (4) OFTEN ☐ (3) SOMETIMES ☐ (2) RARELY ☐ (1) NEVER

10. How often do you refuse to take photos or have them posted on social media?
    ☐ (5) ALWAYS ☐ (4) OFTEN ☐ (3) SOMETIMES ☐ (2) RARELY ☐ (1) NEVER

Total Score:

_____

Date:

_____

Score Sheet
30–50 | Your body deserves a raise in love tokens!
20–30 | You're learning how to accept your body, nice job!
10–20 | You're exiting the body shame train.

What Is Body Image?

A healthy body image reflects who we are because how we look is a profound identifier of who we are. The way we look is the truest form of ID. Nothing says you more than your face. Your face and body are both a picture of the soul and a mirror to it.

We get to see the invisible soul through the visible body.

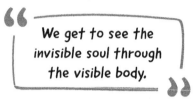

> We get to see the invisible soul through the visible body.

A healthy body relationship allows us to feel good in the skin we're in and take care of it. Confident. Bold. Even if we're wearing our chubby suit, we're not bound or hidden in it because a healthy body relationship allows us to be more willing to go places, do things, reach our goals, and take risks.

Body image is multidimensional like weight. How we look holds societal importance and impacts our perceived self-worth. Multiple studies show that body image influences our self-esteem, sexual intimacy, work confidence, health, eating decisions, and mood.[3] Body image also affects how well or how poorly we treat the body as a sacred vessel of the Holy Spirit. Hello, body imagine impacts every area of our lives.

Body image is made up of four areas:[4]

1. How we perceive our bodies visually

2. How we feel about our physical appearance

3. How we think and talk to ourselves about our bodies

4. Our sense of how other people view our bodies

Do you feel driven to be thin or muscular? Do you hate looking in the mirror? Most of us have what body image activist Dr. Renee Engeln, PhD, calls "beauty sickness," which she describes as the syndrome of body shame or the obsessive self-consciousness stealing our confidence in all areas of life.[5]

We constantly worry: are we thin enough, muscular enough, or pretty enough?

I hope you and I agree: enough is enough.

A body image spray-painted with shame manifests in several ways, such as extreme unhappiness about how we look, distorted self-perception (i.e., we believe we're bigger or smaller than reality and feel unsure about how we look to others), harsh attitudes and language toward our bodies, excessive body checking (i.e., tugging, pulling, or pinching parts), and thoughts about how we look dominating our minds.

There's a difference between acknowledging a flaw and obsessing over one. It's one thing to acknowledge a feature you wished were better on occasion. It's another thing to be significantly dissatisfied to the point of feeling shame, hatred, and contempt for how you look.

Is this you?

Your Body is Like a Donkey

Do you shame and criticize your body excessively? Body shame reminds me of a donkey in the Scriptures. Balaam, a man of God, went on his donkey to meet Balak, a Moabite leader who was against God's people. It angered God that Balaam was willing to go against God to speak to Balak. So, God caused the angel of the Lord to block the donkey's path.

Frustrated, Balaam beat on the donkey to get it to go.

"Go donkey! Move it!" Balaam said, slapping it's rear.

The donkey started to go again, only it was stopped a second time.

Angry, Balaam forced his donkey to go, whacking it more.

"I said go!" Balaam yelled.

It went a little more and a third time was forced by the angel of the Lord to stop. Balaam went ballistic and beat the donkey abusively.

What happened next shocked Balaam.

"What have I done to you that you have struck me these three times," said the donkey. Yes, the donkey spoke.

"Because you've abused me. I wish there were a sword in my hand because I'd kill you right now!" said Balaam, completely missing what God was doing through the donkey.

So the donkey said to Balaam, "Am I not your donkey on which you have ridden, ever since I became yours, to this day? Was I ever disposed to do this to you?" (Numbers 22:30).

That donkey is your body.

Are you like Balaam, completely missing the message that God brings to you through your body? Doesn't your body serve you your entire earthly life? Just like the donkey was a vessel for the angel of the Lord, your body too is a vessel of the Holy Spirit.

Body shame sounds like this:

- I hate my stomach!
- I'd be a fox if I didn't have this big butt.
- I can't go sleeveless. Have you seen my arms?
- My nose ruins my whole face. I need a nose job.
- My thighs can light a fire they're so thick.
- I have chicken legs. I can't wear shorts.
- I can't be seen bald. Where's my toupee?
- Do I look fat?

How many criticisms do you have about your body each day? A Whole & Free Health course participant admitted to twenty-one times that she had to stop her thoughts from criticizing her body within one day. Imagine your boss giving you twenty-one criticisms about your work each day. Would you want to work for that person?

Probably not. You'd quit, switch departments, or get promoted. Unlike your boss, your body isn't fire-able. You're the boss of your body. You can't escape your body. You can't move from it. And you certainly can't switch it for someone else's.

Since your body and soul is an until-death-do-you-part relationship, you might as well learn how to enjoy and care for it.

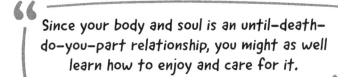

Since your body and soul is an until-death-do-you-part relationship, you might as well learn how to enjoy and care for it.

Body Image Facts

About 90 percent of us have some area of negativity around our bodies.[6] The problem isn't wishing your nose was smaller or lips were bigger. It's having a strong preoccupation about how we look that negatively impacts life, work, relationships, eating behaviors, and food choices.

Psychology Today partnered with eating disorder director Dr. David Garner, PhD, to find insights into body image health factors by performing a study of 3,453 women and 548 men in a famous Body Image Survey.[7]

Fifty-six percent of women were unhappy about their overall appearance with most dissatisfaction about the belly, weight, and backside.[8] Whereas 43 percent of men were unhappy with their overall appearance with most dissatisfaction about the belly, weight, muscle definition, and chest.[9]

Take a look at the Body Worry Chart. Which body parts upset you the most?

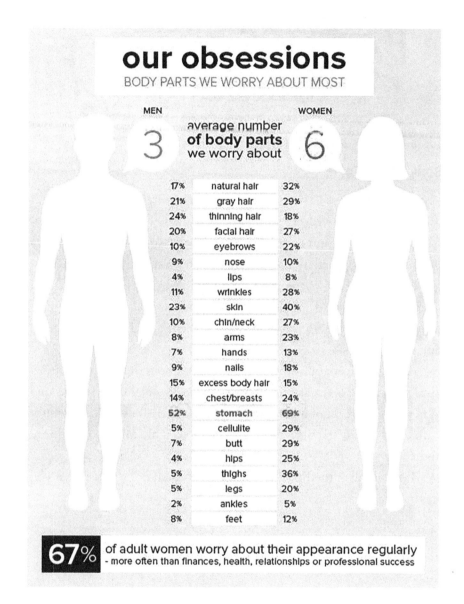

our obsessions
BODY PARTS WE WORRY ABOUT MOST

MEN	average number of body parts we worry about	WOMEN
3		6
17%	natural hair	32%
21%	gray hair	29%
24%	thinning hair	18%
20%	facial hair	27%
10%	eyebrows	22%
9%	nose	10%
4%	lips	8%
11%	wrinkles	28%
23%	skin	40%
10%	chin/neck	27%
8%	arms	23%
7%	hands	13%
9%	nails	18%
15%	excess body hair	15%
14%	chest/breasts	24%
52%	stomach	69%
5%	cellulite	29%
7%	butt	29%
4%	hips	25%
5%	thighs	36%
5%	legs	20%
2%	ankles	5%
8%	feet	12%

67% of adult women worry about their appearance regularly
- more often than finances, health, relationships or professional success

Illustration 26.1   Body Worry Chart[10]

Sixty percent of body dissatisfaction came from body weight.[11] But the study proved that the more unhappy with our body we are, then the more we'll struggle with a higher body mass index. Those who were fifty or more pounds from their ideal weight struggled with body image the most versus those within a five-pound range who struggled the least. [12]

Not surprisingly, most women wanted to lose body fat, but men wanted to gain muscle.

The struggle with body image begins early. Fifty to 80 percent of young women and 25 percent of young men start to feel dissatisfied with their bodies as teens and even pre-teens.[13]

Like adults, young men want toned and defined muscles, whereas young women want thinness. And 81 percent of young women fear fatness which causes weight problems, strengthening the shame-diet-binge-weight gain cycle.[14]

In a study of 1,196 teenage girls, researchers found that the ones who weren't concerned about their weight and had a positive outlook about their bodies fared well with their weight well into adulthood.[15]

However, 59 percent of those who thought negatively about their weight and bodies, despite a normal weight, ended up becoming overweight or obese in adulthood.[16] So the proof is in the pudgy beliefs per Chapter 17. The fear of fatness or self-perception of fatness usually leads to more, not less, fatness.

Body image concerns are growing amongst youth, leading to sad projections in areas of mental, emotional, physical, and spiritual health.

Where Does Body Image Come From?

Body image is created by multiple sources, but the Standard American Diet or Satanic Addictive Deception is behind the scenes again.

Let me explain.

The media is the top source of body shame thoughts for all of us. Fifty-seven percent of women feel more insecure after engaging with social media or watching television.[17] We cannot help but compare ourselves at times to those who make it to the big screen or the social scene.

Media is a large part of the problem. Seeing underweight women, extra buff men, and food porn commercials makes for our severe discontentment with our bodies. Since the big screen is so difficult to get on, actors, actresses, athletes, news anchors, and others are naturally assigned more value because they are the one percent of society who get to be seen by everyone. And those one-percenters look far more glorious than the rest of us toads (in our minds) because they've made it.

Then we watch, comparing ourselves to the finely sculpted echelons of society, get depressed because we don't measure up, see a commercial for cheesy bread, order it, and sulk in our feelings of fatness.

Watch, eat, sulk, repeat.

Reduce visual media (television, internet, magazines, and social) and you'll get an immediate boost in self-esteem.

The sulking in fatness and food temptations leads to poor body stewardship, which is the next major source of body shame. You know this from Chapters 6–13. If we exercise, eat well, and sleep well, we'll increase a positive body image. Those who exercise report increased self-esteem, confidence, and positive feelings about their bodies.[18]

We drop weighty guilt when we do the things that we know we should do like drink water instead of pop, get rest instead of staying up late, and take a walk instead of sitting on the couch. We also know our problem foods create a downward emotional spiral with a not-so-fabulous pity party for our body image sentiment.

Youth are battered by media from an early age to perceive lean as worthy of love and value. Studies show nearly 66 percent of television shows and movies portray lean men and underweight women to have positive traits such as love and joy, while 75 percent of television shows and movies associate those who are heavier with negative traits such as sadness, aggressive attitudes, or laziness.[19] This further supports weight biases and body image dissatisfaction.

Do you see the Satanic Addictive Deception at work?

A non-media source of body image formation are words spoken about your body. Negative words spoken to us like Sheila received, "You have horse lips!" or Frank received, "You're a double wide taking up the whole street" promote body shame.

Word attacks on our bodies from other adults or kids stick with us as does a lack of affirming words about our bodies from parents, peers, or siblings. And if we don't have positive references about our bodies, we'll fail to see our bodies as positive aspects of who we are.

If the negative words are spoken from a love interest that's especially brutal on our body image because another major non-media source of body image is how our love interest makes us feel about our bodies and what they say. We feel special when someone we love thinks we have a beautiful smile or nice backside. We seek out positive body opinions of the one who gets to touch us intimately. Lord knows we all secretly wish to be worshipped for our sexy bodies by our spouses even if we're not so sexy or spouse-less at the moment.

Criticism from our love interest deeply damages self-esteem, like Marie whose husband made snide comments about what she ate and wore or George whose wife refused to be intimate with him because of his size.

Fat jokes or constant requests to lose weight from our loved ones, especially a spouse, require clear boundaries and a desire to change for oneself, not anyone else.

Lastly, we learn from our parents. If our father or mother shamed his or her body, we more than likely will shame ours. At least 80 percent of children of parents who have eating disorders will also have one, and the same is true for body shame.[20]

Children by nature adopt their belief systems from their parents. If a child sees his or her parents dieting or professing that they're not thin enough, the child will gather his or her self-worth from those things the parent approves of, such as thinness.

In other words, body shame like obesity usually transfers from generation to generation if not overcome. We'll work on undoing the damages done in Part Two.

Looks'ology: Psychological Roots of Body Image

I've seen several clients in my therapy practice who've performed daily self-floggings in their critical attitudes toward their body, and I've found that there are psychological, spiritual causes as well. I call these psychological roots of body image, Looks'ology.

Looks'ology
(Looks-o-lo-gee)
is the made-up, psychological name for why we use
looks to distract us from maturing spiritually and emotionally

Masked Negative Emotions

Masked negative emotions can affect how we feel about body parts. An obsession on a body part can divert our attention from negative emotions happening in deeper areas of life.

In other words, we mask negative emotions by focusing on physical criticism or by the over attention to looking good.

Elle chronically picked at her acne and obsessed with the flaws of her face in the mirror. After we dug deeper, she found her impulsive body shaming masked her deep insecurity of not knowing who she was and what she was to do with her life.

As a twenty something, she was dependent on her parents and afraid to grow up. After addressing these fears in therapy practice, her chronic body (face) shaming disappeared, and she resolved her deep insecurities about her future and her abilities to face it.

Look for ways that you're overcritical of an outward body part when you're upset with something else. Emotional Fitness practices can help you to get to the heart of your negative body criticism. Do the actions in Chapter 18.

Ungratefulness

We have an extreme lack of gratitude with our Creator's make of us. Ungratefulness has its roots in covetousness or jealousy. We want more and are unhappy with what we have.

Gia was a healthy weight. She worked out often, ate well, and was filled with the Holy Spirit, but she was plagued with body shame in her mind. Despite being a small size, she insisted that she was heavy and obsessed with cellulite and other features of her body that she deemed unattractive.

Her body shame was most pronounced on an island vacation. Each time she went to the pool, her thoughts slung whips at her body, making harsh comparisons to every other women's body shape. And she felt the chronic insecurity that theirs was better than hers despite her beautiful, lean, and healthy body.

When someone was bigger, she felt superior.

Often, Gia pinched at her thighs and condemned herself for cellulite, thinking everyone was thinking about it too. In her frustration, sometimes she'd punch the body parts she hated.

Gia's low self-esteem was projected onto her body. Instead of feeling worthy of peace and freedom from body shame, the shame kept her bound in her thoughts.

We're to be thankful, content, and prayerful in all things, including when we feel inadequate, insecure, or jealous (1 Thessalonians 5:16–18, Ephesians 5:20, 1 Corinthians 4:7, Philippians 4:11–13, 1 Timothy 6:6–8, and Proverbs 14:30).

Self-Rejection

We can reject ourselves and our appearance because we may not know, like, and trust who we are. Sharon hated her nose so much that she declined socializing opportunities because of fear of others looking at her. She couldn't be herself since her obsession with her schnozzle took the time that would otherwise be used to get to know herself and others.

Our body is a beautiful expression of God's design of us and our ancestry. Our looks magnify the beauty of the family members who have gone before us. To reject a part of us is also to reject some aspect of who we are.

Unworthiness

Unworthiness shows up as vanity or neglect of our looks and appearance altogether. We can attempt to cover our low self-worth with expensive name brand clothing or material things, an over-attention to appearance (excessive mirror time), or excessive makeup.

Vanity is a stronghold of believing self-worth is how we look and causes us to strive for false ideologies of beauty perfection. Unworthiness is deep in one's soul that manifests as a cause of shame, including body shame and weight and eating bondage.

The other side of unworthiness is poor hygiene and dingy, ripped, or ill-fitting clothing. Unworthiness is healed best by crying out to God and allowing His soul surgery to heal it. It's not healed with more makeup, calf implants, or longer workouts.

Looks'ology helps us to see beyond the distraction of hating our looks to find spiritual and psychological roots for wholeness and freedom.

And sometimes the deficit of truth extends body shame into a class of its own—body dysmorphia disorder.

An Introduction to Body Dysmorphic Disorder (BDD)

If you suspect your body image concerns are extreme, you're not alone. In the United States about 2.5 percent of females and 2.2 percent of males have body dysmorphic disorder (BDD).[21]

Abused and neglected individuals develop BDD at a higher rate, making past childhood-trauma a considerable risk factor along with genetic and physiological predispositions.

Body Dysmorphia Disorder Examples

Remember the lady I saw at the gym who needed to get to Kentucky Fried Chicken ASAP? Well, many anorexics couldn't be that way unless there was a true perception of their body image that was distorted. They think they're fat, and the image in their head is believed more than the actual image in the mirror.

In the same way it's possible for an obese person to have a perception of thinness in their minds. Any mental body image distortion will cause eating portion distortion—too little food like in the case of anorexic or too much food as in the case for morbid obesity.

In a simple Google search, you can see how body dysmorphia disorder and the spirit of vanity caused good looking folks to become unnatural looking with plastic surgery.

For example, Pixie Fox had ribs removed to reduce her waist and at least seventeen surgeries and counting to look like a Barbie doll.[22] And Rodrigo Alves' search for perfection caused him to pursue at least forty-seven surgeries to become the human Ken doll. He has since decided to become a woman and changed his name to Jessica.[23,24]

And you that thought you had problems.

I wish medicine were holistic with mental, emotional, and spiritual health treatment as this kind of drive for beauty is a supreme health risk, a call for deliverance, and a clear mental health matter.

Body Dysmorphic Disorder Check [25]

YES (X)	BODY DYSMORPHIC DISORDER (BDD) CRITERION
	Do you have a preoccupation with one or more perceived defects in physical appearance that are not observable or appear slight to others?
	At some point during the course of the disorder, do you experience repetitive skin picking, mirror checking, excessive grooming, and other things?
	Do the behaviors or thoughts cause distress or impairment in occupational, social, or other important areas of functioning?
	Do you have constant concern about your appearance?

Muscle Dysmorphia Check [26]

YES (X)	MUSCLE DYSMORPHIA CRITERION
	Do you meet the Body Dysmorphic Disorder Criterion?
	Do you have concerns that your muscle build is insufficient?

Important: This check is not a diagnosis. Please see a professional for help if you believe
you have body dysmorphic disorder for a full evaluation and treatment plan.

BDD is a form of obsessive-compulsive disorder and has a high suicidal rate and risk in those who suffer from it. If you suspect you have an obsession or a distorted image of yourself, please seek professional help today. I've observed those who continually gorge with food and fatten their bodies have a deep form of BDD.

God, The Master Artist

BDD and body shame hijack God's messages about our bodies. If we don't change this relationship we have with our bodies, we'll be in a never-ending Weight & Eating War.

Body stewardship coach, Jackie Dixon, a Christ-centered model who has also fought the battles with food and weight, said, "We don't realize in the Christian church how much the culture has infiltrated how we treat and love our bodies. Most of us buy into the cultural attitudes in the media. And these attitudes are so saturated that our families, friends, and churches continue to reinforce the world's perspective on how we look and feel in our God-given bodies."[27]

Isn't this so true? When have we studied what God has said about our bodies? Why are we taught so much about God owning our money in tithes and offerings but not much at all about the fact that God owns our bodies too?

Paul said, "Or do you not know that your body is the temple of the Holy Spirit who is in you, whom you have from God, and you are not your own? For you were bought at a price; therefore, glorify God in your body and in your spirit, which are God's" (1 Corinthians 6:19–20). And our bodies are to be "a living sacrifice, holy, acceptable to God, which is your reasonable service" (Romans 12:1). This includes a reasonable service of proper body stewardship.

God is the Master Artist who painted us in various colors, shapes, and sizes. His definition of beauty is the uniqueness of each one of His masterpieces called people. Each person carries a beautiful expression of God's craftmanship.

Let's walk through the Manufacturer's creation.

"Let Us make man in Our image, according to Our likeness ... So, God created man in His own image, in the image of God He created him; male and female He created them (Genesis 1:26a, 27). The word image here means the reflection of the invisible God because God is Spirit (John 4:24).

God's breath of life is in every living thing. We're to be fruitful and multiply His image. We are made in His image, and no one can escape this truth of God's omnipresent spirit.

Let's continue.

Then God saw everything that He had made, and He said indeed it was very good. Like you are when you create something wonderful, God was giddy about what He made!

So much so that He was complete. After He finished the male and female, the Master Artist rested as the work of creation was finished (Genesis 2:1–2).

And ladies, while the world may tell us we're never good enough, John and Staci Eldridge, in the book *Captivating: Unveiling the Mystery of a Woman's Soul*, point out how the woman was the very last thing God created for earth.[28]

How's that for a final touch on the masterpiece of creation of the Earth?

God created us, and we may have enhanced or "added to it" as a Chubby Church member said. But no matter your weight, you're fundamentally beautiful in the male or female form. Since we're from God's artistic brush, both men and women are divinely inspired beautiful.

Take a moment and think about the form and beauty of the male and female form. There's nothing like it. It's truly a beautiful masterpiece. And God made each, together—wholly representing Himself.

He made the male (Genesis 2:7–8).

Then He made the mysterious female from Adam (Genesis 21–22). You've got to love Adam's response when he saw Eve and all her gloriousness.

"This is now bone of my bones
And flesh of my flesh;
She shall be called Woman,
Because she was taken out of Man" (Genesis 2:23).

Or as that corny church joke says, Adam said, "Whoa, man!"

The male and female make up the divine expression of God's image and character.

If we only knew how powerful it is to understand the dynamic duo of the male and female in reflecting God's image together as one, but that's tough to see if we don't embrace our own reflection of God and our unique identity, individuality, and wholeness in Christ, alone.

And they were naked, but there was no shame (Genesis 1:25).

Shame entered when sin (self-harm, obeying enemy, or carnal nature instead of our spiritual man) entered, and Adam and Eve used a fig leaf to cover up their nakedness. With our sin nature came shame and self-consciousness because that's what we get when we listen to the enemy.

I couldn't see what I can see so clearly now.

That the body, the face, is the first way that we are identified in heaven and on earth. When we die, our invisible soul is in a spirit-like shape of a healed, healthy, and whole body. It's the truth of what we've always been.

Our souls know that our heavenly bodies are the truth. They don't have all the ailments, bumps, or bruises of life.

There's no need to fill up with food in the heavens because the presence of God is alive and unhindered. And the food is Life Abundantly Standard at another dimension. There will be no calories or chemicals to concern ourselves with. But here on earth, we just long for that perfection that we know is there, though now we can only see our earthly self with all its imperfections.

We're created by God; therefore, we need to honor God as our Creator, not media, not cultural norms, not our own ideals of beauty or handsomeness, and certainly not the enemy of our souls.

Honor the Creator, Honor Your Body

It's like this: Imagine that you created a meal for your family. You took time to find the right ingredients and perfect the marinade to enlighten their taste buds. You were sure they'd savor the food, delight in the heavenly aromas, and place photos of your meal on Instagram.

But what if they didn't? What if instead of gratitude and pleasure, they complained about every part of your meal—non-stop? The meat wasn't cooked enough, the dessert was too sweet, and your gourmet mashed potatoes tasted like chalk.

Ouch.

The saddest part of this unappreciated meal is that you knew it was good. You tasted it, perfected the recipe, and took extra care in its creation. You knew those countless five-star reviews on Allrecipes.com were right. You made it with love. And you took pleasure in creating it for them to enjoy.

Only, their taste buds were deceived. Maybe it was their toothpaste that blocked the excellence of the meal? Maybe the beverage had some kind of chemical in it that distorted their sense of flavor?

Our heavenly Father feels the same way about our looks. He created something wonderful in us. The Bible tells us so in Psalm 139.

For You formed my inward parts; You covered me in my mother's womb. I will praise You, for I am fearfully and wonderfully made; Marvelous are Your works, And that my soul knows very well. My frame was not hidden from You, When I was made in secret, And skillfully wrought in the lowest parts of the earth. Your eyes saw my substance, being yet unformed. And in Your book they are all written, The days fashioned for me, When as yet there were none of them (Psalm 139:13–16).

It appears that your genetics created you, but ultimately God knew you before you were born. Like Jeremiah, He knew you in the womb (Jeremiah 1:5). Even the hairs on your head are numbered (Matthew 10:30; Luke 12:7).

Since God is not partial and loves all of us, He knew you too! He takes special care in you as His creation. The Word also says, "You are altogether beautiful, my darling; there is no flaw in you (Song of Solomon 4:7 NIV).

And we may be focused on our looks, but the "Lord does not see as man sees; for man looks at the outward appearance, but the Lord looks at the heart" (1 Samuel 16:7).

Several times the Scriptures discuss the beauty of holiness. Our heart and character in Christ are ultimately where beauty comes from.

Paul says, "Your beauty should not come from outward adornment, such as elaborate hairstyles and the wearing of gold jewelry or fine clothes. Rather, it should be that of your inner self, the unfading beauty of a gentle and quiet spirit, which is of great worth in God's sight" (1 Peter 3:3–4 NIV).

God created your body as an expression of Himself. God is the Creator, and we are to worship the Creator more than the creation (Romans 1:25). Psalm 100:3 says, "It is He who has made us, and not we ourselves."

When we're disgusted with our bodies, we send a message to God that we have a problem with His workmanship.

Disdain with our body is also disdain with the Creator who gave life to us through it. To be ungrateful, unhappy, dissatisfied, critical, or harsh toward our bodies is the operation of Satan and keeps us weight and eating bound.

Satan knows that if people hate their bodies, they will remain weight and eating bound. He knows that they'll eat poorly and be subject to poor health that steals energy from laboring for the kingdom of God.

Your face and body make you uniquely you. No two bodies are exactly alike on the outside or the inside. We do further create our bodies in our lifestyle and eating choices, but we get the bone structure, eye color, and body type we have ultimately from God.

> " Disdain with our body is also disdain with the Creator who gave life to us through it. "

Some stockier, some thinner, all beautiful. All unique.

Father God deserves our absolute respect and honor of our God-given looks and bodies, doesn't He? He deserves a thankful heart for being our Creator. We need to embrace our bodies (yes, this includes your face) and the bodies of others, as beautiful as they are, with the knowledge that we can love and appreciate our bodies back to better health.

Let's jump off the body shame train.

Part Two: Win the Body Shame Battle

How To Jump Off the Body Shame Train for Good!

To get off the body shame train we'll need a one-way ticket to God-fidence. We may not be the happiest about how we look today, but as we embrace body honor and heal shame, we're sure to be happier with who we are and how we look in times to come.

We have a big giant to defeat, so we'll use several strategies to do so. Let's get started.

Battle Strategy #1 – Receive Your Uniqueness

Why is it that when we're born into the world, people rub our bums and think we're the most perfect little thing ever. Then we grow up, and we think that we're the worst-looking troll on this side of heaven?

The first stop on the body shame train is to make your only standard of beauty God's standard. God's standard and truth must be the basis for every area of our lives, which includes how we look.

When our definition of our beauty aligns with God's definition, we can heal distorted body shame. His definition is that what He has made is very good, good-looking, and good enough.

Here's the thing: when you're the only one, rare creation that you are, you are perfect immeasurable beauty. The onslaught of media and cultural ideals for beauty cause us to forget the fact that we're divine expressions of our beautiful God.

Yes, you forgot that you're the only one of you created by God.

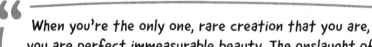

> When you're the only one, rare creation that you are, you are perfect immeasurable beauty. The onslaught of media and cultural ideals for beauty cause us to forget.

There's no one else on our planet of over 7 billion people or in the entire galaxy like you. No one else is you. No one else has your history, experiences, interests, personality, talents, and skills in the exact make up like you. And no one has the exact same body chemistry, fingerprints, hair, voice, or face.

We look at our scars and imperfections and think, *I'm so fat and ugly.* But when you don't feel attractive, you use some basis to judge because how do you know that you're not attractive?

Ask yourself in who's opinion am I not attractive? And if it's your opinion, then ask yourself by what standards? You'll find that you're measuring yourself based on standards unconsciously set for you.

The worlds standards haven't changed much. Worldly standards are about 48 pounds lighter and 6 inches taller than the average women who is 5'4 and nearly 171 pounds as of 2018.[29] And a chest size of 5 inches smaller, biceps of 3 inches smaller, and a waistline of 11 inches smaller than the average male who is 5'9, 199 pounds, and has a 40-inch waist respectively.[30]

The world judges on skin color, ethnicity, height, symmetrical features, hair, body size, chest size (for men and women), skin clarity, and arm size, but who set these standards?

Even experts say our standards of beauty are arbitrary.

Martha Beck said, "Although beauty may be in the eye of the beholder, the feeling of being beautiful exists solely in the mind of the beheld. Standards of beauty are arbitrary. Body shame exists only to the extent that our physiques don't match our own beliefs about how we should look. Good-looking individuals are treated better than homely ones in virtually every social situation, from dating to trial by jury."[31]

She says we mostly measure against our own ideals of beauty. So, we need to shake up those ideals within our minds and from media.

Look at the magazine cover example

WHAT IMAGE ARE YOU LIVING UP TO

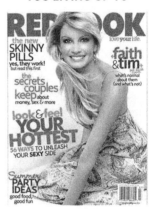

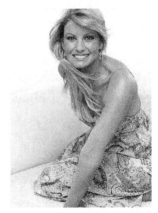

Image 26.2 Cover photo shop example[32]

with Faith Hill. Notice how much thinner her back, arm, and face are in the promoted cover versus her photo.

If you or the world sets standards for how you should look, then you'll never measure up. The world's standard is photoshopped and artificially contrived—also known as a lie. And there we go again listening to the lies and rejecting the truth that what God made is very good.

Since He is the Creator of all people, He also gets to create the standard. And because you are whole, unique, and complete all on your own, the biblical definition of single defined by Dr. Miles Monroe, you are one of a kind.[33]

Something one of a kind is immeasurable because the only thing to measure against is itself.

That means whatever your size or shape doesn't matter.

Your beauty is a nonnegotiable truth of Creation.

God created all things beautiful (Ecclesiastes 3:11). He is the God of beauty. And He is beautiful (Zechariah 9:17a). We're made in the beauty of His image. Therefore, your perception of beauty must be in truth.

There's only one standard, and it's *whatever you are.* Your eyes, your nose, your hair, your bone structure is perfect. Like an oak tree, a red rose, the North Star, or a snowflake are perfect, so are you. Appreciate all your nooks, crannies, life-lived, and other unique attributes that make you—you.

> There's only one standard, and it's whatever you are.

You are beautiful. You are handsome. Are you willing to stop the world's standards? Will you accept your body and looks as His gifts to you? And accept your looks are your gift to others? Yes, your perfectly imperfect package is a beautifully wrapped gift to others too.

> Appreciate all your nooks, crannies, life-lived, and other unique attributes that make you—you.

Are you willing to let go of your own standards for ideal beauty?

From now on receive your God-given uniqueness and accept that the only true standard of beauty is God's. Pray after me, "Father, I receive my uniqueness and beauty. Thank you for every part of how you made me."

Battle Strategy # 2 – Live the Body Honor Manifesto

Our next stop is the body honor manifesto because the opposite of body shame is body honor. Each principle is also a strategy as well. Repeat the following confessions often to heal body shame.

The Body Honor Manifesto – 9 Principles To Increase Body Respect, Love, and Confidence

Principle #1 – Talk kindly. "I only talk kindly to my body."

If we're kind to our body, it will be all the more kind in return. When we offer compassion to our insecurities, our emotional body feels safe to release all that's unwanted from our lives, including unsupportive mindsets, people, weight, and habits.

Kindness kills criticism.

Kindness is like honey that is sweet

> " Kindness kills criticism. "

to the soul and brings healing to our bones (Proverbs 16:24). Proverbs 18:20 tells us that the power of life or death is in the tongue.

Words thought and spoken to us have power in shaping our body image.

Body image is largely formed as a child. In one study among female students, 80 percent of them claimed that their body shame started with negative remarks made by friends and family.[34] And 73 percent of women and 57 percent of men believed their negative body thoughts began from being teased.[35]

We're soul's inside of our human body, and we only know what we look like based on people's comments and our own image in the mirror, especially as small children. By nature we listen to what others say about how we look; therefore, to heal we need to consider not only our own thoughts but also what others have said about our looks.

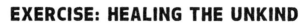

EXERCISE: HEALING THE UNKIND

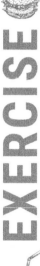

Step 1: Make a list of all the negative things told to you about your body and that you've thought about your body. List your approximate age at the time.

Here are a few examples that contributed to my body shame:

Age 7: "You're getting fat." (my grandmother; I was far from fat)

Age 8: "You're so boney! Get off my lap." (my aunt)

Age 9: "You're skin and bones, I'm calling you Twiggy!" (my grandfather)

Ages 10–12: "Twiggy!" (my grandfather, when referring to me countless times with roaring laughter)

Age 13: "You need to lose some weight to be a model with us." (a modeling school)

Age 13: "You jolly green giant." (a popular peer in my class; you know how that ended)

Age 14: "You're spreading." (my grandmother, right in front of my boyfriend)

Age 15: "Nothing looks good on me. I wish I was skinnier." (me, getting ready for a school dance). The shaming of others now internalized.

Step 2: One by one, share those negative thoughts and comments with the Lord in prayer. Ask the Holy Spirit to heal you from the lies about your body. Simple prayers like: "God, I ask you to remove every hurt and damage done when I was called Twiggy. Heal me, Father."

Step 3: Repent to God for the critical words, thoughts, and treatments you've done toward your body. Also apologize to your body by saying, "I'm so sorry, body, for treating you harshly and saying that you're ugly and unhealthy."

Step 4: Make a list of all the positive things said and thought about your body/looks.

Step 5: Go to a bathroom mirror and look at yourself. Start with saying, "I love you," in the mirror to begin to build a stronger relationship with yourself and your body. Ask God for help to see you as He sees you.

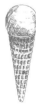

In a study by *Hope College*, it was concluded that those who repeat Scriptures over themselves have an improved sense of body confidence.[36] So, speak Psalm 139:13–14 over yourself and other Scriptures that resonate. Then, for every negative thing on your list, speak something positive over yourself.

How would your body image have been different if affirming words were spoken? Every time you look in a mirror speak truth and affirm yourself. Do this Healing the Unkind exercise to heal body shame any time. Talk often to your body to build a positive, strong relationship with it.

Principle #2 – Thank it. "I'm thankful for my body."

A woman in a Bible study asked me, "What is it you're doing to lose weight?"

My response, "Being grateful."

In my early attempts at weight loss, even when I achieved the target weight, I was ungrateful evidenced by obsessing over my body's imperfections. Oftentimes we look at old photos and wish we would've appreciated ourselves more at the smaller size, am I right?

As discussed, gratitude with our body is also gratitude to God. Gratitude is also an amazing antidote for body shame because gratitude opens the gates of heaven and draws us nearer to God (Psalm 100:4). When we draw nearer to God, we break the enemy's body shame stronghold.

Choose to be thankful for the outside and the inside of you.

Don't just see your eyes looking around doing their thing. See that your eyes see the beauty of your grandmother's smile or daughter's joy. Your heart pumps blood all day every day. And your intestines stretch their digestive muscles with every meal.

Thank your body for all its hard work.

Thank God for every part of the body and what that part allows you to have in your life. I walk you through this in *The Body Love Prayer* in Non-Edible Goodies in Book 1. That prayer did wonders for me to heal my distorted body image and increase my gratitude for it. Keep a simple practice of thanking God for each part as you bathe or dress.

Principle #3 – Accept it. "I accept my body as it is."

Dana Christmas had beautiful skin, a smile that lit up the room, bright eyes, and stylish haircuts. Twenty-four hours later she was unrecognizable. She had severe second and third degree burns on 60 percent of her body, including her head and face.[37]

A horrific fire at my university killed three students and injured fifty-eight people.[38] As a resident assistant, she was burned in her heroic attempt to rescue other dorm students from the greedy flames. In one crazy night all that mattered was that she was alive. Nothing else was important—not her weight, her looks, her hair, or her hand that was deformed because of the fire. This puts things into perspective, doesn't it?

Do her scars of heroism make her any less beautiful? No, because her scars show the beauty of who she is and what she did to help so many others.

We can stop self-rejection when we get our perspectives straight.

Somewhere in the world someone wishes to have a body or features like yours. People are dying right now who can only dream of another chance to better treat their bodies to see their legacy.

Reflections on perspective help stir acceptance. It feels counterintuitive to appreciate your body when you've gained significant weight. But the weight gained could be double or triple in today's food addictive culture.

It really could be worse.

When you feel rejected, unappreciative, demanding, or harsh toward your body and its features, take a moment to reflect on how much worse it could be to cultivate more acceptance of your current appearance.

Principle #4 – Enjoy it. "I enjoy life in my body."

Enjoyment is an extension of our gratitude by practicing active acknowledgement and appreciation for our body as a companion. You're in partnership with it. And you want to enjoy the work you do in it. Cleaning, driving, walking, sitting—all of it can be done with enjoyment.

It's like that house with no paintings on the walls. When we hang up the artwork, it's a sign we've settled in, that we're making a home a home. How can you settle into your body? What can you do to be at home in it?

To enjoy your body is also to take some healthy pride in your appearance. Your clothes express your personality. But sometimes body shame can make us wear boring, revealing, baggy, or black clothing all the time.

So, for the love of God and all things beautiful, don't wear so much black. I do think the grief of body shame shows up in enormous amounts of dark clothing, especially black to look slim.

Your body's like, "Geez, another funeral today."

Help it out.

Dress in a way that brings out your joy. Try out new styles or colors and adjust the fit to get the size right. Match your clothes to match the Whole & Free you, not the old broken and bound version. Could you use a makeover?

 Match your clothes to match the Whole & Free you, not the old broken and bound version.

We feel enjoyment when we take time for adventure, workouts, or sports to get our hearts pumping and muscles moving. We're meant to live. We feel alive as we express physical energy. Brenda felt every part of her body when she went ziplining at age sixty! And Carolyn took on running and ran a half marathon at forty-three. How can you experience more life in your body?

To practice enjoyment is also to be present in your body. Those who have experienced physical or sexual abuse may have trouble being in their bodies. They dissociate from it. To dissociate is to disconnect from feeling grounded and connected to your body.

If you feel like you're out-of-body at times or floating, check out *The Body Keeps the Score* by psychiatrist Bessel A. van der Kolk to heal any post-traumatic stress disorder (PTSD) to better enjoy life in your body.[39]

Principle #5 – Trust it. "I trust my body."

A relationship of trust is the foundation for any positive relationship. Do you trust your body? Have you felt betrayed by it?

We've had to rely on our bodies to act right when giving birth or climbing a ladder.

Incidents we've had when our bodies seemingly failed us, like a birth going wrong or a back going out, can feel like betrayal to us, not to mention when we've experienced abuse, injuries, sickness, disabilities, or accidents.

Yet the body gives frequent signs that something is off nutritionally, emotionally, or spiritually in our lives. For many of the physical ailments and injuries we attract in life, there are emotional reasons too.

 The body gives frequent signs that something is off nutritionally, emotionally, or spiritually in our lives.

Somatization is the technical term for when we manifest health concerns due to unresolved emotional issues. When in chronic pain, we need to also route out the soul pain as even chronic pain has a higher resolution success rate when we deal with past trauma and get psychotherapy.

So, we can trust when the body isn't working properly. It's using pain or the experience to tell us something about how our inputs nutritionally, emotionally, or spiritually need attention.

Reflect on your trust or mistrust in your relationship with your body. Do you trust your body? How can you trust it more?

Principle #6 – Listen to it. "I listen to my body."

Intuitively we know what our bodies need if we take a moment to listen. How well do you listen to what your body is saying?

As we hear and obey the body's still small voice, we can trust that it's leading us to a better wellbeing. It whispers, "Sleep," "Water," "Move,"

"Stand up," "Eat light," or "Please, don't eat cheese; you know how much it hurts me."

As you might recall from Chapter 4, the flesh is our soul's use of the body to carry out its carnal desires for self-harm and indulgence. The body is a miraculous sensory vessel and carries out the soul's will and or God's will.

Your body seeks to be attuned to your soul.

The body and the flesh have different voices.

Your physical body speaks like your soul speaks, only it requests the most basic needs. Intuitively we can hear what we're to eat, drink, and do, but it's difficult to hear when we have a Standard American Diet manipulating it.

But the mind can be conflicted because both brain and taste buds can be manipulated with highly palatable foods. But because the body is scientific in nature, it always seeks your highest good.

Our body doesn't ever want chemicalized non-foods or sugar, fat, and salt-laden foods. It doesn't ask for them. Therefore, it's important to hear beyond your emotional body—and even your beast's addictive voice—to hear the true voice of the body.

It takes practice to hear, but you can learn its voice and intuitively eat your way to better health. As I cleaned up my Standard American Diet, I heard it more clearly.

Pauline decided to listen after a binge episode. She found that her body needed a balanced meal and rest instead of taking on more projects. She wanted to bulldoze past her physical needs, but not listening triggered bingeing.

Amber complained for months about her exhaustion. After taking a few moments to listen to her body's needs, she knew that she needed to stop her protein bars and eat real food. She also figured that electronics at night stole sleep quality. So, she put her phone in another room to charge and focused on an earlier bedtime to honor her body's voice properly.

Check in with your body more often. As we listen to its requests, a beautiful relationship with it emerges that will manifest more body, soul, and spirit freedom in our lives.

Principle #7 – Heal it. "I heal my body."

Imagine that you were taking a shower, and before you could finish cleaning up, mud was thrown on you. So, you started the water again to get the mud off, only it happened repeatedly, which made it difficult to get cleaned up so that you can go to relax. After some time, a guard went up around the shower to protect you from the mud splash so that you can finally get to relax.

Well, the body is turning on the shower itself. It's constantly looking for what's out of order or doesn't belong. It utilizes a sophisticated system to get to its highest degree of health.

The water is the right habits—eating well, exercising, and so on that support the natural cleansing process of the body to heal itself.

The mud is all that doesn't serve you. It's the Standard American Diet and lifestyle we're engaged in daily that prevents us from healing.

The guard is the boundaries you need to put in place to protect your body from unnecessary harm—physically, emotionally, and spiritually.

The Body H.A.B.I.T.S. have a direct impact on a positive body image and heal your body. Hydration (H) reduces negative feelings and bloating. Activity (A) directly boosts body positivity immediately after exercising.[40] Move your body to remove body shame.

Balancing (B) hormones helps because 75 percent of women feel body shame around their cycles due to water retention and less active happy chemicals in the body.[41] Nutrient Loading (I) pours love into our minds and cells. Detoxing (T) gets unloving stuff out of them. And sleep (S) boosts happy brain chemicals and weight reduction.

Refresh with *The Chubby Church Book 1* to continue to apply new tips for implementing the Body H.A.B.I.T.S. in your life. (Reference Chapters 6–13.)

Principle #8 – Look at it. "I look at myself with appreciation."

Validate a healthy body image by looking at yourself. In the thick of my disorder, I couldn't look in the mirror. I looked down when looking at other humans. Body haters have a difficult time looking in the mirror without a slew of thoughts about how upset they feel about their image staring back.

If I passed a mirror in office buildings, stores, or hallways, I'd scurry quickly by it. I piled on my makeup to protect others from seeing the ugly I felt inside.

Do the opposite.

Smile at yourself when you walk past the mirror. Stop the "oh no, don't take a photo" drama when someone wants to snap a shot. Don't pretend your body isn't there or doesn't matter, hide when there's a video camera, or allow your body shame to hold you back from sharing your message on social media.

Expose the shame.

For some of us it would be the most horrendous thing to wear a bathing suit in the open. A lady pastor posted herself in a revealing bathing suit on Facebook. At first, I judged the immodesty, but she shared about her body shame that had plagued her throughout her life. Her post helped her to get free of body shame. Despite anyone else's negative judgment, she healed her own. Most cheered her on to support her liberation.

Sometimes we need to expose the shame for it to heal. For me, I felt my thighs were too fat to wear shorts for a long time. To heal I had to start wearing shorts with confidence. It helped to have a friend take a photo of me in shorts so that I could see that shorts looked fine. No one noticed or cared about the flaws I saw.

You know people are too worried about their own big butt to worry about yours. Several clients were afraid to go sleeveless because of flapping arm fat, but to hide in shame is to wear a long-sleeved shirt in the middle of blazing summer heat.

It doesn't make sense.

Wear the sleeveless shirt and expose the shame. So what, a flapping arm in the wind never hurt anybody. Embracing flawed parts gets the shame out. Shame loves hiding and covering up. So, be sure to talk about your body shame with your accountability partner or a friend like I did with my shorts issue.

Once exposed, shame has no more power.

Show parts of your body that you've hidden due to body shame. To continue to heal the shame take great care of yourself too. Sixty percent of people felt their body shame was due to excess weight.[42] We need to both accept where we are and actively pursue prosperous health and freedom.

> **Once exposed, shame has no more power.**

Also, just because we can wear something, doesn't mean we should. Modesty is a virtue, and even though we have admirable parts, it's a virtue to not to have to show them off. So, be mindful because pride puffs up as much as shame hides.

Principle #9 – Love it

"My body is sacred and special. I love it." Do you feel your body is sacred? Holy? Special?

How do you treat something precious? Do you nurture it? Do you take special care?

Our bodies are the temple of God. Take a moment to ponder being a vessel of the Holy Spirit. How precious that we get to be in bodies that bring life.

We're vessels of the wine of the Spirit. We're filled with the love, peace, and the power of God.

Let's grow out of the body shame-based dieting, workout forcing, and body manipulation to embrace our sacredness, specialness, and preciousness.

Let's work the Body H.A.B.I.T.S. from a motive of divine love and wisdom for our sacredness, not worldly harshness to force the body into change.

As we learn to love our bodies, we'll value them as vessels of the souls and spirits they hold within them.

Have you ever broken a glass with your favorite beverage in it? We're upset that we didn't get to enjoy the beverage. We value the container because we value what's in it. Your container, your body, is so precious. Treat it like it is.

Let's honor our sacredness, the beauty of holiness. "Oh, worship the LORD in the beauty of holiness! Tremble before Him, all the earth" (Psalm 96:9).

Eat like you love yourself too.

Standard American Diet fare has no love in it. It doesn't heal the body. It steals from the body and mind. Because these foods are built on profit and taste motives only, when we eat them, we're sowing this all-take-rude nature into our bodies as well. These foods harvest shame—body shame.

We reap what we sow. Sow love into your body with what you eat and how you care for it. Food made with light and love give light and love to the body and mind as well.

> Food made with light and love give light and love to the body and mind as well.

Battle Strategy #3 – End Comparisons

Bonita, a talented, successful career woman struggled with raging comparisons of her body with everyone else's bodies. She thought, *I'm not as fit as Christy, or I look much slimmer than Pat.*

Body comparison is a source of pain because the Bible calls it envy. And James said, "For where envy and self-seeking exist, confusion and every evil thing are there" (James 3:16).

This jealousy is a constant inner thought war of how we're perceived by others or look in comparison to others, possibly causing disorder in how we eat.

Bonita wouldn't have been able to move forward to emotional

wholeness or freedom if she didn't admit that she was harassed by comparisons.

I took Bonita to the mirror.

She looked into her own eyes. I guided as she spoke acceptance to each part of her physical appearance and thanked it for what that part did for her and how the body part made her special.

Mirror work is the fastest way I've seen my clients grow in self-acceptance.

Do the same. Go to the mirror, look into your eyes, and speak the truth. Do the mirror work to validate yourself and let go of comparing and judging others in their bodies.

Claim inside your mind, *I am beautiful and so are you* to others. While you're at it say, "I have a beautiful body." As we discussed, God made each man and woman, and each is his or her own beautiful.

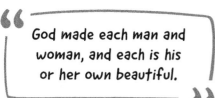

God made each man and woman, and each is his or her own beautiful.

And our own beliefs we hold about our looks impact body shame the most. It's important to believe that you're good looking enough and your body is beautiful enough. Even on your worse hair day, validate your body with thoughts like *I am beautiful* and *I am beautiful no matter how I look at the moment.*

Another way to stop comparing is to give and receive compliments. Receive compliments well by saying a simple thank you. And please don't follow up a compliment with how bad your skin looks or how little you paid for your outfit.

When tempted to feel jealous or superior, share an encouragement with the one you want to compare. Be generous with kind words by giving compliments more. When you think a kind word about someone, tell them.

No more hater'ade against your body or anyone else's body.

Battle Strategy #4 – Magnify Your Soul's Qualities

When the prophet Samuel searched for the next king of Israel, he didn't think that David was God's choice since he was ruddy and young. But God said not to look at the outward appearance because He looks at the heart (1 Samuel 16:7).

God highly values your character beyond how you look. What if you took the energy focused on the body's flaws and put it toward growing your character? To magnify your soul's qualities is to value who you are more than your looks.

When we acknowledge our accomplishments and who we are, we can heal body shame. Keisha's body shame reduced when she acknowledged that she was a loving spouse and mother. She also celebrated that she started a company, was an incredible swimmer, saved her money well, and gave birth.

As we value our life's meaning, our character, and soul qualities, we'll reduce the power of our looks as the sole measurement of self-worth. And we'll be more confident in our bodies. In other words, we'll focus less on the zit and more on the beauty of the whole face. We need to stop getting stuck on our physical flaws and instead magnify the eternal, powerful character of our evolving souls. Make a list of all of your soul's qualities, accomplishments, and character strengths.

What do you value about who you are? What accomplishments in your life support your confidence? What other areas of life can support more meaning?

> We need to stop getting stuck on our physical
> flaws and instead magnify the eternal,
> powerful character of our evolving souls.

Battle Strategy #5 – Reduce Media

The Standard American Diet is supported by the media that gives a Satanic Appearance Deception as well. God gave Adam and Eve everything they needed in abundance, yet the deceiver's advertisement was, "You need more."

Media's the same. Media says, "You're too big, so buy this diet pill." But the Body H.A.B.I.T.S. will lead you to your natural size. Or "You're hungry for dinner, you need this bacon cheeseburger with secret sauce," when you have an honest meal in the fridge.

Media impacts distortion and depression around our bodies and food behaviors. Eighty percent of women admit that watching television makes them feel insecure.[43]

Media shows women who are slightly underweight. The average Victoria Secrets fashion model is a size 4, while the average size of women is U.S. is size 14.[44] Female models are 5'10" and 114 pounds (and probably a tween!) on average.[45] Male models are 6'0" and 167 on average.[46]

As a culture, we watch an insane amount of television and movies and consume a great deal of social media. We create an ideal image to compare ourselves to. The problem is that we don't, and we won't, ever measure up. The standard or bar is too high, which creates a constant sense of failure and low self-esteem.

Instead of trying, let go—not of your body care but of media and the constant self-berating, apologizing, and isolating because of body shame against an ideal that isn't possible except by manipulation of images. Reduce social media, television, and movie watching, and body-esteem will increase.

Pay attention to your body shame feelings after engaging with media to see how it affects you. How much television and social media do you watch? How can you reduce this to support a positive body image?

Battle Strategy #6 – Adjust Your Lenses

Noemi, a beautiful Mexican mother and grandmother, struggled her whole life with her body image. She was made fun of for her weight and her face by peers and loved ones. She was told to wear her hair long to cover up her "ugly face."

After much turmoil, she decided to talk to God about it. She prayed, "Lord, help me to see me like You see me."

And God showed her a vision of herself happy with short hair. She saw herself for the first time as God saw her, and she wept.

She was beautiful. Everything else she believed was a lie.

She cut her hair and felt joy about her looks.

Take note that the best counselor on body shame is the Holy Spirit. He can give you new eyes.

Have you been a healthy weight but still see yourself in your mind's eye at your heaviest weight? Or you can't seem to shake the fat girl or boy image inside?

Sherry in the Whole & Free Health course was an athlete in high school. Back then, she was able to eat whatever she wanted and didn't gain a pound. Fast forward twenty years ... she ate the same, but she saw herself as a teenage athlete. Her body image distortion saw herself as thinner than reality.

We can do the following to adjust our body image goggles:

- Look in the mirror (say something kind while you're there)
- Weigh yourself (limit to once per week, day, or month)
- Take measurements and date them
- Compare past and present images of yourself to gauge how you felt about your body at the time of the photos
- Take exercise classes so that you can see yourself amongst other people in the mirrors to get a better handle on your body size
- Take consistent action to create a healthier body, soul, and spirit

These steps help to focus on internal self-image to the external reality. As we work on our body honor, God will adjust our lens.

Take Action

Gather images of yourself from the past and reflect on how you felt about yourself. Were you happy with yourself, or were you still feeling insecure about your body shape and size?

Final Destination: Welcome to God'fidence!

Fantastic Work! Your final destination is God-fidence! And it's a beautiful place. Are you feeling the renewed energy that comes from receiving God's truth about your body? These steps will ensure you get off the body shame train for life!

Remember to have a dedicated prayer time to take this battle to the Lord. See, body image is the last thing to go. You can change how you eat, your clothing style, your workouts, and your body composition. But body image is in a hard-to-reach box in the crevasse of the attic, and it's difficult to get in there and clean it out. It's a heavy box too.

So, it requires some help to get it out of there and into the trash.

Holy Spirit, help.

For me, body shame took a tremendous amount of prayer, which is always our fundamental defense in everything. I was plagued with body shame at my smallest and certainly at my heaviest. Prayer delivered dreams (night) to help me heal as well as my practicing all these strategies. Other clients and students also had miraculous healings as well.

> **You can change how you eat, your clothing style, your workouts, and your body composition. But body image is in a hard-to-reach box in the crevasse of the attic, and it's difficult to get in there and clean it out.**

The Potter's House

To write a book called *The Chubby Church*, I had no shortage of body insecurities. After all, who has the nerve to tell the church that they're chubby? While most chuckle, some take this as me calling them or the church fat. I am the first member and the pastor of this powerful, hungry congregation. I am certainly not shaming anyone.

It was my students who named the book. It was catchy, and they loved it. After much prayer the title was decided. I felt it was a bit edgy because the Holy Spirit wanted it to stand out to my market—Jesus lovers who struggle with weight and eating.

The title may deter those who have less of a sense of humor. But it also propels those who know they belong to this congregation and want to be ministered to in this crucial area of life.

One reader was on her way to her book club and had *The Chubby Church Book 1* in her large purse. She stopped at the shoe store, and the salesman noticed it and said, "I need that book!" And he proceeded to order it right away.

So, I trust that God put the right title on the book to reach those He wants to reach through it. And of course, I want you to resonate with Whole & Free Health because Whole & Free is the true identity of *Chubby Church* members.

Identity is what this is all about.

Naturally, I thought, *I'm too big to write this book.* I also thought, *I'm too big to teach on eating disorders.* But let me tell you about our faithful, awesome Father.

At my highest weight, God spoke to me about teaching on eating disorders. I was healing, only my physical manifestation hadn't manifested. As you know, the journey is a bit up and down in weight as we're learning to let go of the foods, thoughts, feelings, and behaviors that are the cause of the problem.

The Potter's House Denver ran a counselor center that I interned at for my clinical hours for my counseling psychology program. They also ran a robust lay counseling program which had a variety of speakers.

Well, the day that I felt the most insecure about being too big to teach on eating disorders, my supervisor, Barb, called me into the conference room.

"Jendayi, would you be willing to teach on eating disorders? The instructor scheduled had to cancel," she said.

I couldn't believe it. *Did I hear her correctly?*

"You want me to teach on eating disorders?" I asked with eyebrows burrowed.

"Yes, you seem passionate, and I believe you can do it," she said.

"Wow, of course," I said in awe of our loving Creator who opened a door for me.

He knew that I had what it took to heal and teach. He knew who I was beyond my current size. He knew I wasn't that pizza or cookie binge girl I thought I was. He knew my true identity. He knew I was going to write, not one but at least two books on this very topic. And He knew I'd have the boldness to call it *The Chubby Church* and the personality to tell everyone about it.

He knows His church. He knows *this* church. And you are the church. He knows what we don't. He knows the truth about how we've been deceived about who we are. When I speak to the Chubby Church, I speak to the Whole & Free church, His church, His beloved one who is waking up to his or her true identity in Him.

If I had allowed the absolute horrendous bombardment of my body insecurities to stop me from writing the book, promoting the book, or speaking about the book, I wouldn't have been able to deliver this message of hope, healing, and strategies to block the enemy's victory in your life!

God knew exactly what He was doing when He told me to speak on this subject for the ten years at the Potter's House of Denver.

And what body size and shape should I be to write a book like this? If I were too small or naturally thin with no struggle, would I have understood to this depth? And if I were too big, would you have trusted this content? Today, I am free. I've come a long way to be body confident.

Don't let your body image block your destiny. You may be called to help others in this very area like I am. Get started today. Helping others is the best way to motivate yourself.

One last thing: our self-image is our beliefs about how we see ourselves in our own minds, and it also needs to adjust with our body image. We can't continue to see ourselves as lazy, unhealthy, fat, addicted, and tired.

How we see ourselves limits or expands our biggest dreams for our lives.

You must embrace the transition from the old version of yourself, including the "insecure, heavier" you, to the new "secure, lighter" version of yourself.

> " Don't let your body image block your destiny. "

Otherwise, we will regain back up to the image that we believe we are.

We act in direct accordance with who we believe we are. If you believe your unattractive and don't have value, you'll demonstrate that through actions of self-harm like promiscuity, fornication, or desperation to anyone who'll take you. You wouldn't get a job that pays enough or develop your skills to increase your value in the marketplace since you feel doomed to failure. You wouldn't eat well because why bother if you think your unattractive anyway.

> " How we see ourselves limits or expands our biggest dreams for our lives. "

This type of thinking is an attack on your identity and destiny. The Father of Lies wants you to self-destruct and sin against God. His agenda is simple: if she hates herself, then he can move on to someone else because self-hatred will breed much sin.

The Father of Lights wants you to self-direct.

To self-direct is to shift the words inside to those words that can bring life. Get into alignment to what His words

> " We act in direct accordance with who we believe we are. "

says about you and His transformative power in you. He is the Potter, we are the clay, and we're all the work of His hands (Isaiah 64:8).

For more support, check out Christ-centered life and marriage coach Robyn Coffman's helpful online program Beyond Skin Deep (*https://www.thecoffmancompany.online/beyondskindeep*).

Healing body shame is a major victory toward weight and eating freedom. Next, we'll deal with shame itself.

REFLECT & SHARE

1. How has a negative body image impacted your life?
2. What are some of the things that were said about your body that you need to heal?
3. Which Battle Strategy most resonates for you?
4. How often do you judge and compare your body with others?
5. How can you better value who you are?
6. How does media influence how you feel about your body shape and size?

PRAYER

Dear Lord,

Thank you so much for my body! Thank you for helping me to get off the body shame train and land in your richness of confidence that I am fearfully and wonderfully made by my beautiful Creator!

Thank you for making me in your image. Thank you for making only one of me! I choose to go forward unapologetically in my divinely created image and likeness of you.

I am your child, and I'm honored to carry your Holy Spirit in my sacred vessel. Thank you for revelation and healing in loving my body. Help me to honor it with what I eat and what I do.

I break the stronghold of body shame now in Jesus's mighty name. Fill me with your love to help many others break free too.

Thank you!

In Jesus's name, amen!

CHAPTER 27

DECLINE DATES WITH ICY ISOLATION

Battle #6 - Soul Shame

"A man who isolates himself seeks his own desire;
He rages against all wise judgement"

–PROVERBS 18:1

"Oh, I can't make it."

"Why not?"

"Because I'm feeling fat and bloated
don't want to be around people."

Part One: Understanding Soul Shame

Isolation is all too familiar for those in weight and eating bondage. Isolation is to keep to oneself in obedience to shame. Shame from feeling overweight, too ugly to be seen, ashamed about brutal binges, your body, or simply to be alone with binge foods.

Isolation is also from the shame-based belief that you don't deserve real love but a conditional love based on your body size and a false love with food not people.

Isolation is not normal for human beings. The Bible says that an isolated man seeks his own way and rages against any wise judgment (Proverbs 18:1).

257

We're not in our best mental state when we choose the behavior of isolation. Isolation is to be far away, remote, or set apart. It's meaning comes from the Latin word *insula* which means island.[1]

Do you feel like you're on an island?

As I write this, we're in isolation as a society. We're told to practice self-quarantines and social distancing because of Covid-19, a type of flu that has swept the world and caused governments to mandate staying home.

When I was petting my sweet potato and playing pretend soccer with broccoli, I knew I had to write this chapter.

Isolation is strongly correlated to depression, anxiety, and bipolar disorder.[2] Those who are more isolated increase their death rate by 30 percent.[3] Isolated people also have an increased risk of health concerns such as inflammation, heart disease, and diabetes.[4]

Isolation is a manifestation of our next battle, soul shame.

Soul shame is the core emotional issue of weight and eating bondage

In this chapter, I'll highlight basics of soul shame and coming out of it. While soul shame and body shame operate together, soul shame goes deeper in its affects. Soul shame affects our identity. Identity is about who believe we are, what we believe we can receive in life, and what we believe we're capable of accomplishing in life.

Isolation is only one manifestation, but so are other areas that were covered in all you've read so far.

> " I fed my soul shame when I should've starved it. "

See, I fed my soul shame when I should've starved it. For me, my soul shame manifested in the pattern of food addictive behaviors and dates with icy isolation. Icy isolation is the cold, lonely, empty feeling that a lack of identity feeds. Some may call it cocooning.

Hiding away I fed the shame-guilt-repent-repeat cycle.

I also didn't want to go anywhere because I was embarrassed by my body shape and size that these problem foods created. I preferred to keep to myself when bloated or overweight with tight-fitting clothes or a swollen, inflamed face.

Events, no thanks.

Pool parties, never.

When we feel fat, binge eat, or want to hang out with food addictions instead of connecting with others, we stay inside in shame instead of going out in glory. We don't want to go out because we don't feel confident. We hide behind work, duties, or hobbies.

Isolation is a side effect of all types of bondage.

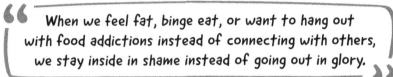

> When we feel fat, binge eat, or want to hang out with food addictions instead of connecting with others, we stay inside in shame instead of going out in glory.

When isolation strikes, we may avoid calls or cancel meetings. We may sulk in emotions of shame, pity, guilt, or avoidance. We definitely don't shower or comb our hair. It's okay to retreat for time for yourself. You may need to if you've poured out or have had a busy week. But when you feel the need to hide your body because of binge embarrassment or to be with problem foods and depressive emotions, shame is the motive.

Isolation behaviors may cause one to:

- Decline events due to poor body image or feelings of fatness
- Decline events due to desire to be with your problem foods
- Dread being in front of people or attention for any reason
- Avoid conflicts
- Avoid people, including in-person and phone conversations, gatherings, or meetings

- Sneak or hide food
- Eat in secret
- Eat one way when with people and another way when people aren't around
- Have poor hygiene
- Skip church

I must ask: are you making dates with icy isolation? If so, how often? What if you just need alone time?

Before we get into understanding soul shame, let's look at the differences of introversion, isolation, and solitude.

Introverted or Isolated

The introverted personality refuels by being alone. Introverts think before they speak, take more time to emotionally process, and thrive when they have time alone.[5]

Extroverts, not so much. They speak their thoughts, openly express emotions, and refuel by being around people.[6]

Therefore, extroverts tend to be more naturally active, expressive, social, and interested in many things. Introverts tend to be more reserved, private, cautious, and interested in fewer interactions but with greater depth and focus.

Check the attributes that best describe you. Which one do you lean toward? Extrovert or introvert? Ambiverts are balanced in their extroversion or introversion, but there is one that's more dominate.

Isolation happens for anyone bound in shame, food addiction, and a lack of self-awareness on what refuels and depletes their energy. And both introverts and extroverts will need to recharge without addictive foods or intense feelings of fatness.

Chart 27.1 Introversion versus Extroversion

INTROVERTS OFTEN	EXTROVERTS OFTEN
☐ Have quiet energy	☐ Have high energy
☐ Listen more than talk	☐ Talk more than listen
☐ Think quietly inside my head	☐ Think out loud
☐ Think, then act	☐ Act, then think
☐ Feel comfortable being alone	☐ Like to be around people a lot
☐ Prefer to work "behind-the-scenes"	☐ Prefer a public role
☐ Have good powers of concentration	☐ Can sometimes be easily distracted
☐ Prefer to focus on one thing at a time	☐ Prefer to do lots of things at once
☐ Are self-contained and reserved	☐ Are outgoing and enthusiastic

Despite extroversion or introversion personality traits, the need for solitude is within all of our souls. We can honor this need without using food.

Solitude is an intentional time with our thoughts in quiet and alone with God, not with problem foods. Solitude is a virtue and spiritual discipline. Daniel, Moses, Elijah, and Jesus took time to be alone with God.

We all need time to be still to hear what our soul is saying and what the Spirit is whispering without distractions.

What Is Soul Shame?

Shame relentlessly gropes at those who struggle with disordered eating. Shame is the core identity battle of any addiction-based struggles, especially food addiction.

Shame is defined as something that brings censure or reproach, a painful emotion caused by the consciousness of guilt, a condition of humiliating disgrace, or humiliating distress caused by the consciousness of wrong or foolish behavior.[7,8]

Everyone with a healthy conscience has shame. Shame is a universal experience that can only exist in a relational context. Shame exists because of our own beliefs and judgments.

Through our relationship with God, we have a moral consciousness or awareness that guides us to what's right or shameful behavior. We feel badly about things we know we shouldn't do. This is a good thing.

However, we can take on toxic shame because we don't believe we're worth freedom from bad habits. A bad habit reinforces shame because the shame needs validation to stay alive. So, we eat, feel bad (shame), repent (feel guilty), and wait until the next emotional trigger of shame. That's what I mean by the shame-guilt-repent cycle.

Our internal soul shame makes us believe that we're unworthy, unlovable, and defective ... that we are fundamentally bad, flawed, or wrong in some way.

Shame causes despair about who we are and what we've done. It doesn't seem to be able to forgive. And it makes us feel like we don't fit in or belong, so we hang out with the misfits of ever-accepting muffins.

Internal shame shows up in our critical thought life. External shame shows up in relationships. It's how others view and see us. If we don't feel like we meet societal norms, such as being a certain body weight, we feel the judgment, biases, and condemnation of our own judgments and those of others. Shame says, "You're a big slob," and then you go ahead and act accordingly.

Brene Brown, shame researcher and author of *Daring Greatly* and *The Gifts of Imperfection*, said, "Shame needs three things to thrive. They are secrecy, silence, and judgment." She said, "It will grow and creep into every corner and crevasse of our lives."[9]

When shame lives in our souls, it'll eat away at our lives. I've had clients admit their shameful acts with food, like stealing it from roommates or hiding it from a spouse. One got in trouble on the job for spending more time with her snacks than working on her assignments.

We do things like stuff ourselves with food then feel the weight of our shame and guilt. We don't tell anyone because shame loves to hide. And sin and shame are synonymous. Therefore, we're urged to confess our sins one to another that we may be healed in order for shame to die (James 5:16).

Our isolation keeps our shame gremlins in the closet. Think about the last time you isolated. Were you embarrassed about what you did with food?

Shame is the root of our dysfunctional relationship with God, ourselves, food, and others.

Study the chart below that illustrates a false belief system and shame-based identity.

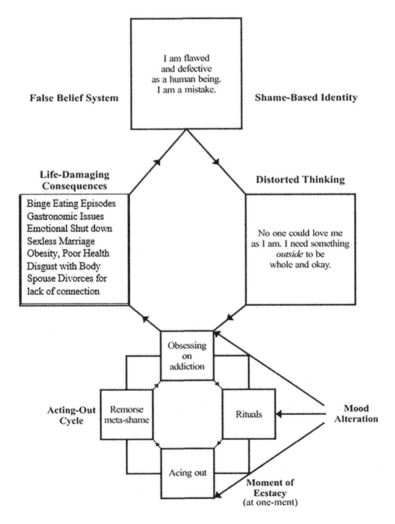

Illustration 27.2   Shame-Based Identity Cycle[10]

In the illustration, can you see the enemy at work to keep your life stuck in a cycle of shame? I hope so. A shame-based identity must be healed to experience the abundant life in Christ.

A few ways that shame manifests are below:

- ☐ Addictions. Food addiction, drugs, alcoholism, and addictions to emotional states such as rage or grief.
- ☐ Mental health problems. Eating disorders as well as other psychological disorders.
- ☐ Poor posture such as slouched or feet pointing inwards, a lack of uprightness.
- ☐ Poor eye contact. When one feels ashamed, he or she may not look someone in the eye and tend to look away or down more often.
- ☐ Lying. Fear of telling the truth or being upfront because of a fear of rejection may cause one to lie and create a web of deception. We may lie about food intake or hide snacks.
- ☐ Difficulty receiving love in relationships. A tendency to push love and kindness away because you're not used to receiving honest love and care.
- ☐ Over-giving. Extreme generosity at the expense of one's own ability or giving more to others than to the needs of your own life and health.
- ☐ Over-dependence. Unable to care for oneself and get life together and tend to take without the resources to give.
- ☐ Self-sabotaging acts against one's highest good.
- ☐ Ways we sabotage due to Chubbological threats are manifestations of shame (Chapter 16).
- ☐ Ways we engage inner glutton, diet nut, or the beast are manifestations of shame.
- ☐ All body shame is an extension of soul shame.

Soul shame drives the behaviors listed. Behaviors driven by soul shame also are laden with condemnation and self-ridicule. There's no grace or love in them. It's either black or white, all or nothing, or in and out of control. What behaviors do you engage in that are motivated by soul shame?

Table 27.3 Shame In-Control and Out-of-Control Cycles[11]

CONTROL	OUT OF CONTROL
Dieting	Overeating
Hoarding	Compulsive Spending
Depressive	Manic
Stoic	Hysterical
Teetotaler	Alcoholic
Sexual Anorexia	Sexual Compulsivity
Perfectionist	Slob
Self-righteous	No Good Sinner
Overly Critical	Self-critical
Blaming	Self-blaming
Over-functioning	Under-functioning
Overachiever	Underachiever

Soul Shame Roots

Soul shame derives from many factors, but we'll narrow down to the most frequent offenders.

The Human Experience

Once Adam and Eve disobeyed God in the garden of Eden, they felt the onset of shame. Shame is a part of the human experience because we have moral conciousness.

The Spirit of life in every human being brings a sense of morally righteous or wretched behavior. We feel shame when we know that we've done something wrong. Toxic shame is when we believe we *are* something wrong. It's when we see ourselves as defective.

Trauma

Trauma is experienced anytime we've gone through a
shocking or difficult time

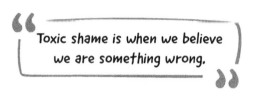

> **Toxic shame is when we believe
> we are something wrong.**

emotionally. It's a primary cause for toxic soul shame. When you've been through trauma such as a loved one passing at a young age, a caregiver who was abusive or abandoned you, divorce, or poverty, we can interpret the meaning of these events into a belief about who we believe we are as well as what we deserve in life.

John's mother was so explosive growing up that when he was ten years old, he was hospitalized from her physical abuse. This traumatic event caused him to believe his life wasn't worth living.

It's no surprise that John wrestled with suicidal thoughts most of his adult life. Since his own mother abused him, it was difficult for him to believe that he could be worthy of life. And since he didn't feel loved and cared for, he cared for himself with binges with his chocolate goodies snuggled up with his favorite action movies, which added to his weight distress. He thought, *If my own mother mistreats me and doesn't care for me, who would?*

We wear our unresolved trauma in the form of our chubby suits and shame. We store the pain as fat. Out of the pain we eat poorly and compulsivey.

Trauma and shame are interconnected because by nature trauma brings shame. Have you experienced trauma? A loved one's absence, abandonmnet, abuse, addiction, or adultry? Or harm from a stranger?

Whatever the trauma—it needs to be thoroughly resolved from a variety of angles; otherwise, it may still live inside. As we learned from Book 1, feelings can be buried alive.

We must heal who we were at the time of the trauma so that we can be fully restored in whom we are now. As I mentioned in Chapter 18, the trauma of my father's death at twelve-years-old stayed with me and manifested as my inner glutton until she was healed at age twenty-eight. Our inner glutton is the inner child who acts out of her trauma, and she needs healing.

The healing for your soul shame comes from you and your little child inside. You offer your own love to your unhealed little self at that time in your life. Therapy and working with the Holy Spirit to receive God's love and truth heals who we are or have been from the trauma. Healing is a necessary part of the journey to wholeness and freedom for life.

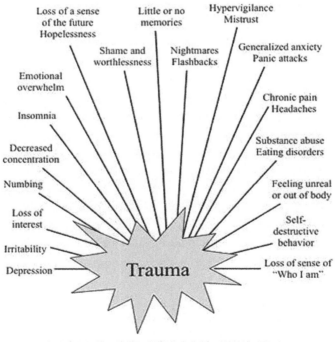

"Trauma survivors have symptoms instead of memories" [Harvey, 1990]

Adapted from Bremner & Marmer, 1998   Copyright 2007 Janina Fisher, Ph.D.

Illustration 27.4   Trauma's Effects[12]

Ancestrial Sin

We're generationally affected by sin that's unconfessed, unrepented for, or unresolved. It's like this: if previous generations don't deal with their wrongdoings, the next generation struggles with it.

In the Bible we hear about generational curses, basically that God will bless those who obey Him for 1,000 years and curse (cause hardship) for those who disobey Him from the third to fourth generation following the generation of disobedience (Deuteronomy 5:9).

Abraham, Isaac, Jacob, and Joseph dealt with a generational sin of lying. Yet God chose Joseph to stop the generational sin of lying (Genesis 12:10–29, Genesis 20:1–18, Genesis 26:6–11, and Genesis 37:21–35).

Could God be using you to end family generational sins?

Stella's mother had her when she was only sixteen years old after running away from her tyrannical father into the arms of the first man who offered her a place to live. Years later Stella had a child at sixteen and endured much relational, financial, emotional, and spiritual hardship causing her to often go on dates with icy isolation.

It wasn't until years later that she found out this pattern of running away and getting pregnant as a teen went three generations back. Stella's daughter was the one God chose to break this pattern.

John Bradshaw, author of *Healing the Shame That Binds You*, says it this way, "Shame-based people will find other shame-based people and get married."[13]

Shame-based couples tend to raise shame-based children. So, instead of feeling supported and encouraged in whom each child is, children graduate from the home feeling inadequate, alone, and co-dependent (too needy to succeed abundantly in life).

Shame-based people deter genuine emotional intimacy because if we believe we're defective or flawed, we can't feel safe or close to others. A lack of intimacy with people is exactly why we continue to use food to fill the voids that shame created. We'll discuss generatoinal issues of obesity and more in the next chapter.

The Unknown Self

The unknown self is the identity crisis that causes us to mistake a hamburger for our mom and dad. We don't know who we are. We don't know how Whole & Free we are. We've missed impartations of love and truth because our upbringings had much shaming in them.

We've been entangled with the sin of gluttony and self-abuse because we've not known how we can escape the cultural ideals, ways, and habits that limit us. If we don't learn our true identity in Christ, we'll be deceived into thinking a false identity is our true identity. Without knowledge of who we are, we won't grab hold of where we are going – or destiny.

Soul shame carries with it a twisted identity that's dysfunctional in his or her coping techniques because he or she doesn't believe her soul is strong enough or spiritual enough to endure the challenges of daily life.

You are enough. You can endure the challenges of daily life. You have the ressurection power of the cross in you.

We get to know who we are through the Word of God and through fellowship with His people who speak life and truth into our souls to rid us of the lies of soul shame.

Which cause of shame is unresolved most for you?

Other Manifestations of Shame in Weight and Eating Bondage

I'm super proud of you for getting to this point in the book. You have the tools and practical instructions to heal all the ways that you've partnered with darkness to perpetuate shame in your life. See, in the kingdom we're free. In Jesus we're free indeed!

We've targeted many manifestations of soul shame already! In fact, both *Chubby Church* Books are a direct blow to soul shame in our lives! Since we've covered isolation, let's take a nibble on a few other manifestations of soul shame that affect weight and eating.

Feeling Fat

Feeling fat is a psychological phenomenon that causes shameful eaters to wallow in feelings of insecurity. It's the same phenomenon as with *Looks'ology*. Just like with body shame, feelings of fatness are shame-based emotions, such as guilt displaced into feeling fat.

Despite having water weight gain, actual excess weight (being overweight), or temporary setbacks, I stopped feeling fat altogether after progress healing soul shame. This felt remarkable because for much of my life that's how I felt. I realized that feelings of fatness are yet another manifestation of unhealed soul shame in the weight and eating bound.

Weight changes day by day and moment by moment. Feeling fat is a form of emotional shame, usually from the guilt-ridden behavior of over-eating or eating the wrong stuff, but it can be unrelated to food.

The shame-based behavior hides the shame-based emotion that triggered it and traps the actual emotion in false feelings of fatness.

Take Delisa for example. Delisa isolated herself because she felt fat. After doing an Emotional Fitness Workout™, she discovered that she felt badly about mistreating her husband instead of comforting him. While she was bloated, she understood why she felt ashamed, and her feelings of fatness disappeared.

Notice your feelings of fatness and dig for emotions with an Emotional Fitness Workout™. Feelings of fatness tend to take over any shame feeling that we have difficulty getting in touch with.

Lack of Emotional Support

When we depend on food for comfort, we're not utilizing enough emotional support in our lives. We need emotional support. After all, who wants to admit that the real lover in our lives is a piece of candy?

This should not be so.

A lack of emotional support keeps the excuse for emotional eating alive and causes us to eat over the emotional waves of life. Furthermore, the waves of loneliness or depression make us feel like we don't belong anywhere or matter to anyone. Can you feel the cold shivers of icy isolation?

I'll be loud about it and say, "You matter! You're important."

It's the Satanic Addictive Deception that deceives us emotionally with the chemical effects of the ingredients on our emotions discussed in Chapter 22.

We all need and deserve real emotional support to replace our fickle, temporary support from problem foods. To get more emotional support, I'll give you strategies for building and keeping relationships. But know that great emotional support comes from being a safe person yourself.

Be someone whom you can trust and confide in when you feel down. Then you'll attract people into your circle whom you can trust and confide in—even about the desire to sneak away with croissants. At the very least, we need to utilize the skills in Chapter 18 (yet again) to become our own best emotional support.

And there's no shame in paying for emotional support through a trusted coach or counselor until you've created enough support in your life. Where (other than food) can you gain more emotional support?

People Pleasing

Are you a yes person? Do you believe you can't say no? Do you have trouble standing up for what you want or believe? Or are you always being the nice guy or gal? People pleasing is living for the approval of others, and it's a sure sign of soul shame.

People pleasing is a good quality that can get out of hand when we're scared of rejection. In my shame I was overly nice and always giving to the point that I was a doormat and constantly being taken advantage of. At that time, I felt resentful of giving so much without progress on my own goals. I still focus on others but with better boundaries, honesty, and self-care.

Do you agree that being nice is pretend behavior to appease others?

Think about it: are you going to tell super nice Shirley that you don't want her highly fat cooking? No, you'll take her food and throw it away behind her back, and she'll continue to waste money and time giving you food you don't want—all because she's so nice and so are you.

People-pleasing, nice folks are often overweight or obese because they're eating their real feelings and don't have ability to stomach solid boundaries or feedback because of their soul shame.

Bradshaw said, "Being nice is primarily a way of manipulating people and situations. By doing so, he (the nice guy or gal) avoids any real emotional contact and intimacy. By avoiding intimacy, he can ensure that no one can see him as he truly (feels he) is shame-based, flawed, and defective."[14]

Essentially, people pleasing and being nice is a form of lying to ourselves and others to placate a fear of rejection (shame) and to avoid criticism or tough conversations. The fear of man can cause a snare (Proverbs 29:25). All fear is bound in shame, and all shame is bound in fear.

> **Shame is a cancer to the soul.**

Biblical View of Shame

Shame is a cancer to the soul. Soul shame is the ultimate destructive force that Christ wants to heal in us. You can see why when you reflect on the damage that shameful feelings of worthlessness have cost you. And how about the damages of food addiction, over-eating, unclean eating, fleshy fasting, and body shame? All of these issues beg us to embrace our healing and deal with the past.

It's soul shame that causes us to sin repeatedly. As you may recall from Chapter 15, sin is synomous with self-harm. Paul said, "Awake to righteousness, and do not sin [self-harm]; for some do not have the knowledge of God. I speak *this* to your shame" (1 Corinthians 15:34).

Paul saw that sin came from shame, so he spoke to the shame. We awaken to righteousness with a right attitude about who we are in Christ.

God's heart is to free us from every broken and bound part. It's your duty to work with God to get the shame out of your soul so that a fleshy soul doesn't cause you to sin (self-harm). It's our shame that condemns us. "*There is* therefore now no condemnation to those who are in Christ Jesus, who do not walk according to the flesh, but according to the Spirit" (Romans 8:1).

We have a responsibility to do whatever it takes to to renounce "the hidden things of shame, not walking in craftiness nor handling the word of God deceitfully, but by manifestation of the truth commending ourselves to every man's conscience in the sight of God" (2 Corinthians 4:2). We do this through confession, learning, and relationship.

Coming out of shame is the message of Jesus Christ!

Jesus came to heal our soul shame so that we can be Whole & Free in Him. Jesus Christ's mission was to heal us from shame and save us from its deathly acts to ourselves and others.

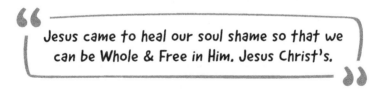

Jesus came to heal our soul shame so that we can be Whole & Free in Him. Jesus Christ's.

Coming out of shame breaks the shame-guilt-repent cycle that keeps us weight and eating bound.

Shame and guilt are the emotions that fuel weight and eating bondage. Therefore, weight and eating bondage cannot exist without shame and guilt.

Shame and guilt are married. You can't have one without the other.

For me, shame was the friend underneath the food. Guilt was the antagonist that brought on the shame. The cycle continued until I was willing to face the ultimate root of the emotional side of the battle—shame and all of its causes rooted in trauma of the past.

It's God's desire that we eat in plenty and be satisfied in order to praise His name and never to be put to shame (Joel 2:26).

Jesus wants us healed because to be in shame invites demonic spirits.

Then they came to the other side of the sea, to the country of the Gadarenes. And when He had come out of the boat, immediately there met Him out of the tombs a man with an unclean spirit, who had his dwelling among the tombs; and no one could bind him, not even with chains, because he had often been bound with shackles and chains. And the chains had been pulled apart by him, and the shackles broken in pieces; neither could anyone tame him. And always, night and day, he was in the mountains and in the tombs, crying out and cutting himself with stones. When he saw Jesus from afar, he ran and worshiped Him. And he cried out with a loud voice and said, "What have I to do with You, Jesus, Son of the Most High God? I implore You by God that You do not torment me" (Mark 5:1–9).

I don't know what this man's shameful acts were that could've invited a reported 2,000 unclean spirits, but we know this man was bound in shame (Mark 5:11–13). The town was amazed as this man's sanity was restored. He was dressed normally and gave the glory to God for his healing (Mark 5:14–16).

Jesus is the light and the Dayspring who has visited us to be set free. "Through the tender mercy of our God, With which the Dayspring from on high has visited us; To give light to those who sit in darkness and the shadow of death, To guide our feet into the way of peace" (Luke 1:78–79).

Jesus came to the cave to get this man free from the demonic forces that infiltrated his soul shame. Jesus also is coming to you right now to heal your soul shame to walk in your identity for your highest purpose and calling. Receive His healing touch. Will you give your soul shame to Him to restore your identity?

Love Heals Shame

God is love. And He and His love are the answers to heal our soul shame. Soul shame heals in the context of relationship with God, yourself, and others.

Receiving His love heals us from soul shame and restores our identity (1 John 4:16). Since shame hinders connection, relational connection is the antidote. Study the illustration on the three stages for coming out of shame.

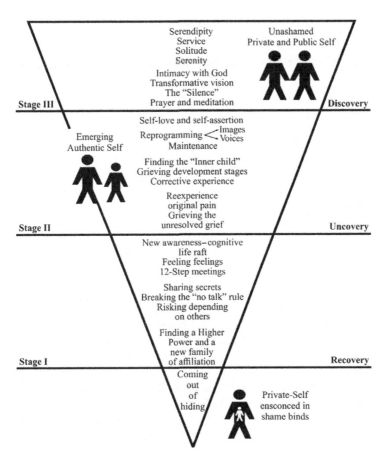

Figure 27.5 Coming Out of Soul Shame[15]

Love God

Notice at the top of the illustration that *Intimacy with God* is in Stage III. That's because to come out of shame is to have a close relationship with Christ. God holds our hands and walks us through the healing journey of love required for intimacy with Him.

Notice how coming out of shame is about coming out isolation and into real relationship in Stage II.

We need to know who He is so that we can know who we are. We get to know Him through His Word and His Spirit, which both speak His voice.

It's from His love that we're able to love other people and ourselves. I don't know if you've ever had the experience of falling short in loving another human, be it a spouse, parent, child, or difficult colleague, but I have. My own lack of love is so evident that at times it has brought me to my knees.

Catch this: we can only love truly from Him, not ourselves. When we practice receiving His love, He gives us the grace to love others more fully. We fill up on His love and then pour it out onto others.

> "Catch this: we can only love truly from Him, not ourselves."

God said to love Him is to obey Him which brings wellness (John 14:24, 1 John 5:3, and Jeremiah 7:23). To love Him is to hate evil (Proverbs 8:13).

To obey Him is to fear Him. Fear means reverence and great respect. To fear Him is the beginning of all wisdom (Proverbs 9:10). We need wisdom to navigate relationships, don't we?

When the fear of God lives in us, we don't continue to sin because to love God is also to love others and prevent sin (self-harm).

For example, God said don't commit adultery. We don't commit adultery not just to be faithful to a spouse but because of our fear of God.

If one doesn't fear God, he or she doesn't have a sound ability to love in a godly way or to respect others or self with the highest integrity. If we love God, then we're known by Him (1 Corinthians 8:3). And even better, "We know that all things work together for good to those who love God, and to those who are the called according to *His* purpose" (Romans 8:28).

Love Him because He knew us and loved us first—God is our first relationship. So, to come out of shame is to get back to the divine order of connected, relational intimacy with Him.

Love Yourself

In Stage II, learning how to love and assert yourself is a necessary part of the journey to discovering your identity in Christ.

We rely on His love and need to come to receive it (1 John 4:16). A relationship with you must be supportive as discussed in Chapter 14. Because we are to love our neighbors as ourselves, we can only love our neighbor or a fellow human being to the extent that we can truly love ourselves.

Face and embrace yourself. Learn who you are, what you need, and what you like and dislike. Discern the truth from the lies of shame.

Relationship conflicts as well as failed relationships offer incredible opportunities to heal from soul shame. It's through relationships that we get to learn more about who we are in terms of strengths, talents, skills, and areas to grow.

From a healthy love for self, you can be authentically you in all your relationships. And when we know who we are, we can build our most successful relationships.

Love Others

To love others is to respect and to serve them from a place of genuine care. It's to make sacrifices as needed to tend to their needs. And we love others to the extent that we know and love God.

Most people will fall short in loving others because there isn't a strong basis for loving self. You've got to be willing to allow others to choose their best paths, even if it affects you. Love doesn't seek its own (1 Corinthians 13:5).

Love is about motive. To come from a place of love is to do things out of love, not out of fear, obligation, greed, or guilt—which all stem from shame. Love motivates, shame shuns, and fear forces.

Let me explain. Would your mother prefer you spend time with her because you have to or because you want to? Would your friend want your compliments because you mean them or because you want compliments in return?

If I give a compliment just to get one back, that's not love, but that's a spirit of flattery and manipulation. If I go to my mom because I'm obligated, then I am doing so out of the fear of her judgment like I owed her something when I didn't. Jesus said to let us owe no man anything except to love him (Romans 13:8). He wants us to have love as the motive in all that we do.

Megan employed Tracey for four years, and the business was busy. But when Tracey had problems with her health, Megan wanted what was best for Tracey, even if it meant more work for Megan or taking the time to replace her.

When Stan wanted to marry Gina, Gina wasn't ready. She wanted to finish school, start her career, and then get married. He waited, celibate, for another two years to marry her. Love waits. Love is patient. Love is kind. Love keeps no record of wrongs. To love others is to want the best for them, even if it costs you.

Our relationship with the Lord is the key to guidelines for relationships. His Word says that we are known by how we love one another. We're told not to covet, murder, disrespect, or get into other people's business.

We're urged to make things right with one another, pray together, pray for one another, and support each other through life's burdens and troubles.

Whoever claims to love God but hates his brother or sister is a called a liar (1 John 4:20). We don't owe anyone anything but love (Romans 13:8).

When we get cleaned up and purified, the love for one another is sincere (1 Peter 1:22). We're to love one another as He has loved us (John 13:34). When we love and do no harm to another, we've fulfilled the law (Romans 13:10).

God is all about relationships and created us for them and for Him to work through them.

Yet, we're not trained in how to build and grow in relationships. Funny, isn't it?

We don't even learn this fundamental life skill in school because it's expected that we'll learn this through our families. But most families lack in basic relationship skills. We can look to 1 Corinthians 13 to learn the keys to a being a healthy person and to have healthy relationships.

Read the below Scripture and replace the word *love* with God, then replace it with the name of someone whom you are in relationship with, and then replace it with your own name.

> *Love suffers long and is kind; love does not envy; love does not parade itself, is not puffed up; does not behave rudely, does not seek its own, is not provoked, thinks no evil; does not rejoice in iniquity, but rejoices in the truth; bears all things, believes all things, hopes all things, endures all things. Love never fails (1 Corinthians 13:4–8).*

Healing, isn't it? Especially when you apply the relationship to yourself.

Shame gives up easily and is rude; shame envies, shame parades itself as pride, and it's puffed up; shame behaves rudely, seeks its own, is provoked, thinks evil, rejoices in iniquity, and ignores the truth; shame loses hope, doesn't trust, easily gives up, and is easily offended. Shame fails.

With love we know that we can heal all issues that pertain to our identity and soul worth. I think you're ready to kick soul shame to the curb. Let's do it.

Part Two: Win the Soul Shame Battle

How To Decline Dates with Icy Isolation for Good!

How much time have you've spent in shame-based thinking and behaviors? Going forward, will you decline dates with icy isolation? Good! Each time you decline dates with shame-based behaviors and thinking, you accept your Whole & Free self. Your true identity and soul worth are in Christ. I'll outline strategies for you to embrace it.

Battle Strategy #1 – Don't Identify with Shame-Based Feelings

Chubby choices stir up guilt, shame, self-doubt, inadequacy, and other shame-based feelings that identify with who we are—a state of being or a way we define ourselves and what we deserve.

I don't eat huge, wheat-based cookies because I don't like how they make me feel. They come with the side portion of shame, guilt, and regret—not to mention the insulin spikes, weight gain, and bloat.

It's not about the cookies. We grow in soul worth to let go of soul shame. Because I don't want to identify as a shame-based person, I don't do behaviors that cause me to invite shame-based emotions like eat poorly.

The Whole & Free soul doesn't want shame-based thinking, emotions, or actions in his life. The Whole & Free identity doesn't identify with doing things that cause guilt and shame to reign in her life any longer.

How has shame permeated your life? Do you feel unworthy? Have you been rejected or abandoned and find it difficult to move past it? My best healing for shame came through crying out to God. I took time to go on a solitude retreat.

And after a while of reading the Scriptures, my soul pressed on the shame that it wanted to release. I got on my knees and started to pray. As I prayed, the Holy Spirit moved through me to heal deep unworthiness. I cried the shame out from the depths of my soul.

God created the soul, so He heals it best. When you're feeling unworthiness or other shame-based feelings, go to Him. Repent and apologize when guilt overwhelms you, and He'll put things into perspective. God knows the devastation we felt when our lover, mother, or father hurt us. He knows the voids and emptiness we fill with food.

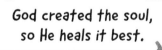

> God created the soul, so He heals it best.

To become Whole & Free we must be willing to do Emotional Fitness Workouts and to process through shame-based emotions. We need to do the work to heal the trauma under the food addiction.

As you reflect on what you've been through, you'll find answers to why you've tolerated so much shame and guilt-ridden behaviors while believing you deserved false comforts and constantly feeling bad.

You don't have to tolerate the shame anymore. Tell your feast beast to shut up so that you can rise up. Stand in the fact that you're a new creation in Christ Jesus (2 Corinthians 5:17). Whether we feel like we deserve to be Whole & Free or not, He's already given wholeness and freedom to us. Receive it.

Battle Strategy #2 – Disobey Shame

Shame wants to continue to thrive in your life, but we're not going to let it. So, you can do the opposite. When you don't want to go somewhere, ask yourself, why? Is it because you've gained weight or feel bloated? If it's the voice of shame, opt to go anyway.

Don't be surprised either if you get the most compliments on days you feel your worst. God has a funny way of making sure you know that He is the God who sees. One Whole & Free Health participant decided to do the opposite and wore a favorite dress without all the nagging undergarments. She was surprised to receive dozens of compliments; it was because she wore the dress Whole & Free.

Disobey the desire to keep impure thoughts inside of your head. When your mind wants to plot a binge or do something harmful, confess to a trusted believer to pray with you to expose the wrongful desire (John 3:20).

When we don't voice it, shame magnifies because it hates the light.

A twelve-step group is a wonderful way to confess in a safe place as well as hold yourself more accountable to directly heal soul shame in your life.

And the best way to disobey shame is to end your food addiction. Food addiction is difficult to accept, I know. We love the idea of moderation but to end the shame-guilt-repent cycle, we need to accept that certain ingredients continue to cause problems for us.

My food addiction was severe. It costs me lots of time and energy. If you're obese, up and down in weight, bulimic, or often go from a slice to the pie within a few days, yours is severe too. When something is severe, we need to sever it.

> **When something is severe, we need to sever it.**

Battle Strategy #3 – Be Your Authentic Self

How much do you feel like you're yourself? How often do you show up as a representative of yourself but not your real self?

Do you act one way at church and another way at work?

Do you feel phony?

You were created to be yourself.

Going forward, be you everywhere you go.

One Whole & Free Health course participant realized that her fake food reflected her fake attitude. She wasn't being herself with people. She would appease them but not really share the truth of her shortcomings, questions about things, or her burdens in life. She felt she needed to hide.

> **Going forward, be you everywhere you go.**

Is this her talking or her shame? You've got it—her shame.

Another believer attended church, but she didn't friend anyone there. She felt judged by the church people and their christianese jargon, so she hung out with worldly people who rejected Jesus but accepted her.

I'm all for a variety of friends with a variety of interests. But the key is to be yourself wherever you go. We need to be real, which includes our love for Jesus and fellowship with other believers to strengthen us.

Your authentic self is the act of being yourself ... the unique, whole, and complete you in all your fullness who you're created to be.

As it's been said, "Be yourself because everyone else is taken." Reduce the divide between how you show up inside of yourself and how you show up to others outside of yourself. When your public and private self are consistent, you've effectively overcome soul shame.

One way we become ourselves is to be honest. Transparency is a blessing. Don't pretend your "blessed and highly favored" when things aren't that great. Don't tell people how to run their lives when you can't manage your own. Be real about things. Be honest with where you're at and your feelings.

> " One way we become ourselves is to be honest. "

Stand in your truth. Instead of hiding what you think or want to do, share it. A friend didn't want to drink anymore but felt pressured by her friends when out to dinner. She decided to stand in her truth and let them know she no longer wanted to drink.

She felt drinking only stirred the alcohol beast, and she wanted to extinguish the beast at the source. Her friends gave her a hard time at first, but as she stood in her truth, protecting her own health, she smiled with victory. As you're okay with your truth, everyone else will be too. What truth do you need to stand in?

I also think it's important to value ourselves. As we value ourselves, we're able to be ourselves without fear of rejection. Value yourself by valuing what you have to offer—your opinions, contributions, and support to relationships.

And finally, to be your authentic self, seek the Father for your identity. Your soul longs for you to know how powerful it is. It's packed with answers. To maximize who you are, you've got to keep learning about who you are. The best way to find out who you are is to pray, *Who am I?*

The labels we've given ourselves—big, fat, obese, struggling, sloppy, or lazy—have accumulated what we know of who we are. Change negative beliefs. The real you isn't these things.

For the next several days, meditate on that question, *Who am I?*

Ask this question to the Creator who made you. You'll get answers. By asking, I was informed in 2007 that I was an author and speaker among many other beautiful things, like healthy,

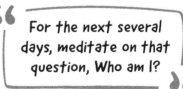

> " For the next several days, meditate on that question, Who am I? "

lovely, smart, good, and whole. I certainly had not published a book yet, but because I heard these words in my spirit, I believed them.

These words transformed me into who I am, my authentic self. Ask, "Who am I?" repeatedly and allow the words to come to your spirit. Keep them close, and they will bear fruit to your soul's authentic expression.

Battle Strategy #4 – Release Judgments

All of the points below create a continuous cycle of shame in our lives because for soul shame to exist we must continue to:

- Feel deeply unworthy
- Do things we judge as wrong (like binge eat)
- Judge ourselves as wrong, defective, or inadequate (beliefs like, I'm broken beyond repair)
- Judge ourselves as powerless, incapable, or undeserving of change
- Judge ourselves as deserving the pain of all of it (I don't deserve freedom)

In *Soul without Shame*, Byron Brown wrote, "Judgment always touches on something we believe is true about us ... and because we believe that there's truth, it can generate self-rejection instead of self-defense."[16] It's okay to release judgments. Simply acknowledge them and let them go.

Even if we believe the judgement is true, it supports your wholeness and freedom to counter it and speak to it as the beast who wants to block and prevent success in your life.

So instead of, "I'll never be able to make changes in my health," you say, "Beast you're a liar. I am Whole & Free. I'm already making shifts in my mindset and my choices."

Each judgment brings with it the validation to your emotional power or powerlessness. Validate the power and let the judgments fly away. Pay attention to the judgments you have about yourself. Review how beliefs work in Chapter 17.

To heal from shame, we must:

- Feel worthy and grateful for who we are and willing to receive God's abundance.
- Do things we judge as right as well as grow from the wrong behaviors we judge for improvement and reduction.
- Judge ourselves as right, whole, and enough.
- Believe we're powerful, capable, and deserving of change.
- Believe we're deserving to receive healing, change, and freedom.

We judge ourselves and others in areas we're the most susceptible to shame or pride.

Pay attention to how you judge others for their body, weight, size, or shape. See how you judge what they eat, how much they eat, or their lifestyle choices.

> **We judge ourselves and others in areas we're the most susceptible to shame or pride.**

Anna judged other women who were thinner, believing they starved themselves to be that size. Her belief that thin women starve themselves caused her to over-eat, believing she would never be able to eat less or starve herself.

How are you judging yourself? Are you labeling yourself as unworthy because you're not in the dress or pant size you want to be? Empathy of the soul and self-compassion are soothing antidotes to shame.

Battle Strategy #5 – Build Healthy Relationships

Many of us isolate because we don't have the skills to build and maintain emotionally supportive relationships.

Let's check your skills now. Take the assessment below and see where you are with your ability to have healthy relationships.

RELATIONSHIP SKILLS QUIZ

Rate yourself on how often you resonate with the statement.

1. I can recognize and express my needs.
☐ (5) ALWAYS ☐ (4) OFTEN ☐ (3) SOMETIMES ☐ (2) RARELY ☐ (1) NEVER

2. I can recognize and meet the needs of others.
☐ (5) ALWAYS ☐ (4) OFTEN ☐ (3) SOMETIMES ☐ (2) RARELY ☐ (1) NEVER

3. I reach out to connect when I need to talk or share.
☐ (5) ALWAYS ☐ (4) OFTEN ☐ (3) SOMETIMES ☐ (2) RARELY ☐ (1) NEVER

4. I genuinely care for the other's wellbeing and highest good. I don't always want something.
☐ (5) ALWAYS ☐ (4) OFTEN ☐ (3) SOMETIMES ☐ (2) RARELY ☐ (1) NEVER

5. I take time to listen well to understand and validate what the other person shares.
☐ (5) ALWAYS ☐ (4) OFTEN ☐ (3) SOMETIMES ☐ (2) RARELY ☐ (1) NEVER

6. I am honest about my thoughts, beliefs, and feelings.
☐ (5) ALWAYS ☐ (4) OFTEN ☐ (3) SOMETIMES ☐ (2) RARELY ☐ (1) NEVER

7. When upset, I can express when I'm hurt without attacking or blaming the other person.
☐ (5) ALWAYS ☐ (4) OFTEN ☐ (3) SOMETIMES ☐ (2) RARELY ☐ (1) NEVER

8. When disagreements and other conflicts happen, I don't end the relationship or avoid or ignore the person.
☐ (5) ALWAYS ☐ (4) OFTEN ☐ (3) SOMETIMES ☐ (2) RARELY ☐ (1) NEVER

9. I'm committed to my relationships for life. I won't just leave the relationship without communication.
☐ (5) ALWAYS ☐ (4) OFTEN ☐ (3) SOMETIMES ☐ (2) RARELY ☐ (1) NEVER

10. I make sure my relationships are mutually beneficial.
☐ (5) ALWAYS ☐ (4) OFTEN ☐ (3) SOMETIMES ☐ (2) RARELY ☐ (1) NEVER

11. When offended, I'm willing to admit it, talk through it, and forgive.
☐ (5) ALWAYS ☐ (4) OFTEN ☐ (3) SOMETIMES ☐ (2) RARELY ☐ (1) NEVER

12. I can talk directly to the person around problematic behavior instead of about them.
☐ (5) ALWAYS ☐ (4) OFTEN ☐ (3) SOMETIMES ☐ (2) RARELY ☐ (1) NEVER

13. I have a life outside of each relationship. I don't put anyone on a pedestal or live my life around anyone.
☐ (5) ALWAYS ☐ (4) OFTEN ☐ (3) SOMETIMES ☐ (2) RARELY ☐ (1) NEVER

14. My commitment to the relationship isn't damaging me. I am not being abused.
☐ (5) ALWAYS ☐ (4) OFTEN ☐ (3) SOMETIMES ☐ (2) RARELY ☐ (1) NEVER

15. I'm honest with others. I don't pretend, flatter, lie, or placate. I confront when needed.
☐ (5) ALWAYS ☐ (4) OFTEN ☐ (3) SOMETIMES ☐ (2) RARELY ☐ (1) NEVER

16. I respect the other person's personal boundaries.
☐ (5) ALWAYS ☐ (4) OFTEN ☐ (3) SOMETIMES ☐ (2) RARELY ☐ (1) NEVER

17. I instill healthy boundaries to protect my wellbeing in my relationships.
☐ (5) ALWAYS ☐ (4) OFTEN ☐ (3) SOMETIMES ☐ (2) RARELY ☐ (1) NEVER

18. There is a proper balance of give and take in my relationships. I'm not resentful for over giving.
☐ (5) ALWAYS ☐ (4) OFTEN ☐ (3) SOMETIMES ☐ (2) RARELY ☐ (1) NEVER

19. I let the other person know that they matter to me. I share that I love them and care about them.
☐ (5) ALWAYS ☐ (4) OFTEN ☐ (3) SOMETIMES ☐ (2) RARELY ☐ (1) NEVER

20. I listen to feedback.
☐ (5) ALWAYS ☐ (4) OFTEN ☐ (3) SOMETIMES ☐ (2) RARELY ☐ (1) NEVER

Total Score:

Score Sheet
20–40 | You're in for great improvements.
40–60 | You've getting there, keep going.
60-80 | You've done some work, and it shows.
80-100 | You're probably a relational rock star, teach others!

If your score was low, don't worry because all skills, including relationship skills can be learned. Practice getting better at behaviors you scored low on with the current relationships in your life.

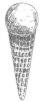

QUIZ

Also, we're going to take inventory of your relationships to improve them, so that we can lean on healthy relationships more than food.

Think about it, how often do you connect and share what's on your heart with others? Do you have people with whom you can be vulnerable and honest without fearing judgment or rejection?

Do you have people who support your best health? What I find is that people pleasers are extra kind and giving. We may be great givers and horrible receivers. We may also be dishonest by being unwilling to express our needs, requests, opinions, and desires.

Instead, we get upset at others and eat over what's eating us. To defeat isolation, we'll have to learn how to connect and balance that connection with the solitude we need.

EXERCISE: RELATIONSHIP INVENTORY

Fill in the chart below or on paper to assess your relationship health. Below list your closest relationships and rate them 1 (hardly ever) - 5 (very much).

Name	Is this relationship supportive and responsive?	Do you feel you can be yourself with this person?	Do you feel safe in this relationship?	Is this person someone whose habits and mindset you feel in alignment with?	Relationship Health Score (Add points) (4) – (20)

EXERCISE

Find Your People

You may need to better build your connections by meeting people whom you can connect with and can mutually build a healthy relationship. Have you tried meeting people based on your values, hobbies, or interests?

Through my passion and calling to write, I've made new friends with Christian and secular writing groups. I also love to hike, so I connect with faith-based hiking groups. To meet people, check out meetup.com, ministry, and church events around your interests.

I encourage us all to have a small group to do life with that meets frequently to defeat isolation and encourage your soul's emergence. Christ called us to fellowship with other believers and to share our issues with one another. See Chapter 19 for more encouragement on how to create a small group.

Reach Out

How did you build your most recent friendships? We build relationships by reaching out and responding back. If you find someone interesting, ask them on a virtual tea date. Explore the relationship to see if values align. A fruitful relationship will reflect Christ.

Friendships need time to build. Make time by following the formula: reach out, respond back, repeat. Your communication and responsiveness are essential to building new relationships.

Connect

Real relationships develop from the art of connection. If you've felt like your relationships are disconnected or not mutually emotionally supportive, increase your connection by active listening and sharing what's on your heart.

Active listening is paying full, focused attention to understand what the person is saying. It's not thinking of what you're going to say next or fumbling around with your phone. Be present. Keep interruptions to a minimum.

Revitalize stale relationships by asking questions and actively listening to the responses.

For relationships to flourish, share what's on your heart, what's happening in your life, what you're excited about, what God is showing you or teaching you at the moment, and what your passions are.

You're worthy of your voice being heard because you are worthy of your needs being met. Say it out loud: "I'm worthy of my voice being heard and my needs being met."

As *Chubby Church* members, we bust out of shame when we allow ourselves to be known and seen.

So have fun. Don't take yourself so seriously.

Lighten up, and your body will follow.

> " Don't take yourself so seriously. Lighten up, and your body will follow. "

Commit

God loves when we show the commitment to others like He does through His covenant relationship with us. In Christ we don't just cut off relationships without communication.

Unlike a contract that cancels when one decides he or she no longer wants the relationship, covenant relationships are committed through the entire lifespan.

God is so faithful (2 Thessalonians 3:3). He commits to us. Who in your circle of friends can you call faithful? How can you show more commitment in your relationships?

Battle Strategy #6 – Develop Relationship Skills

I don't have to tell you that we've missed some valuable life training in two critical skills needed for successful relationships: boundaries and handling conflict.

We tend to eat over what's eating us. An internal conflict, such as not having a boundary, or a conflict can easily move us off track.

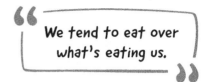

> We tend to eat over what's eating us.

- **Establish Boundaries.** We need personal boundaries. Barbra Russell said in her mighty little book, *Yes! I Said No!* – "People pleasing is not a spiritual gift."[17]

  Books, such as Barbra's for a quick read or *Boundaries* by Drs. Henry Cloud and John Townsend, are sure to help you create better boundaries to strengthen how you want to be in a relationship with yourself and others.

  Cloud and Townsend describe basic boundaries as "anything that helps to differentiate you from someone else or shows where you begin and end."[18]

  Examples include:[19]

  - Our skin
  - Words (i.e., "no")
  - God's truth
  - Geographical (physical) distance
  - Time (time off from people)
  - Emotional distance (when you need to stop sharing with someone unsafe)
  - Other people (not enabling or being around people who are harmful or getting support)
  - Consequences

  They also describe things within your boundaries such as:[20]
  - Your feelings
  - Your attitudes and beliefs
  - Your behaviors (and your presence/where you go)
  - Your choices

- Your values
- Your limits (you set with others, as well as ones set to protect yourself)
- Your resources and gifts
- Your thoughts
- Your desires
- Your love (your heart)

I highly recommend studying their book *Boundaries* if you feel you need more understanding in this space.

A simple way I've set boundaries is a four-step process that I shared in Chapter 16:

Step One: Figure out what you want. "I don't want to feel ignored when I visit."

Step Two: Figure out an appropriate consequence if the person doesn't honor your boundary. "If she ignores me again when I visit, I won't come over for a while."

Step Three: Share your new boundary and its consequence with the person. "I don't want to feel ignored when I visit, so if that happens again, I'll take a long break from visits."

Step Four: Do what you say you're going to do if that happens again.

Boundary creation doesn't have to be hard; it just must be done to manage your own peace well. What boundaries will support you to create healthier relationships?[21]

Get Great at Conflict

If you were to guess, how much conflict would you say you've eaten over? How about isolated over?

All conflict doesn't need to be solved now. However, conflicts that trigger us to overeat and isolate need to be processed.

292

A framework I've created has helped me and clients to deal with relational conflicts at home and at work. Let's face it: to be in any healthy relationship long term, you're going to need get good at handling conflict.

> " Let's face it: to be in any healthy relationship long term, you're going to need get good at handling conflict. "

Step One: Get Your Ego Out of the Way

The ego, as defined by spirituality teacher, Wayne Dyer, is our earth going only self.[22] The ego's job is to self-protect, defend, and preserve all that we think we are.

So, the ego does just that in conflict because conflict is perceived as a threat. A threat may be the loss of relationship, respect, our ideals, or something else. To move the ego out of the way, get to the bottom of how you feel.

An Emotional Fitness Workout™ helps you to figure out what you're upset about so you don't isolate or eat because you're avoiding a tough conversation.

Conflict avoiders act out of their little girl or boy emotional capacity. To mature in love is to put childish things behind us and graduate eating our fears and instead learn to confront them and have the tough conversations.

As adults we need to learn how to confront and deal with things in a way that doesn't bring harm to ourselves or others.

Avoidance is a selfish, childish behavior because it comes from our inner child's fears.

Our families of origin may have swept things under the rug or exploded, but as family in Christ, we opt to learn how to reconcile and communicate. I'm a witness that, not only can you do this, but you can get really good at it.

Step Two: Find the Real Problem

We make many assumptions, so get the facts and figure out about what the actual problem is. Conflicts are best resolved when we can name the real problem clearly.

Toni was angry over a conflict with her spouse about which contractor to use for their kitchen remodel. Toni ate lots of cheesy crackers over this issue. Her ego wanted to eat, sulk, and blame her husband for being a jerk.

Toni's real problem was that she made a verbal commitment to her contractor before she spoke with her husband about it. She felt obligated and was upset that she would have to say no. Her problem wasn't that her husband selected someone else and didn't listen to her. It was that she failed to get her husband's opinion before committing to her contractor about the job.

People pleasing creates conflicts. An Emotional Fitness Workout™ helps you see what your real problem may be so that you can deal with it properly.

To get her angst out, Toni would need to apologize to her contractor for not coming through on her commitment.

Like weight is a symptom and not the problem, so can our conflicts be symptoms of the real problem. Do you have conflicts that may need clarity on what the real problem is?

Step Three: Brainstorm Solutions, Then Solve

We have a funny way of not always seeing the possibilities. Some conflict solutions aren't a win-win. There are other solutions we can uncover simply by brainstorming ideas and checking in with the other party or a mentor on how to handle things.

Perhaps Toni could've spoken with her husband and said, "I'm sorry for being so upset. I told my contractor that I would use him for this job. How do you suggest I handle it? Is there anything else we can do so that I can honor my word?" Or, "Maybe we can use my contractor for the bathroom and yours for the kitchen?"

There may be other ideas that can create more relationship.

Most don't even ask themselves what other possibilities there are, but they just make things this or that. To solve things, we also need to have conversations. I know for me the hardest conversations were the ones that felt vulnerable to my heart, like when I had to admit to feeling jealous, hurt about something, or had to give tough feedback to someone else. I know how intimidating it can feel, but as one who has practiced, I also know that you can get great at speaking your truth in love.

You may need to learn how to have difficult conversations or to learn how to bring up your points. I love the book *Crucial Conversations*. In it the authors strongly suggest that you make sure that the person you're resolving a conflict with knows you care about them, and their goals, first. They suggest establishing what they call "Mutual Purpose" and "Start with Heart."[23]

Be willing to listen and stay in the conversation until a solution that works for all is found. This takes putting the ego outside while you connect from a place of love and desire to keep the relationship intact. Debates happen because we're busy protecting our own desires and motives.

They suggest starting with your relationship's goals being most important. Be quick to apologize if you know you're wrong.

We ought to make things right with our brother as not doing so can cost us eternal life (1 John 3:15). Look out for my future course and book called *Reconciled* for Christ-centered conflict Resolution.

The Shame Healer

The best way to come out of soul shame is to come to Jesus Christ. Fully and completely. Shame is rooted in deep unworthiness.

Christ redeemed our souls because they have value. The value of the priceless, precious blood of our Lord and Savior Jesus Christ.

We love our Lord because He first loved us.

He first saw us as worthy because He made us.

We have purpose and life through Him. On the journey of wholeness and freedom, we grow in our soul's worth.

Asking a question, "What am I worth?" helps us to see that we're worth more than a big mac and fries, life and mood damaging foods, and poor treatment. You are worth so much more than what you've settled for.

Whole & Free journey is more than food. It's your fullness and wellbeing. Your total wellness.

You're a child of the King. You're worth letting the shame-based identity go. You're worth your total Wholeness & Freedom in Christ it's time to go for it.

REFLECT & SHARE

1. How often do you isolate? Describe how isolation shows up for you.
2. How does shame-based behaviors, thoughts, and emotions show up in your life?
3. How has the feeling of fatness affected your decisions?
4. What relationship skills do you need to develop?

PRAYER

Heavenly Father,

I come to you now to give you all my soul shame. I give you my traumas, hardships, and my past. I give you my desire to isolate with my food addictions that cause shame and guilt to perpetuate in my life. Severe these things God. I ask you to deeply purge me from shame-based emotions and I know that I can handle them, I won't be overcome by them.

I trust you that I can fully overcome! I can do all things with Jesus Christ who strengthens me.

Let me overcome so much that I love, value, and appreciate who I've become and every part of the journey of life that got me here.

Stop me from associating myself with the father of lies. Deliver me from all evil.

Remove guilt, regret, fear, and self-doubt far from me. I bind every wicked spirit of rejection from me now. Every demonic presence of emotional burden I command you to get out now!

I choose to accept myself. I choose to walk in the soul worth you've died and rose to give me!

Thank you for choosing me. Thank you for healing my soul deeply and completely! Thank you for giving me courage to deal with conflicts and not eat over them. Give me courage to apply all that I've learned in these books and your Holy Book.

Thank you for new and renewed healthy relationships in my life. Help me to get where you are calling me to go, help me to be a pillar of faith and love in my family. Thank you, Lord, You are good and you are GREAT!

In Jesus mighty name, I pray, amen.

CHAPTER 28

RESIZE FAMILY FAT GENES

Battle #7 – Genetic Predispositions

---

*"But showing love to a thousand generations of those
who love me and keep my commandments"*

−EXODUS 20:6, NIV

Some hand-me-downs, I'd love to return.

Part One: Understanding Genetic Predispositions

After my grandfather's funeral, my family did our usual funeral thing. We got together, ate food, and took photos. I thought one photo was particularly cheery, so I put it on Facebook.

The photo had twelve family members all dressed up in funeral best. It was sure to get likes. And it did. But one Facebook friend (I use the term *friend* loosely) commented, "Wow, this photo has a bunch of people who look like they eat too much."

Oh, yes he did.

Needless to say, he was unfriended.

Some people don't have any tact. But he was right. Just about everyone in the photo was indeed obese.

Genetics play a role in our weight struggles. Thankfully, our DNA doesn't determine our destiny. Our habits do.

299

The giant we're defeating in this last battle is our genetic predispositions.

Is Your Weight & War Generational?

Oftentimes we want to give up at the very end of the Weight & Eating War because we don't think we can defeat our fat genes.

We think, *My mama's fat, my grandmama's fat, my granddaddy's fat, and my aunts are all fat, so I'm destined to be fat too.*

Fiona's family had the fat genes so bad that her mother died early at 500 pounds, and her sister followed at 300 pounds. Fiona was scared to be morbidly obese like her family members and became a fitness instructor to stay slim and trim.

But over time the food addiction as well as her genetic predispositions caught up, and she yielded to the food crazies. To exacerbate her struggle, her conditionally loving and not-so-bright husband left her under the terms, "I don't want no fat wife."

The struggle is real.

Obesity has three classes: class 1 (BMI range 30–34), class 2 (BMI range 35–40), or class 3 (BMI range of 40 plus). Over the past eighteen years, class 1 rose over 12 percent and class 3 severe obesity rose from 4.2 percent to 9.2 percent.[1] See graph.

If parents grow in body mass, children grow too. Fiona's not alone in the more difficult weight and eating struggle; many families succumb to the Standard American Diet lifestyle that negatively impacts genetic factors.

Your Weight & Eating War, like mine, may be generational. Genetics, as indicated by my family photo, may truly be against you like they are against me.

So how is someone like Fiona, me, or you to overcome a fifty-year war of family obesity?

The answer is Jesus Christ, through and through.

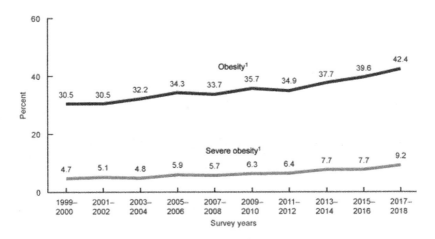

Graph 28.1 Obesity Trends[2]

The last time I checked, God searches for the ones who take what they've been given and make it effective and impactful on the earth. "For the eyes of the Lord run to and fro throughout the whole earth, to show Himself strong on behalf of those whose heart is loyal to Him" (2 Chronicles 16:9a). He searches for the overcomers (Revelation 12:11).

Obesity is a sickness to be overcome. Overweight is pre-obesity. Overweight is the sniffle before the full-fledged flu takes hold. Overweight and obesity genetics can be overcome by your daily habits, faith, and determination to change you and your family's trajectory for the better.

In Part One we'll start with understanding the issues facing families. And in Part Two I'll provide you with strategies to defeat genetic predispositions.

Why Genes Matter

Our family is a set of people who love us no matter what. Even if they're shame-based, critical, or annoying as all get out, they're ours. We belong. I see the family unit as the people chosen for our best spiritual growth in life.

Our health influences the health of the family.

Family health is a big source of worry. We worry about our parents, siblings, children, nieces, nephews, aunts, and uncles. We care because it's encoded in our hearts to care.

It's a blessing when a parent takes care of herself because it's less of a burden on us. And few things are more painful than when a child of any age kills their health with junk food and sweet drinks.

But do genetics or chubby choices matter most? Our DNA? Or the bins of buttery popcorn whenever we watch a family movie? Research repeatedly proves the chubby choices matter more than genetics.[3]

You're not victimized by your genetics. And your DNA is not your destiny.

So, you can return your family fat genes for a right-sized pair with your habits. Yes, you have the control to resize family fat genes into your right-sized jeans.

Bound Parents, Bound Children

Heavy on my heart are the issues that affect children. Parent or not, we influence the next generation. The way we eat and live impacts everyone around us, including our children and their health.

Forty-eight percent of kids with overweight parents become overweight and 80 percent of children from obese parents become obese.[4,5] Whereas only 13 percent kids of normal weight parents become overweight or obese.[6] An obese child has at least a 50 percent likelihood of obesity in adulthood.[7]

The National Center for Biotechnology Information researchers found that 25 to 40 percent of obesity is inherited.[8] And the World Health Organization calls childhood obesity "one of the most serious public health challenges in the twenty-first century."[9]

In 2016, 18.5 percent of children in the United States were obese or 13.7 million kids, and 60 million worldwide were obese.[10] For perspective, in 1980 this rate was 10.4 percent.[11] And it has more than tripled since 1970.[12]

We have our hands full.

Think about the long-term impact of a society that is too big. What would be the impact on our military? Health care system and costs? Self-esteem and wellbeing? Or longevity?

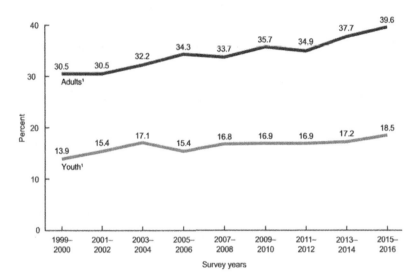

Graph 28.2 Childhood Obesity Trends[13]

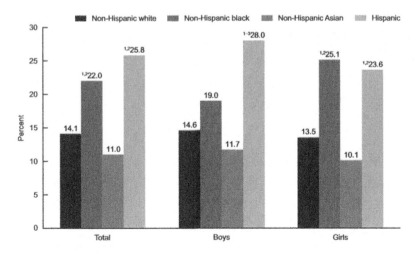

Graph 28.3 2015–2016 Obesity rates in Girls and Boys by Ethnicity[14]

As you can see from the chart, minority families and children have it worse for a variety of reasons. One is that urban areas have what Dr. Joel Furman, author of *Fast-Food Genocide,* calls food deserts. In these areas people eat only 5 percent real foods because they don't have access to them.[15]

Government both subsidizes and incentivizes fast food development over other types of business growth in minority communities.[16] Therefore, there are triple the amount of fast-food venues in minority communities.[17] And fast-food brands seduce families to believe it's more expensive to be healthy. Without access to healthy food or strong nutritional information, what can we expect?

Because of poor diet, African American youth contract adult diabetes, hypertension, and strokes earlier than their counterparts. Hispanic males are far more affected by obesity and diseases than their counterparts.

Is it okay to allow our children to grow obese when we influence the food choices they make?

What if we were held responsible for the poor health of our children? In 2009, Jerri Gray was persecuted for the felony of childhood neglect because she allowed her son to grow to 555 pounds by age fourteen.[18]

Brady Kluge was fifteen years old and 220 pounds when he was featured in *Fed Up*, a documentary highlighting issues affecting the childhood obesity epidemic. He so wisely said, "I've done what my parents done; my parents have done what their parents done, it's passed on from generation. Once you start overeating, it becomes the worst habit and just grows."[19]

It was sad to hear Brady's struggle because not only does obesity set children up for a lifetime of prescriptions and self-esteem struggles, it sets them up for a harsher world of scrutiny and emotional health issues such as depression.[20]

Brady's peer ridicule began when he was eight. Girls in his class wanted to see his fat shake while running, so they insisted he run so that they could laugh.

The Obesity Action Coalition reports 24 percent of boys and 30 percent of girls who are overfat are teased at school.[21] And over 50 percent of overweight kids report peer victimization.[22]

One repeated study showed other children prefer a child in crutches with one leg in a brace, a child in a wheelchair with one hand missing, or a child who has a disfigured face to a child that's obese.[23]

Studies show educators, medical professionals, and employers are all biased toward an overweight or obese child compared to a normal weight one.[24] Parents are also negatively biased unfavorably toward their own larger child than the normal weight one.[25]

Concerns and Causes for Childhood Obesity

A major reason for childhood and adult obesity is that many believe the lies we've been told about how it's our fault that we're fat. As I said, it's not your fault.

We're in a fatty food obsessed culture that brainwashes us to think exercise more and eating less makes us lose weight. As a society, we've promoted exercise but missed the memo to not eat food porn, so we've all gained weight.

If exercise worked, we wouldn't have as much of a problem. But exercise maintains weight. What, when, and how you eat reduces weight.

Exercise only contributes to 5 to 10 percent of weight outcomes. Eating contributes to 90 to 95 percent of all health outcomes, including weight. Exercise promotes more eating and hunger.

Maggie Valentine at twelve years old weighed over 200 pounds yet exercised as much as is suggested to lose weight, but the scale never budged.[26]

Her parents fed her processed foods, focusing on specific ingredients like fat or sugar but missed the insulin-resistance-causing processed foods themselves. Processed foods are refined despite what they advertise. They lack real fiber and nutrients and are the cause of disease.

Makers of processed foods want us to be confused. They highlight ingredients so that we're distracted from the fact that it's not real food, which deceives parents from the food truth of fruits and vegetables.

So, dear young ones like Maggie go through severe emotional pain over efforts to lose weight despite doing everything she's told to do. It's emotional pain that we know all too well.

Because the eat less move more lie is widespread, neither parents nor doctors know how to help children. And children are faced with decisions about gastric bypass surgeries and other dramatic measures to control weight, which we know also have a high failure rate if the soul isn't addressed. Sad.

As discussed, all calories aren't the same. The Lord knows that we don't have time to do the exercise required to burn off the Standard American Diet each day.

The misinformation is killing us.

One major reason for childhood obesity is the Satanic Addictive Deception. Another is its infiltration into school lunch programs.

How difficult it must be for these young ones to go to school where they're bombarded with unhealthy choices.

By 2006, 80 percent of all schools had exclusive contracts with major beverage and fast-food companies.[27] As discussed, we and our children, grandchildren, nieces, and nephews do not need any of their products.

In *Fed Up*, former President Bill Clinton said, "We can cure literally 80 percent of the problem for children in school, if we went back to school cafeterias where they prepare the food in the school."[28]

Childhood obesity is also affected by advertisements to children. Food advertisements condition children as young as babies to see big brands as trusted food experiences, which sets up children for weight and eating bondage for a host of proven psychological reasons.

Namely, children are vulnerable to believe what they see. And foods advertised are chemicalized and loaded in fat, sodium, and sugar, which causes children to learn to listen to food from the brain (food addiction) and not the needs of the body like we talked about in Chapter 26.

And these addictive foods foster food addiction and overeating.

One study showed that kids who watched television with food commercials ate 45 percent more snacks while watching than those who didn't watch commercials.

Marketing to children is another devious act of the Satanic Addictive Deception (S.A.D.) because it seeks to addict children to health demoting foods that sets them up for prescriptions and even early death, yet their big food brands are excited to have lifelong customers.

Another contributor to childhood obesity is food funded research.

Fed Up highlights research deceptions and funding conflicts of interest. To name one of many examples, the American Academy of Family Physicians was funded by Coca-Cola. Their research falsely stated that soft drinks aren't a cause for obesity and don't affect children's health when science indicated it did.[29]

When facts are lies, we've fallen into the quagmire of confusion with no results for our efforts.

The biggest lie from the food industry and reinforced by the medical industry is to eat less and move more.

But the food industry failed to recommend eating less of their foods.

We're to eat little to no refined ingredients—namely sugar, flour, saturated fats (in burgers, cheese, and fries), or processed foods whether we exercise or not to reduce the damaging health effects—whether skinny, chubby, or somewhere in between.

Yes, we're watching the Satanic Addictive Deception distribute research directly opposed to nonbiased research on what we should eat.

One of the effects of this deceptive research is counting tomato paste like you would find in ketchup as a vegetable. This is a sad diversion from food truth. With laws that allow pizza and fries to be vegetables, we can't expect industry or government to care more about our children and future lineage than us.

And it starts with us.

No one shapes a child's health more than the adults around, especially the parent who buys and prepares the food. Women do 93 percent of the grocery shopping and 84 percent of the food preparation in their homes.[30]

But the biggest factor in childhood obesity is a caregiver's willingness to continue their food addiction, which only doubles the pain for the child's food addiction. Daily lifestyle and health matters for children, and it starts in the womb.

Health in the Womb

Genetics kick in before children are born. The Standard American Diet has profound effects on our metabolic health in the womb, and in the future, matter.

Researchers found that "the environment provided by the human mother is more important than her genetic contribution to birth weight."[31]

Metabolic imprinting is the term that describes how the mother of the child's metabolism affects her child's metabolism and obesity chances.

In *The Case Against Sugar*, Gary Taubes reports, "The higher the blood sugar of the mother, the greater the supply of glucose to the fetus. The developing pancreas responds by overproducing insulin-secreting cells."[32]

This makes the baby more likely to grow obese due to the womb environment and a genetic predisposition to glucose (blood sugar) and insulin sensitivity.

The quality of the father's health does also matter too, but the mother's health matters more since she dines with the child in her womb for several months. Research has found that the current state of insulin-resistance in mothers impacts generations to come.[33]

A study found children born of the obese moms had "higher rates of inflammation and three times the risk of severe obesity" in a third of cases.[34]

The same moms who delivered babies after weight loss significantly reduced rates of inflammation and risk of severe obesity down to a tenth of cases.[35]

The mother's nutritional health desperately matters to the long-term health for her child. Not only does sugar or glucose matter, but the larger the amount of meat mom eats during pregnancy increases the overweight probability in her children.[36]

Have you noticed the next generation has an even bigger struggle indicated by a larger size? Gary's research shows that "each successive generation includes more and more children predisposed—preprogrammed, in effect, to become obese and diabetic adults and obese and diabetic mothers."[37]

Weight status of the mother can stretch as far as her grandchildren. Michael Gerber puts it this way, "Obesity begets obesity."[38]

If not corrected, our insulin resistance created by the Standard American Diet begets insulin resistance in our children as well as bigger and less healthy children, and it makes obesity a predetermination in the epidemic we're experiencing.

For this reason, children born into processed food-oriented homes have a greater chance of dying before their parents. Processed foods are also causing parents to die before they see their children's life milestones.

Do you know how your mother ate when pregnant with you? My mom admitted to an enormous amount of pizza when she was pregnant with my younger brother, and he came out a little cute gorilla with loads of hair everywhere and was about ten pounds.

Rise To Resize

Epigenetics is the science of gene alteration. Epigenetics literally means above genetics.

You can rise above your genes.

Those of us who gain weight at the thought of a sugar granule have genetic factors working against us.

Genes work like a dial. You can turn them on, turn them off, speed them up, or slow them down based on your food and lifestyle choices.

I love this because we have the power to generate health.

There are about 175 total possible gene combinations that can lean toward larger body mass.[39] Sixteen specific genotypes can affect our weight and eating.[40] In addition we have genotypes that also affect our vulnerability to addiction itself.

George Mateljan, bestselling author of one of my personal favorites, *The World's Healthiest Foods,* said, "The nutrients in the foods we consume communicate with our genes, delivering information that alters which aspects of our genes—those that promote health or those that engender dysfunction and disease—will be activated."[41]

One diet fad right now is high fat. Only my face puffs up whenever I eat too much fat. For me, during a single day of high fat consumption within normal caloric range, I'll gain two pounds. See, based on genes, a calorie isn't an equal calorie employer for some of us.

Well, it turns out I have a variant in the FADS1 gene that affects fat metabolism. My ideal way of eating is lower fat intake. I discovered this through learning my body, but the test confirmed it. I also reluctantly canceled my membership to the International Butter Club.

Donna struggled with her weight for thirty years. It was a revelation to her when she discovered she had MCR4, the gene that causes some not to have a strong sense of fullness, also called the appetite gene.[42] I have this one too.

Trish gained insight about several genes working against her weight efforts, including one that helped her to see that the long days in the gym weren't going to work for her. She changed her diet to lower fat intake and changed her workout routine from long cardio workouts to short high intensity interval training and weight workouts. She knew she would have to put in more effort to see results. She did. And she reaped the benefits.[43]

Genes indicate why we don't tune into hunger easily, why we can't stop craving sweets, and why we're sensitive to addictive eating.

In the chart, look at sixteen genotypes that can affect weight and eating struggles.

Genotypes that affect Weight & Eating

1	FABP2	Fat Absorption	Affects how well we process fat intake.
2	ADIPOQ	Weight Regain	Adiponectin promotes energy expenditure (caloric usage or caloric hang outs). Predicts susceptibility to weight regain.
3	APOE	Age-Related Metabolism Fatty Acid Sensitivity	Promotes normal or abnormal fat and cholesterol metabolism. If this shows up, then more interval workouts could help.
4	APOa2	Fat Metabolism	Another variant of the above.
5	DRD2	Food Reward	May cause us not to stop binging mistakes because this gene makes the reward of the binge greater than the pain of the binge.[44]
6	INSIG2	Insulin/ Cholesterol	Supports lipid/cholesterol regulation and synthesis of fatty acids.
7	KCTD10	Cholesterol and Lipids	Can promote higher or lower levels of HDL cholesterol.[45]
8	LEPR/LEP	Appetite	Supports normal appetite function, feeling full.
9	MC4R	Obesity	Causes more appetite stimulation.
10	PPARG	Monounsaturated Fat	Found in 87 percent of the population and controls the storage of fat.[46]
11	TCF7L2	Sugar Sensitivity	About 61 percent have no major sensitivity to sugar metabolism. Those with this gene do have a predisposition to sugar's negative effects.[47]
12	PCKS1	Insulin Resistance	Insulin utilization.
13	FADS1	Fatty Acid Response	May cause higher cholesterol and trouble with fat digestion/consumption due to metabolism.
14	FTO	Feeling Full	Higher chance of being overweight because one may not feel full after a meal affects 40 percent of population.[48]
15	NMB	Hunger	Three percent of population have a higher chance of being overweight, higher body mass index, increased food desire, and increase in less discretion around food.[49]
16	SLC2A2	Sweet Tooth	High cravings for sugar, lower carbohydrates, and reduced simple sugars. Affects 8 percent of the population.[50]

Chart 28.4   Genes Affecting Weight and Eating Bondage[51]

Interesting, huh?

Proper genetic testing does wonders for aha moments. Before factory farming, food additives, genetically modified organisms, fast-food abundance, and processed food, we didn't have manifestations of our fat genes so abundantly. People ate real food that was clean and didn't struggle with chronic health the way we do today.

We can flip the switch from a Standard American Diet over to the Life Abundantly Standard for new results.

What would it look like to bring honor to God in your health, diet, and family?

Furthermore, some families have it extra tough. Hispanic, Native American, and African American families are subject to more health concerns.

African Americans are twice as likely to die from heart disease, strokes, and cancer than Caucasian Americans and 50 percent more likely to have hypertension.[52]

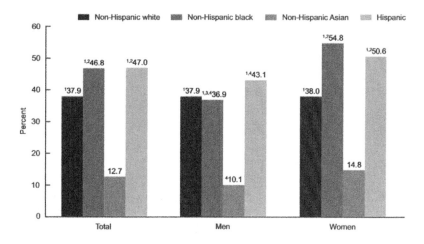

Chart 28.5 Obesity by Ethnicity[53]

There are other alarming stats, but I'll spare you.

We're dealing with significant barriers to health education, access, and resources. In addition, we're also less open to change.

And we can be the family wellness advocate.

I mentioned Chef AJ in earlier chapters.

As the author of *The Secrets to Ultimate Weight Loss,* Chef AJ personally knows the effects of food addiction that runs in families. Her Jewish family had an edge up in eating clean from a biblical perspective but partook in the Standard American Diet's processed and addictive ingredients.

She is passionate about food addiction because she's seen the havoc it can do in families and has lost several family members from it. Check out her books, recipes, and programs at *www.chefaj.com.* Like Chef AJ, you too can overcome. Let's talk about how.

Part Two: Win the Genetic Predispositions Battle

How To Resize Family Fat Genes for Good!

Great news! You've got all you need to Resize Family Fat Genes. We've covered much ground throughout both books. You've already learned how to defeat the biggest giants that make gene expression unfavorable. Here are a few suggestions to further support winning genetic predispositions.

Battle Strategy # 1 – Get Tested

We don't need to look far to know we have a genetic predisposition. But knowledge is power. It's good to know what specific genotypes are affecting you. Several companies such as Orig3n Noom DNA, Metabolic, or Hunger DNA tests or GenoPalate as well as many others allow you to check your genes with mailing a saliva test.

You send it back, download an app, and a few weeks later your results will be posted on the app in a full report with nutritional recommendations based on your genes.

You can also find tests that look for addictive genotypes. Alcoholic families, obese families, and dieting families are clear evidence of addicted brain tendencies that make eliminating problem foods more difficult.

If you don't want to spend the money, you really don't need to. Look around at the next family gathering and you already know that you'll need to put in the work of learning how to eat to defeat genetics.

Battle Strategy # 2 – Come to Acceptance

The hardest thing to accept is that we're not normal eaters. We can't do what it seems like everyone else can when it comes to food. Our families may have addicted brains, or at least we inherited one.

As I've said before, the best way to become a normal eater is to fully accept that you are not a normal eater.

We need to understand that we can't eat like everyone else if we want to be our best for the Lord. We can't just shove any ol' chemicals and fattening ingredients into our mouths and think it's okay.

It's not. And He certainly wants better for us.

But we've got to come to acceptance of the fact that our brains and genotypes are vulnerable to the Standard American Diet fare more than our neighbors.

Will you come to acceptance?

Will you accept that, as disappointing as it may be, we can't continue to eat the way we want to eat without taking our brains into account?

Will you accept that you may need to put in additional effort to learn and manifest results?

We need to make different choices because, friend, it only gets worse if we don't.

And much worse.

Imagine your life outcomes if you don't make changes. Decide today to accept that you'll need to do things differently in our Satanic Addictive Deceptive culture to escape Satan's Agenda of (early) Death due to the Standard American Diet.

Then, get in community with others who are ending this Weight &

> Decide today to accept that you'll need to do things differently in our Satanic Addictive Deceptive culture to escape Satan's Agenda of (early) Death due to the Standard American Diet.

Eating War. And come to Jesus with the grief of not being like everyone else. I understand, but you still win!

Battle Strategy # 3 – Be Healthy

Keep things about health, not weight. As we've learned, focusing on weight only brings about more weight problems. A health focus is more fruitful for making change.

You're an example of health for your family because you've taken ownership of your health. Your willingness to win the Weight & Eating War is remarkable. It shows that you're focused on being healthy for life.

Your soul wants to prosper in health. "Beloved, I pray that you may prosper and be in health, just as your soul prospers" (3 John 1:2).

While it's easy to be battered and bamboozled by shame-based families who don't want you to change, we know from the last chapter that we can stand in our truth to overcome the soul shamers we face.

All that's required is that you believe well. Believe for the best health outcomes for yourself and family members. Believe that your actions matter no matter how small the healthy choice is.

Your efforts count. Faith without works is dead (James 2:26). And it's the faith of a mustard seed that moves the weight and eating mountain (Matthew 17:20).

Focus on your own health even if others around you refuse to make change. I know from personal experience that living with a food addict is challenging. Whether it's a parent or spouse, you cannot change or control them.

But you can inspire them. Like Josh Lajaunie who grew to 400 pounds as he indulged in the supremely palatable real food of his home state of Louisiana.

In early 2011, he decided to divorce the Standard American Diet and adopt the Life Abundantly Standard. He also became a long-distance runner and left his 200-pound chubby suit in the dust.[54]

Since then, he's inspired his own family (and many others) to stop food addiction by transforming to plant-based eating. Read his inspiring book *Sick to Fit* and check him out on social media.

You are an inspiration to others. As much as it burdens us to see others struggle when we have answers, focus on being an example every day. Like Abraham in the Scriptures, it only takes one to make effective change for many.

Battle Strategy # 4 – Be the Wellness Advocate

Every family needs a wellness advocate. The God-appointed wellness advocate is the one reading this chapter. You! Congratulations!

A wellness advocate is the person who coordinates wellness activities like healthy family get togethers or nutritional education movie nights where you enjoy healthy treats while watching movies like *Fed Up, That Sugar Film,* or *Forks over Knives.*

You can email them the wellness tips you find, online events, or healthy and easy meal recipes to try. Or simply bring a delightful health promoting dish to your family gatherings. You can be the one to encourage them in health, and as the Scriptures say, those who are generous will themselves be watered (Proverbs 11:25).

If you feel another family member is more suitable to be the wellness advocate, then support them to do so, and ask them to take an active role in your pursuit of greater health.

I find that as I give to others, I've stayed motivated in my own health.

You'll find the same.

Your family needs someone who stands for 1 Thessalonians 5:23, that He will sanctify us wholly in body, soul, and spirit. Let it be you!

Encourage your family by speaking life in areas of health and body image. A body positive environment can be cultivated by making sure others, especially children, know that they are beautiful.

You can speak life into the younger generation and even the ornery old folks. Do your best to leave a seed of encouragement and positivity with everyone you encounter. In our families this area of health needs much encouragement.

Always invite green vegetables to your table, which helps others to know that healthy, God-grown foods are welcome.

Either way, be mindful not to project your own issues with food or body image onto others. As the wellness advocate, you certainly don't need to be the food police. Let them do what they do as you do what you do.

Battle Strategy # 5 – Support Children

I know it seems like we love our kids when we give them cakes and candies, but these tasty takers will set them up for food addiction, overeating, and body image problems.

Tasty takers only promote our ever-growing rates of chronic diseases, which are happening younger and younger because of these foods. You've read the stats, so support the children close to you by loving them with loving food. Loving food is food that gives back. Foods like fruits and vegetables.

My nephew loves when I make him green smoothies. A child that seems extra hungry is more than likely dealing with malnourishment already and food addiction. Recall that the thylakoids in greens as well as the fiber in plant-based foods and fruits will support nourishment and reduce cravings for adults and kids alike.

Obesity is a disease of malnourishment.

Make the time you enjoy with children count. Play sports and games or take walks, which makes things less about junk foods.

Studies show that when children are taught nutrition, they choose better. When they are shown how to make healthy food, they'll have fun and eat well.

Also, healthy lunch program advocates found that when healthier options are in front of children before the junk options, they'll choose the healthier options. Keep a fruit bowl in sight if you have kids at home. You can write your state officials to advocate for children's health programs in your area.

Most of all share your love for God with the children in your life (Matthew 19:14). Michelle Adams, author of a sure family uplifter called *Family Strong:7 Gifts of a Lasting Legacy,* advocates family wellness on multiple levels. She said, "It's important that our children believe in a Power that is greater than themselves—a Source they can turn to for comfort and strength provides stability in a world that can often seem chaotic."[55]

Make it your business to support children in all forms of health— especially spiritual.

Battle Strategy # 6 – Develop More Health-Conscious Friendships

Harvard medical researchers analyzed the Framingham Heart Study for social aspects of obesity or "obesity contagion."

With over 12,000 participants, researchers found our chance for obesity increases by 57 percent when we socialize with a friend who is obese and 71 percent if it's the same gender friend.[56] It's about a 40 percent increased chance of obesity for us if our siblings gain weight.[57]

If a spouse gains, we increase our chance of gain by 37 percent.[58]

Other studies show that weight gain will affect us the closer we are to the one who has gained weight. So, there is a proven social affect for a variety reasons of becoming like whom we hang out with.

Healthier friends have a dramatic reverse affect. Studies show that our health outcomes can improve depending on the healthfulness of our social circle.

We need and love our family and friends no matter their size.

However, for health transformation we'll need to get out of our comfort zones to connect with healthier circles to support a transition into a healthier life.

A faith-based fitness community can do wonders, and as the wellness advocate, you can center social interactions around healthier food and activities. Find or build health-conscious friendships who support your transformation.

With God All Things Are Possible

We're to overcome natural and spiritual strongholds by the blood and testimony of Jesus Christ. You've gone to the doctor's office. Don't they ask every time, "Does anyone in your family have heart disease? Diabetes? Cancer?"

Just like we have medical issues, families have spiritual issues to check for too.

We need to check for spiritual strongholds as well because we transfer genetic dispositions from a natural and a spiritual place to the next generation.

What we don't overcome, our children will struggle with all the more.

Is God's promise of long life through family honor or more specifically honoring our mother and father? To honor is to place value and hold in high regard. "Honor your father and mother, which is the first commandment with promise: that it may be well with you and you may live long on the earth" (Ephesians 6:2–3).

But right after this promise we're informed of spiritual battles with unseen things, also known as spirits. "For we do not wrestle against flesh and blood, but against principalities, against powers, against the rulers of the darkness of this age, against spiritual hosts of wickedness in the heavenly places" (Ephesians 6:12).

Spirits of fear, hatred, rejection, rebellion, iniquity, sexual immorality, the little girl or boy (wicked immaturity/tantrums), witchcraft (control), and the occult amongst others discussed, like gluttony, taunt families.

Take a moment to review the demonic interference discussion in Chapter 19.

But like Abraham all God needs is you. When God/Yahweh called Abraham out of his father's house, Abraham didn't know what to expect. All he had was an instruction and a hope. And he put one foot in front of the other and walked to his personal promised land in the Lord.

I say to you, trust that you're reading all these words for a reason.

You are transforming. Continue to surrender all things, including genetic predispositions and unbelief to the Lord.

We may need to do more work than others who don't have genetic predispositions, but we can trust that we can do all things through Him who strengthens us (Philippians 4:13).

We may have to come up with alternatives to problem foods or be more rigid with our personal food plan, but we're worth the abundant life, even if it takes more effort in the short term to transition from the not so abundant one.

If we look to another or ourselves to win the Weight & Eating War, we'll continue to struggle. Partner with the Creator of the universe. The God who took Abraham and transformed a nation. The Father who took the Son and redeemed us all.

We've defeated many giants in the past seven battles.

We're moving onto our personal promised land.

There is rarely a day that won't require our commitment to our best life.

Don't give up.

"With God all things are possible" (Matthew 19:26).

REFLECT & SHARE

1. How has my family influenced my chubby choices?
2. How can I lead by example in health in my family?
3. What can I do to be a wellness advocate?

PRAYER

Heavenly Father,

Thank you for revelation and wisdom about my genes. I know you are stronger than my genes. I know now that my choices are the biggest predictor of my health outcomes. Help me to choose wisely.

I am an overcomer by the blood of the Lamb and the testimony of Christ Jesus. Have mercy on me and my family to change our health for the better. Please give me the courage to apply the strategies outlined in The Chubby Church books for my victory.

Open my family's hearts and ears to listen to me about health and wellness. Provide a way for me to show them your transformative power by my own spiritual, physical, emotional, and mental health transformation.

In Jesus's name, amen.

CHAPTER 29

KEYS TO WHOLE & FREE HEALTH

"It will come to pass when you come to the land which the Lord will give you, just as He promised, that you shall keep this service"

−EXODUS 12:25

Some foods we run from like we just saw an ex from high school.

W e've taken every giant down. You've made it; enter your promised land! Remember that God uses weight and eating bondage to mold and shape you into whom He's called you to be—Whole & Free in Him. He knows you can win all seven battles because He already won them. You just need to walk out your salvation, your healing, and your deliverance. And you can do that, too, because His Spirit is with you.

Our job is to believe well and put action behind the Whole & Free us instead of the broken and bound version.

In this Chapter, I wanted to give you a few ways to make the transition a bit smoother from the old to the new for weight and

> " Our job is to believe well and put action behind the Whole & Free us instead of the broken and bound version. "

eating freedom for life. Some points are reemphasized because they're important.

All in all, you have two books full of keys to clarify the meaning of Whole & Free Health. Each chapter seeks to elevate you mentally, spiritually, physically, and emotionally for the upward call of Christ Jesus.

Jesus Christ is the Key to Whole & Free Health. Honor Him as Lord to defeat your giants and win the Weight & Eating War. Persist until you win—until you are in the personal promised land you know is yours.

Your personal promised land is the biggest miracle of health transformation that you can see for yourself. It helps to keep your personal promised land vision from Chapter 5 in front of you.

Did you do that yet?

If not, go to *www.TheChubbyChurch.com* and download your Call to Weight & Eating Freedom Action Plan to get clear on your vision. Trust God and work the Battle Strategies for your victory.

Keys to Whole & Free Health

The following guidelines are a mix of insights to embrace our wholeness and freedom. You no longer have to believe the lies about your body, yourself, or your food issues. Take heed to the keys as they will guide you to the full manifestation of the health that you're believing God for.

Transition to the Life Abundant Standard

God created food for us to enjoy. Big Food created food for us to be enslaved. God created food for us to eat in abundance. Big Food created food for us to pay them an abundance in money. Think about it: to be enslaved to sugary soda or a crunchy chicken sandwich is all the evidence we need to know that we've been exploited.

> **We cannot truly enjoy food that has enslaved us.**

We cannot truly enjoy food that has enslaved us.

Foods that make us sick and tired have devastating consequences. They make us feel hopeless and powerless to change. In no way can these foods be claimed as God's best. It's the Satanic Agenda of Death.

We have a very real enemy who wants you to worship him (Satan) through your stomach.

> **We have a very real enemy who wants you to worship him (Satan) through your stomach.**

Paul was clear when he said, "For many walk, of whom I have told you often, and now tell you even weeping, *that they are* the enemies of the cross of Christ: whose end *is* destruction, whose god *is their* belly, and *whose* glory *is* in their shame—who set their mind on earthly things. For our citizenship is in heaven, from which we also eagerly wait for the Savior, the Lord Jesus Christ, who will transform our lowly body that it may be conformed to His glorious body, according to the working by which He is able even to subdue all things to Himself." (Philippians 3:18–21).

God wants this area transformed. This book is an order to win, not to dilly dally along. We're to come out of the Standard American Dietary ways that are killing us.

We cannot persist to obey our cravings for food that steal, kill, and destroy the body, mind, and spirit. The Standard American Diet is 84 percent processed, highly processed, and unclean foods based on both biblical and health principles, with only 16 percent fruits and vegetables. We're to increase our intake of real foods according to Genesis 1:29–30.

To transition out of this way of eating, we let go of false and fake foods and eat real and honest ones. S.A.D foods cause and create weight and eating bondage just as much as toxic shame does. It's important to reduce processed and fast food in our lives no matter our size or goals for the sole purpose of obedience and alignment with God's advice.

We enjoy more of the abundant life when we align with God's abundant food. We're to be a strong, healthy army for the Lord, sanctified wholly in spirit, soul, and body (1 Thessalonians 5:23).

> " It's important to reduce processed and fast food in our lives no matter our size or goals for the sole purpose of obedience and alignment with God's advice. "

Here are some reiterated ideas on how to transition from the S.A.D to the L.A.S.:

- Start right away or set a date to transition off a problem food or ingredient.
- Focus on what to eat, instead of what not to eat.
- Grow your amount of life abundant food intake over time.
- Find a new, non-media hobby to avoid food commercials and attacks on your body image that make us eat more.
- Replace problem foods with alternative versions.
- Increase the quality of your foods, especially your meats.
- Eat whole instead of refined grains.
- Focus on real foods.
- Prepare and eat more at home.
- Eliminate fast and processed foods.
- Never beat yourself up or condemn yourself for slip ups; they're to be expected.
- Keep learning.
- Don't expect to never overeat; stay away from extreme expectations with yourself.
- Take things one meal at a time.
- Set your intention by planning what to eat each day.
- Know that sometimes your inner glutton or beast wins; keep going.
- Enjoy nurturing your body, soul, and spirit by applying Books 1 & 2.

Watch for All or Nothing Dieting Mindsets

A lifestyle change means daily efforts for the long haul. Diets are all or nothing—either on or off. All or nothing mindsets stem from unhealed trauma and a need to control. In Cognitive Behavioral Therapy (CBT) the all-or-nothing mindset is called a thinking distortion.

Do we need another diet? No.

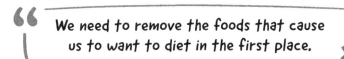

We need to remove the foods that cause us to want to diet in the first place.

We need to remove the foods that cause us to want to diet in the first place.

Earlier I said that the Standard American Diet is an eating disorder in itself. It's our addiction to this way of eating that causes us to want to diet (stop) eating it, but then we go back to it because it's addictive!

Therefore, our overarching goal to reduce and remove the foods is a lifestyle change that happens right now or over time if you need it to.

For freedom you'll need a defined food plan to be successful.

Explore food plans from Bright Line Eating, Food Addicts Anonymous, Chef AJ, Never Binge Again, or Mastering Diabetes to enhance your bio-individual food plan to have clear guidelines for what healthy eating looks like for you.

Pay attention to how you interact with problem foods. For example, if bread makes you revert to a full-fledged processed food lifestyle or you've had an on again off again relationship with it, try the whole grain option instead of the white refined option. Or eat two slices instead of the loaf. Or have bread once a week instead of daily.

If you find it to be nearly impossible to eat a portion once a week, then you know it's got to go. You'll be more successful in a healthy lifestyle if the ingredients of the bread are totally out of your system than you will doing an on again off again diet thing.

Diets are a distraction from true health transformation.

Most people swing from diet to diet or this tidbit of nutritional information to that tidbit only to get themselves all confused. Then they circle the mountain instead of casting it into the sea.

Watch out for the temptation to start new diets or fall into traps of this or that nutritional information like eat plums don't eat plums type of propaganda. Adhere to tried and true food truth to deter confusion and delay. Choose to adopt God's food truth in the Life Abundantly Standard for life.

Dieting behaviors are a sign of mental health problems as is untreated food addiction. Focus on daily health one meal at a time. Revisit Chapter 17 to Adopt the Freedom Mindset.

Heal Food Fear

When we're scared with anxieties around food, we have food fear. Some foods we run from like we just saw an ex from high school. If you feel like you can't trust yourself alone with a bag of cookies for example, you have food fear. In no way should any food make you feel afraid: "For God has not given us a spirit of fear, but of power and of love and of a sound mind" (2 Timothy 1:7).

Food fear shows up as:

- Fear of going out to eat
- Fear of being overwhelmed by your temptation to eat, overeat, or binge
- Fear of processed foods
- Fear of unhealthy foods
- Fear food groups (like carbs)

Take a moment to list out the foods that intimidate you—the ones that sit on the table and whisper your name in a creepy way. It's creepy because we know that cookies don't talk, so that voice comes from within.

Our fear of food is a sign of food addiction.

Food fear can be overcome through healing your inner glutton's needs (see Chapter 14), identifying the erroneous belief (see Chapter 17), or disobeying your beast (see Chapters 22–23).

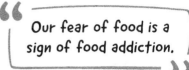

> **Our fear of food is a sign of food addiction.**

See, your inner glutton is really your inner child who doesn't believe she can hold up when faced with temptation, yet. She needs more healing to strengthen her resolve in who she is. Your healing words encourage her to know she doesn't have to go crazy and eat everything for fear that she won't be able to say no or stop. An Emotional Fitness Workout™ helps at the onset of food fear feelings.

Fear has an irrational belief under it too. An acronym is False Evidence Appearing Real (F.E.AR). Another one is Face Everything and Rise (F.E.A.R.). When you feel food fear, ask yourself, "What am I believing?" Then replace it with an affirmation that brings peace and causes you to raise your game.

Food addiction has a funny way of making us feel fearful of food or fearful of becoming out of control with it, especially during holidays and vacations. That's because we know it's our Pig. As Dr. Glenn Livingston would say, "We can cage the Pig!"

You have tools now. You don't have to be in fear about any food, nor do you need to harbor anger at the Standard American Diet.

Food fear can turn into another mental issue when we experience anxiety around foods. If you suspect you're overly health conscious, orthorexia nervosa is when health becomes rigid in your life.[1]

Orthorexia nervosa symptoms include:[2]

- Perfectionist, extremely rigid food control
- Inability to handle tricky food situations
- Undereating or restrictive eating
- Anxiety when faced with foods not considered healthy
- Self-imposed anxiety based on what they feel they can or can't eat

We want to get the problem foods out but not be overly rigid or filled with food fear.

For example, it's not never, ever eating a brownie again. It's not ever eating a brownie that's made from wheat and refined sugar because your addicted brain makes you eat more and more wheat and sugar.

It's also not being afraid of eating the brownie but choosing not to eat it due to your experience and history of eating brownies and their effects. Or you can decide to eat the brownie, enjoy it, and move on or to have less of it.

To get the S.A.D. out is good. Notice whether life revolves around being alone with our healthy foods, just as it can revolve around being alone with our unhealthy ones. We don't want to live for anything but the Lord.

Trust that you can make great food decisions even amid poor options.

Protect Your Environment

Food fear is one thing, but to protect your environment from temptation is wise. As Chef AJ says, "If it's in your house, it's in your mouth!"[3]

We do need to be mindful of tempting foods in our environment. We underestimate how protective it is to keep the binge foods and ingredients out of our homes.

> We underestimate how protective it is to keep the binge foods and ingredients out of our homes.

If a food is tempting, get it out. Make it super inconvenient to attain it.

Your environment is powerful. See, when we're vulnerable from a long and tiresome workday, it's easy to ravish all the highly palatable food that's there.

Humans can't help but choose the most densely energetic food in the environment.[4] We're wired to find the highest caloric food in the least amount of effort in the least amount of time.[5] Research proves that if given the option between a carrot and piece of celery, we'll choose the carrot. If given the option of a carrot or a piece of cake, we'll choose the cake.

I don't know a clearer explanation for wasted produce.

Keep the junk out so that you choose optimally. For more insights on living with a food addict, check out my blog on *www.thechubby-church.com*.

How can you better protect your environment from foods that don't support your wellbeing?

Be Patient

Many desire to be healed and whole this instant. They do one or two therapy sessions and kick themselves for not being how they think they should be. I've seen dozens of people get frustrated with themselves and God because they're not healed yet.

God is perfecting us and will finish the work in us until He comes (Philippians 1:6).

There is no end date on healing. It's a lifelong process with God.

There are only levels or phases of healing. And to be frustrated because you need more healing in an area you thought you solved is soul shame. Soul shame always lets us know we're not good enough—that we should be done with the granola bar binges already.

If you've been in weight and eating bondage for years, give healing some time. It takes time because to come out of weight and eating bondage is also to come out of bondage—period.

Be patient with yourself as you learn your needs. As the soul heals,

> **To come out of weight and eating bondage is also to come out of bondage—period.**

our eating habits adjust and weight stabilizes. You love your body and soul right out of shame.

If you feel the need to rush to lose weight, you've fallen into a dieter's mindset. So, don't make attempts to drop ten pounds in a week. Instead put in place actions that support change. There is no end date on healthy living. As you make healthful daily choices, you'll manifest your healthiest body, soul, and spirit.

Celebrate All Along the Way

Celebrate the progress you're making and have made all along the way. When soul shame tempts you to beat yourself up over the mistake you made, your Whole & Free you is cheering you on for all of your efforts, big and small.

Celebrate:

- Your binges shrunk in calorie load (You've gone from 2,000 calories to 250 calories.)
- You no longer wallow in self-pity or beat yourself up for mistakes.
- If you do wallow in self-pity and beat yourself up, you don't do so as long.
- You don't manifest your inner glutton at the same frequency.
- You no longer diet or get duped by get-skinny-quick ads.
- You're on track more often.
- You no longer use food to cope and don't emotionally eat over things you used to.
- You identify your addictive voice and more times than not you don't listen to it.
- Every time you don't listen to your addicted voice.
- You went from a binge daily to bi-weekly.
- Your sugar demon is quiet.

- You wear clothes that fit.
- You've upgraded your food quality.
- You downsized from the family-sized portion to a personal-sized one.

Bust out your theme song and dance. You're changing! I'd love to hear that you're celebrating all your successes in every area of life. Increase the amount of celebration for your life, and you'll have a life to celebrate!

Focus on Health Not Weight

Keep your focus on health. *Be healthy.* When you believe you're healthy, you do healthy actions and manifest healthy results.

> " Increase the amount of celebration for your life, and you'll have a life to celebrate! "

What we give words to we give life to. We don't want to be controlled by our weight, so we need to reduce its influence in our lives and give it less of our thought life attention as a problem. Think about what you think about. If health, weight, or food takes up most of your thought life, it will pose to be most of our life's problems. As you reduce your thoughts on weight and food and instead do actions to meal plan and take great care of yourself, weight and food will become less of a problem.

What we focus on expands.

You can reduce your focus on weight by not saying things like, "Oh, I'm so fat," or, "I need to lose weight." Talk about all you're doing to live into your identity in health. Keep your healthy actions focused on health, not weight loss efforts.

On the flipside, if weight discussions have been a taboo part of soul shame, be bold and share more about what's really happening for you in your weight.

Weight fluctuates up and down all day long. It's a very complicated metric and can limit us psychologically if we get stuck on it. To measure changes, use measures that make sense, such as body fat, before and after photos each month of progress, waist or hip measurements, or clothing size.

Keep your focus on doing healthy actions, believing that you are a healthy person and being healthy.

Make Time To Sit and Eat

You've been there, driving with your knee, managing to get a bite of that delicious bacon cheeseburger while manually shifting gears with fallen crumbs in the crevasses that even the best car detailers can't seem to get to. Or is that just me?

You know my Burger King story, but McDonalds, Wendy's, and Chick-fil-A have hung out in my car too. The car should be *the car*, not the table, restaurant, or picnic, but for many of us it's our dining space.

The National Highway Traffic Safety Administration reported 80 percent of accidents and 65 percent of near misses are caused by foods, with burgers and coffee being involved most often.[6]

We make time to eat when we eat less in the car, bus, or—if you're really a rebel—the motorcycle. Imagine that.

Certainly store (non-binge inducing) healthy options in the glove compartment so that you don't get over hungry when having a long drive or one of those hectic days. Better on-hand options prevent ravished eating later.

But yes, you can make time to eat mindfully by eating more at home. I realize at home could mean in your bed, on the couch, or in your home office. But do consider eating at the table.

Take a moment to sit down and eat.

When we eat at the table, it's an act of nurturance. When you eat, do it consciously and slowly. Sit your bum in a chair and savor the flavors.

Furthermore, dining with others helps us to be more mindful to sit and eat. It also helps us to focus on connecting with people more than food. Eat a few meals with the family each week or invite friends over to sit at the table and enjoy the fellowship. Also invite the Lord because He likes to dine with us too (Revelation 3:20).

Help Others

When we help others in an area we struggle with, we'll see the struggle end. Helping others who struggle promotes our best health because we feel accountable.

Help by sharing this content with others. Be the wellness advocate in your family. Host a book club to process through the Reflect & Share questions together. Share a Battle Strategy with someone else. Or become a sponsor of a twelve-step recovery group.

We don't start to help after we implement everything. We start to help now so that everything is easier to implement. As we help others, we heal ourselves. So why not start today? How can you help others to get Whole & Free?

> "As we help others, we heal ourselves."

Pride Puffs Up

After fully defeating the seven battles of the Weight & Eating War, you've made it to your promised land! But consider this chapter a warning before you enter that promised land. Just like Joshua gave a stern warning to the children of Israel, I will do the same with you to avoid recapture.

Have you ever said, "I've been good today," in regard to how you've eaten?

The shame and pride in us make us think that we're good or bad depending on how we eat. And you're not good or bad based on how you eat or what you eat.

You're good, period. But we can be arrogant or humble in our pursuits in health.

Either are a sign of being broken and bound, not Whole & Free. God is stabilizing your identity through your health journey. And one of the best pieces of advice I can offer is to watch out for pride that puffs up (1 Corinthians 8:1). In other words, stay humble.

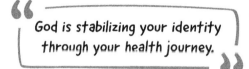

God is stabilizing your identity through your health journey.

Oftentimes we get in our best bodies and act the fool. Have you been there before?

We reveal lots of skin, think we're better than others, or have this *I've arrived* mindset, so we start eating like we used to and come back to the same base of the mountain we were at when we started. God is healing our identity. He wants us to get the arrogance out so that our worth and value isn't based on how we look or what size we wear.

Many wear chubby suits because of the shame of the trauma, along with body and soul shame, but also because of the shamelessness of our eating.

We don't humble our mouths.

Shamelessness is pride and arrogance. Shame and shamelessness (pride) operate together. They both come from a soul of worthlessness,

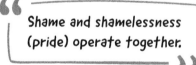

Shame and shamelessness (pride) operate together.

which gathers worth from things outside of Christ. Don't wait to feel worthy or valuable to eat right. Our worth isn't in our size or how we eat; it's found in Christ alone.

Some ways arrogance and pride show up in our weight and eating matters are:

- In denial about the severity of food addiction in our lives
- Continuing to engage in foods you know are an idol
- Too much time in the gym, with mirrors, or social media selfies
- Not satisfied with our bodies how they are
- Obsessed with attaining a smaller and smaller size after achieving healthy weight
- Focus moves from healthy to "skinny" focus
- Over attention to clothing, make up, and looks

- Immodesty, wearing revealing clothing
- Superiority demonstrated by comments or judgments about others viewed as less than
- Judging what others eat
- Conceited comments about looks and body
- Showing off your body
- Not giving any effort because we think we've arrived
- Disobeying what you know God asked you to do regarding food

Any of these items are a manifestation of a soul that needs to heal. When you sense any of them, it's a call to heal. We heal pride by humbling ourselves before God and doing the soul healing work. Get on your knees before God to heal you to avoid weight gain recidivism.

To get comfortable in our right-sized bodies is also to get comfortable in a humble soul. We are tested through our choices as to whether we love the Lord our God with all our heart and soul (Deuteronomy 13:3). Let us make sure that we don't have any food idols or pride there.

Embrace the Whole & Free You

It's a bit weird to go through life without the drama of weight and eating struggles at first. You don't have to get your love and comfort from supremely succulent snacks or rush to the gym to work it off for several hours. It's sweet to just have a drama free, less exciting life in that way.

You get to create your life and its outcomes.

Who are you now that you don't have a weight and eating problem? Who are you now that you can hear your soul speak amongst the beast, the lies, and the emotions?

Who do you want to be?

What do you want to build?

As you move out of the weight and eating struggle, you embrace the Whole & Free you. Review the Battle Strategies and put them in place one at a time until successful.

You've been Whole & Free this whole time. Only the lies—the Father of Lies, to be more accurate, has infiltrated your truth with this smokescreen of a broken and bound identity that you've lived in. You don't have to choose foods that don't serve your highest good. You don't have to eat to fit in at gatherings. You can stand in your truth. You can stand in the truth of what God says about food.

As Dr Seuss said, "Why fit in when you were born to stand out?"[7]

And as Jesus said, "Let your light so shine before men, that they may see your good works and glorify your Father in heaven" (Matthew 5:16).

You're Whole & Free When

- You believe that you're Whole & Free.
- You have nothing to hide, including your soul.
- You have dealt what you need to from the past.
- Your actions, thoughts, and words are aligned and congruent.
- You don't engage with behaviors that bring shame, guilt, and regret.
- You have faith in God and yourself to come through on your word and desires.
- You no longer have an out of control, high control nature, but there's an excellence and rest that you do things out of, not out of a place of striving.
- Your worth is not in how much you weigh, how you look, or any other performance metric but in Christ alone.
- You don't fear man, food, or rejection.
- You can manage your life (financials, household, responsibilities, and possessions).
- You help others to become Whole & Free.

Do the Work

Don't we deserve what we work for? Our truest desires are backed up with actions. And God rewards those actions. People who work toward health will be blessed with better health.

We sow and we reap.

If we sow the wrong way into our bodies, we'll continue to reap depression, emotional instability, body shame, and fatigue. Every time we choose the sweet-deceiving enemy's table instead of God's, we sow the wrong seeds. No matter how much we pray, if we don't change our choices, we'll harvest aches and pains.

> " If we sow the wrong way into our bodies, we'll continue to reap depression, emotional instability, body shame, and fatigue. No matter how much we pray, if we don't change our choices, we'll harvest aches and pains.

We're double minded when we say that we want to be free but treat our body poorly (James 1:8).

When actions align with words, we get results. Faith without works is dead. Faith in health is demonstrated by healthy choices and actions—by sowing well.

Our bodies are the number one thing we sow into. More valuable than money, our bodies are what we steward the most.

Take the parable of the talents: the one rewarded was the one who made the most of the investment given. He took the ten denarii and multiplied it.

He invested. He sowed. He trusted.

All of this is action. "For a dream comes through much activity, and a fool's voice is known by his many words" (Ecclesiastes 5:3).

For the right actions he was rewarded with more.

Action creates outcomes.

We can't play victim and be like the sower who didn't advance the investment. He was kicked out because poor stewardship cannot be rewarded (Matthew 25:14–29).

It would feel like a waste to give the organic dish to the person who doesn't care if they eat organic or not. Why would I waste time and energy giving super thoughtful, health-conscious meals to people who could care less about how they treat their bodies?

> The remedy to end excuses is to choose not to have any excuses.

We give to those who make effort, who sow, and who do what they're supposed to do.

To sow poorly is a disguise for obeying temptation.

Blessed is the man who endures temptation, for when he has been approved, he will receive the crown of life which the Lord has promised to those who love Him. Let no one say when he is tempted, "I am tempted by God"; for God cannot be tempted by evil, nor does He Himself tempt anyone. But each one is tempted when he is dram away by his own desires and enticed. Then when desire has conceived, it gives birth to sin; and sin, when it is full-grown, brings forth death (James 1:12–16).

The remedy to end excuses is to choose not to have any excuses. No more playing victim to temptation. You are victorious. Bless your body. Bless your soul. Bless your spirit.

Hallelujah!

REFLECT & SHARE

1. Which Whole & Free Health keys spoke to you the most?
2. What can you do to protect yourself from eating mishaps?
3. How has arrogance affected you in the past?

PRAYER

Heavenly Father,

You've heard my battle cry! Praise you, Lord, for defeating my giants!

You alone help me to win each battle. Thank you for leading me to my personal promised land.

Please show me a vision for my future so that I may see your purpose and plans for my life. Thank you for helping me to see beyond shame and all of its manifestations in my life. I receive that I am Whole & Free. I am no longer bound by my weight and eating struggles. In you I am free indeed.

You are my joy and my strength. I will walk boldly toward the upward calling of Christ Jesus.

Praise your holy name! And to you I give all the glory!

In Jesus's name, amen.

CHAPTER 30

ENCOURAGEMENT FOR HERE OR TO GO

"For we are His workmanship, created in Christ Jesus for good works, which God prepared beforehand that we should walk in them"

–EPHESIANS 2:10

Where are the harvest workers?
Were they lured away by Papa John's?

I'm so proud of you. Let the finishing of this book be a sign to you that you will overcome weight and eating bondage for good. All of this was so that He may sanctify us wholly in spirit, soul, and body according to 1 Thessalonians 5:23, and I celebrate your commitment to the abundant life in Christ.

However, we must actively work the Battle Strategies.

This book was *An Order To Win the 7 Battles of the Weight & Eating War for Good!*

Let's reflect on the word *good*.

God is good (Matthew 19:17; Psalm 119:68). And what He created in you is good (Genesis 1:31). And you were created for His workmanship for good works (Ephesians 2:10). Throughout the Scriptures we are encouraged to do good works.

See, besides greater obedience to the King, another main point of

343

healing weight and eating bondage was to be of greater service to the King. That service is your heart's truest and highest calling—your good works that you're called to do.

Good works are acts of kindness, mercy, love, teaching, edification, charity, support, and service to others. It's creating that which you are called to create.

Out of who we are, we produce.

We're to be fruitful and multiply (Genesis 1:28). We're to be a tree that yields good fruit (Matthew 7:17–18). This book is about winning the weight and eating battle for good. That good is for God's good purpose as well as good deeds.

The Lord said, "The harvest truly *is* great, but the laborers *are* few; therefore, pray the Lord of the harvest to send out laborers into His harvest" (Luke 10:2).

Let me break Luke 10:2 down for us to understand why it's so important for us to win the Weight & Eating War for good.

The verse is letting us know that many will come into the kingdom and worship the Lord, but they'll be broken and bound. And the Lord needs all of us to be ready to help those who need discipleship, wisdom, understanding, encouragement, and support to transform into who He's made them to be.

The problem is that those who claim Christ are broken and bound themselves. They're stuck in the Satanic Addictive Deception bound by entertainment and food porn, which causes them not to have the energy, discernment, or wherewithal to dig in and help those who are coming in.

The S.A.D. makes them numb, lethargic, and self-focused—a great strategy of the enemy to hinder the workers needed to help fully disciple and grow people of God.

They're watching not working.

His people aren't ready. They've not allowed for sanctification in body, soul, and spirit and, therefore, are not Whole & Free in Him. This can cause much church hurt and damage to one another in the body of Christ. If we're not healed and fully sanctified in our motives, words, and actions, we cause more harm than good.

Many carry shame that weighs them down and makes them think they're not good enough. They haven't healed their daddy absence, mom issues, relationship problems, or personality flaws. Some preach but walk in great hypocrisy.

They've heard what they're to do, but their low self-worth and self-sabotaging bad habits block them from getting it done. Or they don't know what they're supposed to do, so they stay in confusion instead of going before God to figure it out.

Therefore, pray for yourself and your friends diligently to be Whole & Free in Him and get to the front line of their ministries.

The Lord needs us.

He works through people.

He needs us to do what He's called us to do.

I know that too many have a divine assignment and people are perishing because they're too busy playing video games and getting high on junk foods. It isn't right.

And by the grace of God, I pray that won't be you or me in Jesus's name.

I hope you understand that good works don't equate to salvation. Jesus loves you no matter what.

But to be saved and sitting is a kingdom crime.

Our salvation doesn't require us to work. We don't get more saved or more loved by God because of what we do or don't do. He loves you. But out of transformation by His love, we are to be obedient to Him and zealous to do good works. So, when He gives you an assignment, do it.

Good works are the works God has called you to do. They're the works also of applying what you've learned in this book and His book. Jesus modeled an excellent body, soul, and spirit stewardship and served many. We too can take good care of ourselves and do a whole lot of good.

Keep these Scriptures close:

- "Let your light so shine before men, that they may see your good works and glorify your Father in heaven" (Matthew 5:16).
- "For it is God who works in you both to will and to do for *His* good pleasure." (Philippians 2:13).
- "Likewise, the good works *of some* are clearly evident, and those that are otherwise cannot be hidden" (1 Timothy 5:25).
- "Let *them* do good, that they be rich in good works, ready to give, willing to share, storing up for themselves a good foundation for the time to come, that they may lay hold of eternal life" (1 Timothy 6:18–19).
- "Who gave Himself for us, that He might redeem us from every lawless deed and purify for Himself *His* own special people, zealous for good works" (Titus 2:14).
- "This is a faithful saying, and these things I want you to affirm constantly, that those who have believed in God should be careful to maintain good works. These things are good and profitable to men" (Titus 3:8).
- "Beloved, I beg *you* as sojourners and pilgrims, abstain from fleshly lusts which war against the soul, having your conduct honorable among the Gentiles, that when they speak against you as evildoers, they may, by *your* good works which they observe, glorify God in the day of visitation" (1 Peter 2:11–12).

In the beginning, I said that my main mission was to get you spot and wrinkle free because our Bridegroom is coming. It's not about being a size 2. It's about picking up our weight and eating cross, bite by bite, for His highest good in our lives.

Yes, Jesus is coming!

Meditate on Revelation 22.

"And behold, I am coming quickly, and My reward is with Me, to give to every one according to his work. I am the Alpha and the

ENCOURAGEMENT FOR HERE OR TO GO

Omega, the Beginning and the End, the First and the Last." Blessed are those who do His commandments, that they may have the right to the tree of life and may enter through the gates into the city. But outside are dogs and sorcerers and sexually immoral and murderers and idolaters, and whoever loves and practices a lie. "I, Jesus, have sent My angel to testify to you these things in the churches. I am the Root and the Offspring of David, the Bright and Morning Star." And the Spirit and the bride say, "Come!" And let him who hears say, "Come!" And let him who thirsts come. Whoever desires, let him take the water of life freely ... He who testifies to these things says, "Surely I am coming quickly" (Revelation 22:12–17, 20).

Look at the moral decline in our news today. See, all bondage keeps us focused on self when we have greater concerns at hand. There's a country and community that need your helping hands. A kingdom is coming forward but not without great shaking.

You are an end-time soldier for such a time as this.

Let us be a strong army.

Let us be ready for the coming of our Lord.

Let us not become disqualified. We will bring our body, soul, and spirit under the full lordship of our King as Paul said, "I discipline my body and bring *it* into subjection, lest, when I have preached to others, I myself should become disqualified" (1 Corinthians 9:27).

We will not be like those who "profess to know God, but in works they deny *Him,* being abominable, disobedient, and disqualified for every good work" (Titus 1:16).

No, we will be fruitful.

We will multiply His Spirit and truth.

We will hear Him say, "Well *done,* good and faithful servant; you were faithful over a few things, I will make you ruler over many things. Enter into the joy of your lord" (Matthew 25:21).

You are Whole & Free. Walk in it.

REFLECT & SHARE

1. Why did you want to Win the Weight & Eating War for good?

2. How do you feel you've been hindered in sharing good works?

3. How will winning elevate your purpose and calling?

4. How has the Scripture you chose to stand on from Chapter 5 at work in you?

PRAYER

Thank You, Father,

You are a great and mighty King. I bow to you and only you. I surrender my mouth to you, my eating to you, and my being to you. I surrender my past, present, and future. Let my name be written in the Lamb's Book of Life!

Let me see your mighty power break every stronghold of the Satanic Addictive Deception in my life! I will not practice a lie! I will not be put to shame! I will not obey any idols in my life!

Thank you for making me clear with purpose. I will manifest my destiny. I will fulfill my calling.

Thank you for allowing me to be a worker of great works in your kingdom.

I rejoice in you because by your stripes I am healed.

I have won the Weight & Eating War for good. I declare today that it is finished. I receive that I am Whole & Free! All glory to you!

In Jesus's mighty name I pray, amen.

A few actions:

- Please join my mailing list for more insights and goodies at *https:// www.thechubbychurch.com*

- Write a review here: *https://www.amazon.com/review/create-review/ edit?ie=UTF8&channel=glance-detail&asin=0997186704*

- To be notified of more books by Jendayi Harris, follow my Amazon Author page here: *https://www.amazon.com/Jendayi-Harris/e/ B07Q5NMWQM?ref_=dbs_p_pbk_r00_abau_000000*

- And I'd love your prayers. Please pray: Lord, bless Jendayi to write more books quickly and speak powerfully to help the body of Christ usher in your kingdom, protect her and her household, in Jesus mighty matchless name. Amen!

INVITATION TO CHRIST

Oh, taste and see that the Lord is good; Blessed is the man who trusts in Him!

–PSALM 34:8

Jesus is like a football. Hold on to Him through to the end zone of life.

Do you remember a time you tasted a new dish? You may have been skeptical but took a bite anyway. Only when you taste and see what the Lord has to offer, will you see just how delicious life with Him is.

See, in life you'll have troubles. You'll have good times, and you'll have rough times. But the promise in Christ Jesus is eternal life. In Him, we get life with great joy, peace, and hope.

With Christ Jesus we're given a new set of tools to cope. In exchange for our anxiety, we get to talk to our loving creator in prayer. In exchange for our discouragement, we get encouragement. In exchange for confusion, we get the Truth of the His Word in the Bible. In exchange for loneliness, we get communities that come along side us. In exchange for our weakness, we get His Strength.

And the gifts He gives are endless. They give in moments of sadness, celebration, terror, and disappointment.

His tasty spiritual fruit beats the Satanic Addictive Deception.

This is how I liken a holy God—our God, who is love.

Because life is challenging, we need to think of Jesus like a football.

Our goal is to get to the endzone of life, holding on to Him. No matter what the obstacles, fumbles, or offense – we win if we just don't drop the ball.

We get to be adopted to a heavenly, holy Father, through His Son, by the power of the Holy Spirit.

One thing is for sure: "For God so loved the world that He gave His only begotten Son, that whoever believes in Him should not perish but have everlasting life" (John 3:16). God absolutely loves you and is excited about you!

He wants you on His team.

He wants to help you with this thing called life. He wants to teach you how to love, grow, and help yourself, your family, and others.

He gives the free gift of salvation, which is an invitation to His kingdom. He's already Lord, but we just want to acknowledge Him in our lives and come into alignment with the true Lover of our souls.

And because God is so good, all you need to do is bring your words and heart into alignment by confession, then seek out a church to get baptized as soon as possible for the remission of sins in the name of Jesus Christ—who signs the check on our salvation.

Baptism is a sign that you've now entered the kingdom of God and are partnering with the Holy Spirit to bring about your true identity and purpose in the earth.

Will you pray the prayer on the next page to acknowledge the Lord? As Romans 10:8-11 instructs, "If you confess with your mouth the Lord Jesus and believe in your heart that God has raised Him from the dead, you will be saved. For with the heart one believes unto righteousness, and with the mouth confession is made unto salvation. For the Scripture says, 'Whoever believes in Him will not be put to shame'".

DAYSTAR NETWORK'S PRAYER FOR SALVATION[3]

"Dear Lord Jesus,

I know that according to your Word in John 3:3, I must be born again to see the kingdom of God. Father I know I am a sinner. I believe Christ died for me. I believe that you shed your blood, died on the cross for me, and rose again from the dead. I repent and turn from my sins. I need you, Jesus.

I no longer want to be in control of my life. Please come into my heart, forgive me of my sins, and be my personal Lord and Savior from this day forward. Please give me the strength by your precious Holy Spirit to live for you.

Please forgive me of my sins … I want to turn from my sins.

Jesus, thank you for the gift of salvation. I promise to obey you with the help of the Holy Spirit and to follow you all the days of my life. In Jesus's name, amen."

For resources for your confession go to:

https://howtoknowjesus.joycemeyer.org/
http://www.daystar.com/prayer/know-jesus/

Check out various churches in your local area until you find one that feels right for you. Churches are like restaurants: you've got to try them until you find a favorite. Get a good Bible that you can understand and enjoy your new adventure with the Lord!

Congratulations! Your life will never be the same again.

Welcome to the team! If you've prayed this prayer, please email:

info@wholeandfreepress.com.

ACKNOWLEDGEMENTS

I am deeply thankful to the many people that have prayed over this work, contributed to this work, supported me in the work, and who received the work. I could not have done this without your prayers, love, encouragement, kindness, beta reading, proof-reading, editing, teaching, training, patience, coaching, and generosity that saw me through. I'll trust you know who you are. Few days go by that I don't thank God for laying me on your heart for prayer or support to see His plan through.

I love you.

Thank you! Thank you! Thank you!

VICTORY MORSELS

How the Standard American Diet is part of the Satanic Addictive Deception of Satan's Agenda of Death

S.A.D.
[fast/convenient packaged/refined foods, horrifically treated animals (foods)- without life (earth made nutrient density) and rushed lifestyle]

More Slow Kill of: Organs, Hope, Joy, Light, Energy -> Hospital Bound
Ultimately Early Death/Unfulfilled Usefulness for Kingdom
[Cause cravings/prompting more perscriptions & S.A.D. food]

Reduced Energy
[Gives more life (time) to entertainment, craves more "energy dense" SAD food]

The cycle of going to highly palatable foods, produces a lack of desire and taste for natural, whole, healthy, nutritionally dense, healing, life giving foods.

Food doesn't just feed the body, it feeds the mind, brain, heart, and spirit.

The S.A.D. is how the Beast will connect with your Beast (carnal nature) – the lower intention to ultimately cut short God's best destiny for our lives.

Perscriptions
[Drs aren't equipped with dietary advice/nutrition, prompts side effects and causes cravings, more cellular depletion, more perscriptions/ with orginal problem of the same - S.A.D. food]

Food Commercial Exposure
[Seek entertainment - cause cravings/prompts more S.A.D. food]

Sickly/Ailments
[Prompts Dr's visits, low energy, craves SAD food]

Life Abundantly Standard
And God said, "See, I have given you every herb *that* yields seed which *is* on the face of all the earth, and every tree whose fruit yields seed; to you it shall be for food. Also to everything ... in which there is life, I have given every green herb for food" [Gen 1:29-30]

Daily Calorie Intake
50-100% - fresh 'alive' whole plant food, uncooked [Gen 1:29]
0-50% - whole plant and non-plant 'clean' food, cooked [Gen. 9:3; Lev. 11; Duet. 14]

Standard American Diet
Consuming foods and ingredients that create and cause addictive nature in brain, altar taste buds, inflammatory states in the body, disordered eating, or unbalanced, inadequate nutrition promoting disease of body, soul, and spirit.

Daily Calorie Intake
60-100% processed, highly processed foods, refined, 'dirty', 'dead' and animal foods [addictive, dead foods]
0-40% whole plant foods, much cooked

The thief (Satan) does not come except to steal, and to kill, and to destroy.
I have come that they may have life, and that they may have *it* more abundantly. - John 10:10

357

What is the Standard American Diet?[3]

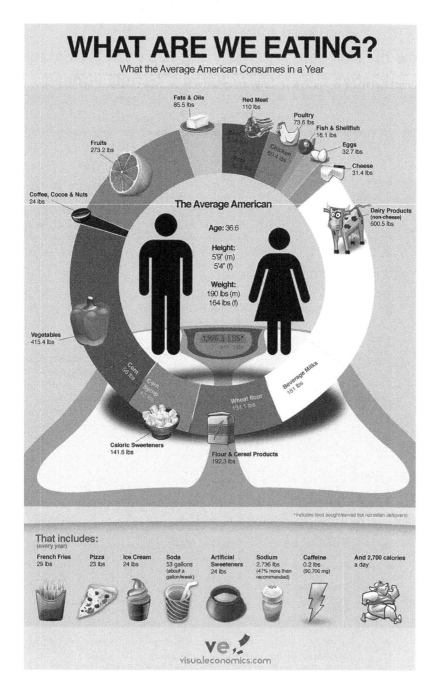

144 Researched Issues Caused by Sugar[1]
By Nancy Appleton PhD & G.N. Jacobs

1.   Sugar can suppress your immune system.

2.   Sugar upsets the mineral relationships in the body.

3.   Sugar can cause juvenile delinquency in children.

4.   Sugar eaten during pregnancy and lactation can influence muscle force production in offspring, which can affect an individual's ability to exercise.

5.   Sugar in soda, when consumed by children, results in the children drinking less milk.

6.   Sugar can elevate glucose and insulin responses and return them to fasting levels slower in oral contraceptive users.

7.   Sugar can increase reactive oxygen species (ROS), which can damage cells and tissues.

8.   Sugar can cause hyperactivity, anxiety, inability to concentrate, and crankiness in children.

9.   Sugar can produce a significant rise in triglycerides (bad cholesterol).

10. Sugar reduces the body's ability to defend against bacterial infection.

11. Sugar causes a decline in tissue elasticity and function. The more sugar you eat, the more elasticity and function you lose.

12. Sugar reduces high-density lipoproteins (HDL) (good cholesterol).

13. Sugar can lead to chromium deficiency.

14. Sugar can lead to ovarian cancer.

15. Sugar can increase fasting levels of glucose.

16. Sugar causes copper deficiency.

17. Sugar interferes with the body's absorption of calcium and magnesium.

18. Sugar may make eyes more vulnerable to age-related macular degeneration.

19. Sugar raises the level of neurotransmitters: dopamine, serotonin, and norepinephrine.

20. Sugar can cause hypoglycemia.

21. Sugar can lead to an acidic digestive tract.

22. Sugar can cause a rapid rise of adrenaline levels in children.

23. Sugar is frequently mal-absorbed in patients with functional bowel disease.

24. Sugar can cause premature aging.

25. Sugar can lead to alcoholism.

26. Sugar can cause tooth decay.

27. Sugar can lead to obesity.

28. Sugar increases the risk of Crohn's disease and ulcerative colitis.

29. Sugar can cause gastric or duodenal ulcers.

30. Sugar can cause arthritis.

31. Sugar can cause learning disorders in school children.

32. Sugar assists the uncontrolled growth of Candida Albicans (yeast infections).

33. Sugar can cause gallstones.

34. Sugar can cause heart disease.

35. Sugar can cause appendicitis.

36. Sugar can cause hemorrhoids.

37. Sugar can cause varicose veins.

38. Sugar can lead to periodontal disease.

39. Sugar can contribute to osteoporosis.

40. Sugar contributes to saliva acidity.

41. Sugar can cause a decrease in insulin sensitivity.

42. Sugar can lower the amount of vitamin E in the blood.

43. Sugar can decrease the amount of growth hormones in the body.

44. Sugar can increase cholesterol.

45. Sugar increases advanced glycation end products (AGEs), which form when sugar binds non-enzymatically to protein.

46. Sugar can interfere with the absorption of protein.

47. Sugar causes food allergies.

48. Sugar can contribute to diabetes.

49. Sugar can cause toxemia during pregnancy.

50. Sugar can lead to eczema in children.

51. Sugar can cause cardiovascular disease.

52. Sugar can impair the structure of DNA.

53. Sugar can change the structure of protein.

54. Sugar can make the skin wrinkle by changing the structure of collagen.

55. Sugar can cause cataracts.

56. Sugar can cause emphysema.

57. Sugar can cause atherosclerosis.

58. Sugar can promote an elevation of low-density lipoproteins (LDL).

59. Sugar can impair the physiological homeostasis of many systems in the body.

60. Sugar lowers the enzymes ability to function.

61. Sugar intake is associated with the development of Parkinson's disease.

62. Sugar can increase the size of the liver by making the liver cells divide.

63. Sugar can increase the amount of liver fat.

64. Sugar can increase kidney size and produce pathological changes in the kidney.

65. Sugar can damage the pancreas.

66. Sugar can increase the body's fluid retention.

67. Sugar is the number one enemy of the bowel movement.

68. Sugar can cause myopia (nearsightedness).

69. Sugar can compromise the lining of the capillaries.

70. Sugar can make tendons more brittle.

71. Sugar can cause headaches, including migraines.

72. Sugar plays a role in pancreatic cancer in women.

73.   Sugar can adversely affect children's grades in school.

74.   Sugar can cause depression.

75.   Sugar increases the risk of gastric cancer.

76.   Sugar can cause dyspepsia (indigestion).

77.   Sugar can increase the risk of developing gout.

78.   Sugar can increase the levels of glucose in the blood much higher than complex carbohydrates in a glucose tolerance test can.

79.   Sugar reduces learning capacity.

80.   Sugar can cause two blood proteins—albumin and lipoproteins—to function less effectively, which may reduce the body's ability to handle fat and cholesterol.

81.   Sugar can contribute to Alzheimer's disease.

82.   Sugar can cause platelet adhesiveness, which causes blood clots.

83.   Sugar can cause hormonal imbalance. Some hormones become underactive, and others become overactive.

84.   Sugar can lead to the formation of kidney stones.

85.   Sugar can cause free radicals and oxidative stress.

86.   Sugar can lead to biliary tract cancer.

87.   Sugar increases the risk of pregnant adolescents delivering a small-for-gestational-age (SGA) infant.

88.   Sugar can lead to a substantial decrease in the length of pregnancy among adolescents.

89.   Sugar slows food's travel time through the gastrointestinal tract.

90.   Sugar increases the concentration of bile acids in stool and bacterial enzymes in the colon, which can modify bile to produce cancer-causing compounds and colon cancer.

91.   Sugar increases estradiol (the most potent form of naturally occurring estrogen) in men.

92.   Sugar combines with and destroys phosphatase, a digestive enzyme, which makes digestion more difficult.

93.   Sugar can be a risk factor for gallbladder cancer.

94. Sugar is an addictive substance.

95. Sugar can be intoxicating, similar to alcohol.

96. Sugar can aggravate premenstrual syndrome (PMS).

97. Sugar can decrease emotional stability.

98. Sugar promotes excessive food intake in obese people.

99. Sugar can worsen the symptoms of children with attention deficit disorder (ADD).

100. Sugar can slow the ability of the adrenal glands to function.

101. Sugar can cut off oxygen to the brain when given to people intravenously.

102. Sugar is a risk factor for lung cancer.

103. Sugar increases the risk of polio.

104. Sugar can cause epileptic seizures.

105. Sugar can increase systolic blood pressure (pressure when the heart is contracting).

106. Sugar can induce cell death.

107. Sugar can increase the amount of food that you eat.

108. Sugar can cause antisocial behavior in juvenile delinquents.

109. Sugar can lead to prostate cancer.

110. Sugar dehydrates newborns.

111. Sugar can cause women to give birth to babies with low birth weight.

112. Sugar is associated with a worse outcome of schizophrenia.

113. Sugar can raise homocysteine levels in the bloodstream.

114. Sugar increases the risk of breast cancer.

115. Sugar is a risk factor in small intestine cancer.

116. Sugar can cause laryngeal cancer.

117. Sugar induces salt and water retention.

118. Sugar can contribute to mild memory loss.

119. Sugar water, when given to children shortly after birth, results in those children preferring sugar water to regular water throughout childhood.

120. Sugar causes constipation.

121. Sugar can cause brain decay in pre-diabetic and diabetic women.

122. Sugar can increase the risk of stomach cancer.

123. Sugar can cause metabolic syndrome.

124. Sugar increases neural tube defects in embryos when it is consumed by pregnant women.

125. Sugar can cause asthma.

126. Sugar increases the chances of getting irritable bowel syndrome.

127. Sugar can affect central reward systems.

128. Sugar can cause cancer of the rectum.

129. Sugar can cause endometrial cancer.

130. Sugar can cause renal (kidney) cell cancer.

131. Sugar can cause liver tumors.

132. Sugar can increase inflammatory markers in the bloodstreams of overweight people.

133. Sugar plays a role in the cause and the continuation of acne.

134. Sugar can ruin the sex life of both men and women by turning off the gene that controls the sex hormones.

135. Sugar can cause fatigue, moodiness, nervousness, and depression.

136. Sugar can make many essential nutrients less available to cells.

137. Sugar can increase uric acid in blood.

138. Sugar can lead to higher C-peptide concentrations.

139. Sugar causes inflammation.

140. Sugar can cause diverticulitis, a small bulging sac pushing outward from the colon wall that is inflamed.

141. Sugar can decrease testosterone production.

142. Sugar impairs spatial memory.

143. Sugar can cause cataracts.

144. Sugar is associated with higher rates of chronic bronchitis in adults.

Food Addict's Anonymous Promises[2]

1. We will know freedom and the promises of a happy and healthy life.

2. Our creativity will flow with the self-discipline we need to put it into action.

3. The chaos inside of us will be gone, so the chaos around us will diminish.

4. Our thinking will become clear.

5. We will be able to learn new information and knowledge and retain what we have learned.

6. We will accomplish complicated tasks with less confusion than before we were abstinent.

7. We will be consistent and dependable.

8. We will no longer fear trying something new and different.

9. If an endeavor is unsuccessful, we will be able to regroup and try it a new way.

10. We will be able to listen to others' ideas and suggestions without becoming defensive or argumentative.

11. We will become present and alert around our friends, family, and significant others.

12. We won't have to shut down, dissociate, or avoid listening anymore.

13. We can be ourselves because we won't allow abuse of any kind to be done to us by ourselves or others.

14. We will no longer attempt to fill our emotional and spiritual needs through our mouths. Instead, we will use our mouths along with our hearts to ask for what we need and deserve as children of God.

15. We will be able to listen with empathy to others' suffering.

16. We will not need to be controlling or insistent that "our way is best."

17. We will no longer be judgmental about everyone we meet.

18. The urge to see all the ways we were less sick than others will leave us.

19. Our self-esteem will no longer be tangled up in our perceptions about our bodies.

20. If on any given day we think we look fat, ugly, or old, we can choose not to lash out in anger or frustration at the people around us.

21. We will be able to hear and feel our Higher Power in our hearts and be still.

22. We will no longer experience the panic, fear, and anxiety of our yesterdays.

23. When presented with multiple choices, we will be able to reach clear decisions and understand what is appropriate for us.

24. We will know freedom from the fear of change in our relationships with the community, our families, and our friends.

25. We will begin to trust our intuition.

26. We will cherish our abstinence as critical to our physical, emotional, and spiritual survival, and we will stay abstinent!

Body Honor Manifesto

Whole & Free Health
Regarding my body, I…

Talk kindly
"I only talk kindly to my body."

Thank it
"I'm thankful for my body."

Accept it
"I accept my body as it is."

Enjoy i
"I enjoy life in my body."

Trust it
"I trust my body."

Listen to it
"I listen to my body."

Heal it
"I heal my body."

Look at it
"I look at myself with eyes of appreciation."

Love it
"My body is scared and special. I love it."

UPCOMING BOOKS

Follow me on Amazon to be notified of upcoming books!

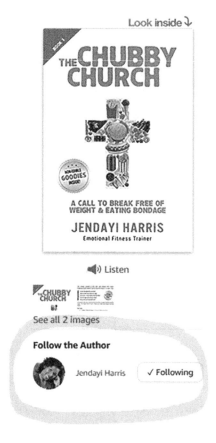

Look up The Chubby Church then click "Follow the Author"
or click the following link:
https://www.amazon.com/Jendayi-Harris/e/
B07Q5NMWQM?ref_=dbs_p_pbk_r00_abau_000000

Are you in need of hope for a close relationship?

After over 20 years of relational conflict between mother and daughter, God did a miracle healing in the life of Jendayi's mother, Joann.

Undiagnosed is a beautiful story of a redeemed mother and daughter relationship in Christ Jesus. In this memoir, Jendayi shares the process of healing and how God answers prayer, heals addiction, and restores family.

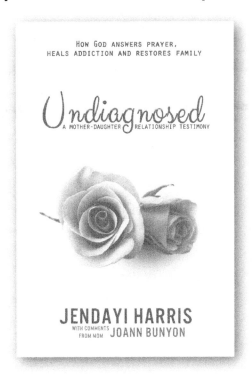

How is your Self-Talk?

- Are you tired of struggling with not doing what you know better to do?
- Do you talk yourself into poor choices that you regret later?
- Do you feel you need to obey the voice in your head?
- The missing foundational link to creating true freedom and wholeness – practically

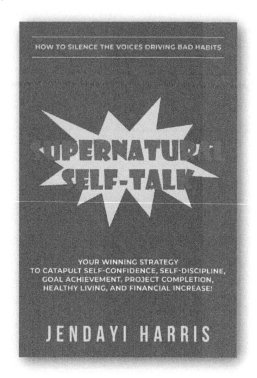

In this short read, Supernatural Self-Talk, Jendayi uses Biblical principles, stories, and practical tips, this book will help build your self-talk to support your best well-being and to develop more supportive, connected conversations within yourself and with others. If you beat yourself, have trouble letting go of things you don't want to do, or have the need for inner healing get this book! It will change your inner world which will manifest in your outer world.

Follow Jendayi Harris on Amazon to be notified of new books.

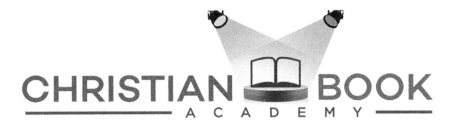

CJ and Shelley Hitz help Christian writers of all genres. Your story matters!

We help make your God-given dream of writing and publishing a book a reality. Your story matters to God and will impact and encourage others as you take this courageous step of faith.

Inside Christian Book Academy, we help you:

- Conquer your fears inside real community.
- Write words that will outlive you.
- Publish books that fulfill your calling.

Join this community of Christian authors and get access to the proven step-by-step plan you can use to write, publish and market your book (even if you have no idea where to start).

Find out more to join our community of Christian writers at:
http://christianbookacademy.com/

Get started with this free training at:
http://trainingauthors.com/formulas/

Too busy to read?
Listen to Jendayi instead on:

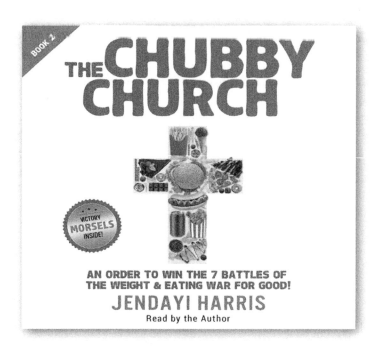

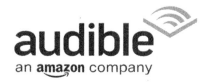

www.audible.com

Did you enjoy *The Chubby Church*?

I need your help to get the word out about
The Chubby Church Books.

Will you help?

Your review helps others decide to purchase this book on
www.Amazon.com.

Thank you!

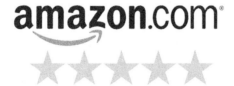

Post your review today!

Join Whole & Free Health to

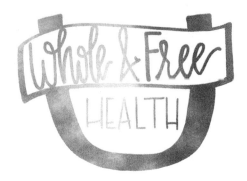

- Share in *The Chubby Church* reading experience
- Have a place to share your successes
- Find products that work for others for cleansing and supplementation
- Share recipes
- Share and receive devotionals, prayers, and encouragement
- Get accountability
- Meet others who share the journey
- Join optional paid courses – Whole & Free Health Body, Whole & Free Health Soul, or Whole & Free Health Spirit. You can choose online and live workshops as available, to focus on applying *The Chubby Church* book contents and more
- Join optional paid audio-visual book club for Jendayi to read to you

It's FREE!

Go to: *www.Facebook.com*
Search: Whole and Free Health

Team JESUS Collection

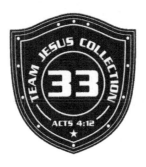

Founder – Josh Buris
Get the book for evangelism:
JESUS vs satan by Josh Burris
(Available on Amazon and Amazon Kindle)

Team JESUS Collection (TJC) is all about sharing the Gospel and encouraging others to share.
We do this in Four Ways:

1. *"JESUS vs satan"* by Josh Burris, This book shares the Truth about JESUS and exposes our enemy satan.

2. JESUS vs satan Soundtrack, A special playlist of songs/artists handpicked by Josh Burris (email below if interested).

3. Inspirational Movies/Videos (email below if interested).

4. Special Clothing Line

Email: *TeamJesusCollection@gmail.com*

Online Store: *https://teespring.com/stores/team-jesus-collection*

Follow Us! Facebook: *https://www.facebook.com/TeamJESUSCollection/*

Follow Us! Instagram: *https://www.instagram.com/teamjesuscollection1/*

JESUS vs satan book link:

https://www.amazon.com/JESUS-satan-There-Only-Teams/dp/0692121358/ ref=sr_1_12?keywords=Jesus+vs+satan&qid=1562001085&s=gateway&sr=8-12

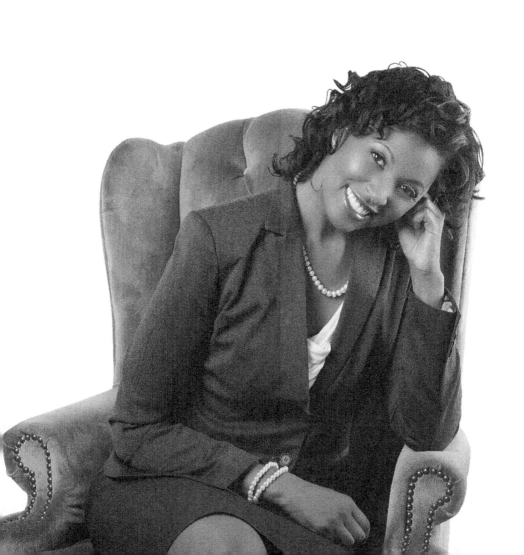

Jendayi Harris is a minister of practical advice on how to do life in Christ well. She has a Bachelor of Science in Business Administration from Seton Hall University as a part of the distinguished Martin Luther King Scholarship Association. She received her Master of Arts in Counseling Psychology from Colorado Christian University. She's a Nationally Certified Counselor, as well as a Licensed Professional Counselor in Colorado. After a health revelation in her early twenties, she became a Board-Certified Health Coach with the Institute of Integrative Nutrition.

From a Ministry standpoint, she has been mentored by Rabbi Ralph Messer of Simchat Torah Beit Midrash, Pastor Tayo Obigbesan of Christ Liberty Restoration Ministries and is now an active member of BridgeWay Church under Pastor Peter Young and Apostle Bill Johnson of Bethel Church.

Jendayi is certified as a DiSc instructor with TTI and a Certified Emotional Intelligence facilitator from industry leader, Talent Smart. In her leisure time she enjoys teaching, writing, family and running.

Her unique background and experience in many areas as well as incredible life experience makes her a source of Godly practical advice and wisdom in an age of information and great confusion.

As a Soul Freedom Author & Teacher, she speaks on a range of topics and issues of soul and family restoration. In her opinion, to love God, your self, and others, is the most productive response to our daily insanity.

To hire her for speaking or to hear about her latest releases, visit her site at

www.jendayiharris.com.

Photograph by Kymora Jaxson Photography

NOTES

Chapter 21: An Order To Win

1. "Scooby Doo, Where Are You!" The Shake Ups, accessed May 23, 2019, *https://www.youtube.com/watch?v=XB1-W4lIla0.*

2. "Adult Obesity Prevalence Maps," Behavioral Risk Factor Surveillance System, Centers for Disease Control and Prevention, accessed September 21, 2020, *https://www.cdc.gov/obesity/data/prevalence-maps.html.*

3. Ibid.

4. Ibid.

5. "Defining Adult Overweight and Obesity," Centers for Disease Control and Prevention, accessed September 17, 2020, *https://www.cdc.gov/obesity/adult/defining.html.*

6. Holland, Kimberly, "Obesity Facts in America," Healthline Media, accessed July 29, 2020, *https://www.healthline.com/health/obesity-facts.*

7. Ibid.

8. "Overweight and Obesity: A Major Public Health Issue," U.S. Department of Health and Human Services, *Prevention Report* (2001): 16.

9. Daniel Sunil, "Obesity and Heart Disease," August 15, 2015, *https://www.obesityaction.org/community/article-library/obesity-and-heart-disease/.*

10. Ibid.

11. Daniel Sunil, 2.

12. Ibid.

13. "Sudden Cardiac Death (SCD): Symptoms, Causes," Cleveland Clinic, accessed May 14, 2019, *https://my.clevelandclinic.org/health/diseases/17522-sudden-cardiac-death-sudden-cardiac-arrest.*

14. Benoit Plourde, Jean-François Sarrazin, Isabelle Nault, and Paul Poirier, "Sudden Cardiac Death and Obesity." *Expert Review of Cardiovascular Therapy* 12, no. 9 (2014): 1099–1110, *https://doi.org/10.1586/14779072.2014.952283.*

15. Kathleen Y. Wolin, Kenneth Carson, and Graham A. Colditz, "Obesity and Cancer," *The Oncologist* 15, no. 6 (May 27, 2010): 556–65, *https://doi.org/10.1634/theoncologist.2009-0285*.

16. American Cancer Society, *Cancer Facts & Figures 2020* (Atlanta: American Cancer Society, 2020), 49.

17. N. S. Mitchell, V. A. Catenacci, H. R. Wyatt, , and J. O. Hill. "Obesity: Overview of an Epidemic," *The Psychiatric Clinics of North America*, 34, no. 4 (December 2011): 717–732, *https://doi.org/10.1016/j.psc.2011.08.005*.

18. Ibid.

19. Himender Makker, "Obesity and Respiratory Diseases," *International Journal of General Medicine* 2010, 3. (October 2010): 335, *https://doi.org/10.2147/ijgm.s11926*.

20. E. Silvestris, G. de Pergola, R. Rosania, and G. Loverro, "Obesity as Disruptor of the Female Fertility," Reproductive Biology and Endocrinology 16, no. 1 (March 2018): 22, *https://doi.org/10.1186/s12958-018-0336-z*.

21. Mirjana Dobrio, "33 Scary Obesity Statistics for Changing Your Life," Loud Cloud Health, accessed May 9, 2020, *https://loudcloudhealth.com/resources/obesity-statistics/*.

22. Ibid.

23. A. Katib, "Mechanisms Linking Obesity to Male Infertility," *Central European Journal of Urology*, 68, no. 1) (2015): 79–85, *https://doi.org/10.5173/ceju.2015.01.435*.

24. D. T. Felson, J. J. Anderson, A. Naimark, A. M. Walker, and R. F. Meenan, "Obesity and Knee Osteoarthritis: The Framingham Study," *Annals of Internal Medicine* 109, no. 1 (July 1, 1988): 18–24, *https://doi.org/10.7326/0003-4819-109-1-18*.

25. Obesity Action Coalition, *Understanding Obesity Stigma* (Tampa, Florida: Obesity Action Coalition, 2016).

26. N. S. Mitchell, V. A. Catenacci, H. R. Wyatt, and J. O. Hill, "Obesity: Overview of an Epidemic," *The Psychiatric Clinics of North America* 34, no. 4 (December 2011): 717–732, *https://doi.org/10.1016/j.psc.2011.08.005*.

27. G. E. Simon, M. Von Korff, K. Saunders, D. L. Miglioretti, P. K. Crane, G. van Belle, and R. C. Kessler, "Association between Obesity and Psychiatric Disorders in the U.S. Adult Population," *Archives of General Psychiatry* 63, no. 7 (July 2006): 824–830, *https://doi.org/10.1001/archpsyc.63.7.824*.

28. Ibid.

29. National Center for Chronic Disease Prevention and Health Promotion (NCCDPHP), "Health and Economic Costs of Chronic Diseases," Centers for Disease Control and Prevention, accessed February 27, 2019, *https:// www.cdc.gov/chronicdisease/about/costs/index.htm.*

30. Ibid.

31. Megan Orciari, "Obesity among American Workers Costs the Nation Billions in Lost Productivity," *Yale News*, accessed November 11, 2020, *https://news.yale.edu/2014/11/14/ obesity-among-american-workers-costs-nations-billions-lost-productivity.*

32. Obesity Action Coalition, *Understanding Obesity Stigma* (Tampa, FL: Obesity Action Coalition, 2016).

33. "Battle," *Merriam-Webster's Dictionary*, accessed January 15, 2020, *https:// www.merriam-webster.com/dictionary/battle.*

34. Obesity Action Coalition, *Understanding Obesity Stigma* (Tampa, FL: Obesity Action Coalition, 2016).

35. Ibid.

Chapter 22: Rebuke the Sugar Demon and Her Cheesy Cousins – Battle # 1 – Food Addiction (S.A.D.)

1. Jeffrey Kluger, "The Hunger That Can't be Satisfied," *Special Time Edition* (January 2019): 30–32.

2. Michael D. Lemonick and Alice Park, "The Science of Addiction," *Special Time Edition* (January 2019): 8–13.

3. Jeffrey Kluger, "The Disease of the Pleasures," *Special Time Edition* (January 2019).

4. "Phein," *Urban Dictionary*, accessed February 12, 2018, *https://www. urbandictionary.com/define.php?term=phein.*

5. The Science of Addiction, 13.

6. Youfa Wang, May A. Beydoun, Lan Liang, Benjamin Caballero, and Shiriki K. Kumanyika, "Will All Americans Become Overweight or Obese? Estimating the Progression and Cost of the U.S. Obesity Epidemic," *Obesity* 16, no. 10 (October 16, 2008): 2323–30, *https://doi.org/10.1038/oby.2008.351*

7. Michael Greger, "How Not To Diet," (New York: Flat Iron Books, 2019), 52.

8. Ibid.

9. Vera Ingrid Tarman and Philip R Werdell, *Food Junkies: The Truth about Food Addiction* (Toronto, Canada: Dundurn, 2014) 71.

10. Kai Tomboc, "Is Food Addiction Real? – A Visual Case Study," Easelly, August 8, 2019, *https://www.easel.ly/blog/food-addiction-visual-case-study/*.

11. "Stages of Food Addiction," Food Addiction Institute, May 3, 2020, *https://foodaddictioninstitute.org/food-addicts/stages-of-food-addiction/*.

12. N. M. Avena, P. Rada, & B. G. Hoebel, Evidence for Sugar Addiction: Behavioral and Neurochemical Effects of Intermittent, Excessive Sugar Intake. Neuroscience and biobehavioral reviews, 32(1), (May 2008) 20–39. *https://doi.org/10.1016/j.neubiorev.2007.04.01*.

13. Barbara O'Dair, "Compulsion without the Chemicals," *Special Time Edition* (January 2019): 22–29.

14. Food Junkies, 24.

15. Michael Moss, Salt, Sugar, Fat: How the Food Giants Hooked Us (London: WH Allen, 2014), xxv.

16. Jason Fung, The Obesity Code: Unlocking the Secrets of Weight Loss (Vancouver: Greystone Books, 2016).

17. Ibid.

18. Federation of American Societies for Experimental Biology (FASEB), "Highly Processed Foods Dominate U. S. Grocery Purchases," *Science Daily*, March 29, 2015, accessed January 20, 2019, *http://www.sciencedaily.com/releases/2015/03/150329141017.htm*.

19. Rick and Karin Dina. Raw, Foods Mastery Summit 2020, *https://rawfoodmasterysummit.com/*.

20. Centers for Disease Control and Prevention, *National Diabetes Statistics Report, 2020* (Atlanta, GA: Centers for Disease Control and Prevention, U.S. Dept of Health and Human Services, 2020).

21. Ibid.

22. "New CDC Report: More Than 100 Million Americans Have Diabetes or Prediabetes," Centers for Disease Control and Prevention, July 18, 2017, *https://www.cdc.gov/media/releases/2017/p0718-diabetes-report.html*.

23. Craig Hales, Margaret Carroll, Chery Fryar, and Cynthia Ogden, "NCHS Data on Obesity," *NCHS Data Brief Prevalence of Obesity and Severe Obesity Among Adults,* United States, 2017–2018, no. 360 (February 2020), *https://doi.org/10.1037/e554432013-001*.

24. Maggie Fox, "Heavy Burden: Obesity May Be Even Deadlier than Thought," NBC Universal News Group, August 16, 2013, *https://www.nbcnews.com/healthmain/heavy-burden-obesity-may-be-even-deadlier-thought-6C10930019*.

25. "Obesity: Facts, Figures, Guidelines," West Virginia Health Statistic Center, accessed February 3, 2020, *https://www.wvdhhr.org/bph/oehp/obesity/mortality. htm.*

26. "Heart Disease Facts," Centers for Disease Control and Prevention, accessed September 8, 2020, *https://www.cdc.gov/heartdisease/facts.htm.*

27. "FastStats – Leading Causes of Death," Centers for Disease Control and Prevention, accessed January 12, 2021, *https://www.cdc.gov/nchs/fastats/ leading-causes-of-death.htm.*

28. American Cancer Society, *Cancer Facts & Figures 2020* (Atlanta, GA: American Cancer Society, 2020).

29. "FastStats – Leading Causes of Death," Centers for Disease Control and Prevention, accessed January 12, 2021, *https://www.cdc.gov/nchs/fastats/ leading-causes-of-death.htm.*

30. "Obesity and Overweight," World Health Organization, accessed April 1, 2020, *https://www.who.int/news-room/fact-sheets/detail/obesity-and-overweight.*

31. Ibid.

32. FastStats – Leading Causes of Death, 1.

33. The Case Against Sugar, 58.

34. Salt, Sugar, Fat: How the Food Giants Hooked Us, 76–80.

35. Alexis C. Madrigal, "When Did TV Watching Peak?" The Atlantic. Atlantic Media Company, May 30, 2018, *https://www.theatlantic.com/technology/ archive/2018/05/when-did-tv-watching-peak/561464/.*

36. Kai Tomboc, "Is Food Addiction Real? – A Visual Case Study," Easelly, August 8, 2019, *https://www.easel.ly/blog/food-addiction-visual-case-study/.*

37. "Bliss Point (Food)," Wikipedia, Wikimedia Foundation, October 20, 2020, *https://en.wikipedia.org/wiki/Bliss_point_(food).*

38. Salt, Sugar, Fat: How the Food Giants Hooked Us, 11.

39. Ibid.

40. "Howard Moskowitz." Wikipedia. Wikimedia Foundation, October 19, 2020. *https://en.wikipedia.org/wiki/Howard_Moskowitz.*

41. Erica M. Schulte, Nicole M. Avena, and Ashley N. Gearhardt, "Which Foods May Be Addictive? The Roles of Processing, Fat Content, and Glycemic Load," *Plos One* 10, no. 2 (February 18, 2015): 4, *https://doi. org/10.1371/journal.pone.0117959.*

42. Gary Taubes, *The Case against Sugar* (New York, NY: Anchor Books, 2016).

43. "Study: Sugar Hidden in Junk Food Eight Times More Addictive Than Cocaine," ABC13 Houston – KTRK-TV, February 25, 2015, *https://abc13. com/sugar-addiction-cocaine-addictive-foods/533979/*.

44. Nicole M. Avena, Pedro Rada, and Bartley G. Hoebel, "Evidence for Sugar Addiction: Behavioral and Neurochemical Effects of Intermittent, Excessive Sugar Intake," *Neuroscience Biobehavioral Reviews* 32, no. 1 (May 18, 2007): 20–39, *https://doi.org/10.1016/j.neubiorev.2007.04.019*.

45. Ibid.

46. Martínez Steele, Eurídice, Larissa Galastri Baraldi, Maria Laura da Costa Louzada, Jean-Claude Moubarac, Dariush Mozaffarian, and Carlos Augusto Monteiro, "Ultra-Processed Foods and Added Sugars in the U.S. Diet: Evidence from a Nationally Representative Cross-Sectional Study," BMJ open – BMJ Publishing Group, updated March 9, 2016, *https://www.ncbi. nlm.nih.gov/pmc/articles/PMC4785287/*.

47. "How Much Is Too Much?" SugarScience.UCSF.edu, December 8, 2018, *https://sugarscience.ucsf.edu/the-growing-concern-of-overconsumption.html*.

48. Ibid.

49. Kris Gunnars, "Daily Intake of Sugar – How Much Sugar Should You Eat Per Day?" Healthline. Healthline Media, updated June 28, 2018, *https:// www.healthline.com/nutrition/how-much-sugar-per-day*.

50. Alex Fox, "The Average American Eats 57 Pounds of Sugar Every Year," The Hill – Changing America, updated November 19, 2019, *https://thehill.com/changing-america/well-being/ longevity/469907-the-average-american-eats-57-pounds-of-sugar-every-year*.

51. Markham Heid, "Is Sugar as Bad for Kids as It Is for Adults?" *Time*, August 1, 2019, *https://time.com/5640428/sugar-kids-vs-adults/*.

52. Jeff Cronin, "New Nutrition Facts Labels To Feature Added Sugars with Daily Value," Center for Science in the Public Interest, updated October 4, 2017, *https://cspinet.org/news/ new-nutrition-facts-labels-feature-added-sugars-daily-value-20160520*.

53. The Case Against Sugar, 13.

54. Centers for Disease Control and Prevention, Long-Term Trends in Diabetes (Atlanta, GA: Centers for Disease Control and Prevention Division of Diabetes Translation, April 2017), *http://www.cdc.gov/diabetes/data*.

55. Centers for Disease Control and Prevention, *National Diabetes Statistics Report 2020* (Atlanta, GA: Centers for Disease Control and Prevention, U.S. Dept of Health and Human Services, 2020), *https://www.cdc.gov/diabetes/ statistics/slides/long_term_trends.pdf*.

56. "CDC COVID Data Tracker," Centers for Disease Control and Prevention. Centers for Disease Control and Prevention, accessed October 10, 2020, *https:// covid.cdc.gov/covid-data-tracker/?CDC_AA_refVal=https%3A%2F%2Fwww. cdc.gov%2Fcoronavirus%2F2019-ncov%2Fcases-updates%2Fcases-in-us. html#cases_casesper100klast7days.*

57. Gary Taubes, *The Case Against Sugar* (New York, NY: Anchor Books, 2016), 49–54.

58. Ibid, 56.

59. William Dufty, *Sugar Blues* (New York: Warner, 1993), 22.

60. The Case Against Sugar, 22.

61. The Case Against Sugar, 22–23.

62. The Case Against Sugar, 71.

63. Ian Stern, "15 Natural Supplements To Stop Sugar Cravings," Dr. Ian Stern, July 18, 2019, *https://drianstern.com/blogs/learn/ how-to-stop-sugar-cravings-with-nutritional-supplements.*

64. Michael Via, "The Malnutrition of Obesity: Micronutrient Deficiencies That Promote Diabetes," *ISRN Endocrinology* 2012 (January 05, 2012): 1–8, *doi:10.5402/2012/103472.*

65. Jayson Calton and Mira Calton, The Micronutrient Miracle: The 28-Day Plan To Lose Weight, Increase Your Energy, and Reverse Disease (Melbourne, Vic.: Black Books, 2016), 26.

66. "Office of Dietary Supplements – Chromium," NIH Office of Dietary Supplements – U.S. Department of Health and Human Services, October 1, 2020, *https://ods.od.nih.gov/factsheets/Chromium-HealthProfessional/.*

67. Ibid.

68. Nancy Appleton, *Lick the Sugar Habit* (Garden City Park, NY: Avery Publishing Group, 1996), 88.

69. *Ibid*, 98.

70. Michio Kushi, *Your Body Never Lies – the Complete Book of Oriental Diagnosis* (Garden City Park, NY: Square One Publishers, 2006), 136.

71. Anika Knüppel, Martin J. Shipley, Clare H. Llewellyn, and Eric J. Brunner, "Sugar Intake from Sweet Food and Beverages, Common Mental Disorder and Depression: Prospective Findings from the Whitehall II Study," *Scientific Reports* 7, no. 1 (July 27, 2017), *https://doi.org/10.1038/ s41598-017-05649-7.*

72. Nancy Appleton, *Lick the Sugar Habit* (Garden City Park, NY: Avery Publishing Group, 1996), 51.

73. Holly Strawbridge, "Artificial Sweeteners: Sugar-Free, but at What Cost?" Harvard Health, accessed February 3, 2020, *https://www.health.harvard.edu/blog/artificial-sweeteners-sugar-free-but-at-what-cost-201207165030*.

74. Stephen D. Anton, Corby K. Martin, Hongmei Han, Sandra Coulon, William T. Cefalu, Paula Geiselman, and Donald A. Williamson, "Effects of Stevia, Aspartame, and Sucrose on Food Intake, Satiety, and Postprandial Glucose and Insulin Levels," *Appetite* 55, no. 1 (2010): 37–43, *https://doi.org/10.1016/j.appet.2010.03.009*.

75. Holly Strawbridge, "Artificial Sweeteners: Sugar-Free, but at What Cost?" Harvard Health, accessed February 3, 2020, *https://www.health.harvard.edu/blog/artificial-sweeteners-sugar-free-but-at-what-cost-201207165030*.

76. Ibid.

77. Betty Kovacs Harbolic, "Artificial Sweeteners: Types, Side Effects, Chart & Benefits.", Medicine Net (September 4, 2020), *https://www.medicinenet.com/artificial_sweeteners/article.htm*.

78. Nancy Appleton, *Lick the Sugar Habit* (Garden City Park, NY: Avery Publishing Group, 1996), 132–133.

79. Michael Moss, Salt, Sugar, Fat: How the Food Giants Hooked Us (London: WH Allen, 2014), 7–8.

80. Satya Sharma, Hea Chung, Hyeon Kim, and Seong Hong, "Paradoxical Effects of Fruit on Obesity," *Nutrients* 8, no. 10 (October 2016): 633, *https://doi.org/10.3390/nu8100633*.

81. Michael J. Morris, Elisa S. Na, and Alan Kim Johnson, "Salt Craving: The Psychobiology of Pathogenic Sodium Intake," *Physiology & Behavior* 94, no. 5 (August 2008): 709–721, *https://doi.org/10.1016/j.physbeh.2008.04.008*.

82. Ibid.

83. Ibid.

84. "A Dangerous White Toxin We Eat Daily – No, It's Not Salt Or Sugar!" Doctor.ndtv.com, October 26, 2018, *https://doctor.ndtv.com/living-healthy/a-dangerous-white-toxin-we-eat-daily-no-its-not-salt-or-sugar-1807879*.

85. "Top 10 Sources of Sodium." Centers for Disease Control and Prevention. Centers for Disease Control and Prevention, February 26, 2021. *https://www.cdc.gov/salt/sources.htm*.

86. Denis Campbell, "Pizzas Contain up to Three Times Recommended Daily Limit of Salt," Guardian News and Media, updated December 17, 2014, *https://www.theguardian.com/lifeandstyle/2014/dec/17/pizza-salt-levels-unacceptably-high*.

87. AJ, Chef, and Glen Merzer, The Secrets to Ultimate Weight Loss: A Revolutionary Approach to Conquer Cravings, Overcome Food Addiction, and Lose Weight without Going Hungry (Los Angeles, CA: Hail to the Kale Publishing, 2018), 11.

88. Monica Reinagel, "How Salty Foods Affect Hunger and Weight Loss," Quick and Dirty Tips – Nutrition Diva, accessed March 17, 2020, *https://www.quickanddirtytips.com/health-fitness/weight-loss/ how-salty-foods-affect-hunger-and-weight-loss?page=1.*

89. Glenn Livingston, Salty-Crunchy Snacks = 300% More Addictive Than Chocolate?, November 23, 2020, email.

90. Michael Greger, *How Not To Diet* (New York, NY: Flat Iron Books, 2019), 124.

91. "You May Be Surprised by How Much Salt You're Eating," U.S. Food and Drug Administration, updated July 19, 2016, *https://www.fda.gov/consumers/ consumer-updates/you-may-be-surprised-how-much-salt-youre-eating.*

92. Ibid.

93. Marie Masters, "103 Hypertension Statistics and Demographics You Should Know." Leaf Group, accessed February 12, 2021, *https://www. livestrong.com/article/13731495-high-blood-pressure-statistics/?utm_ source=newsletter&utm_medium=email&utm_campaign=022021_ curated&utm_content=cta5.*

94. "How Not To Die from High Blood Pressure," NutritionFacts.org, YouTube Video, 5:42, October 17, 2016, *https://www.youtube.com/ watch?v=lupPd8SsZNc&feature=emb_rel_end.*

95. Ibid.

96. Ibid.

97. Ibid.

98. Michael Greger, MD, "The Evidence That Salt Raises Blood Pressure," NutritionFacts.org, updated January 20, 2016, *https://nutritionfacts.org/video/ the-evidence-that-salt-raises-blood-pressure/.*

99. "How Not to Die from High Blood Pressure," NutritionFacts.org, YouTube Video, 5:42, October 17, 2016. *https://www.youtube.com/ watch?v=lupPd8SsZNc&feature=emb_rel_end.*

100. "High Blood Pressure: Why Excess Sugar in the Diet May Be the Culprit," Diabetes.Co.Uk, updated May 5, 2017, *https://www.diabetes.co.uk/in-depth/ high-blood-pressure-excess-sugar-diet-may-culprit/.*

101. Michael Burnier, "Should We Eat More Potassium To Better Control Blood Pressure in Hypertension?" *Nephrology Dialysis Transplantation* 34, no. 2 (2018): 184–93, *https://doi.org/10.1093/ndt/gfx340.*

102. Ibid.

103. Ibid.

104. James DiNicolantonio, Salt Fix: How the Experts Got It All Wrong— And Why Eating More Might Save Your Life (New York, NY: Harmony, 2017),144–145.

105. Alice G. Walton, "Study Suggests Sugar Is Worse for Blood Pressure Than Salt: Really?" *Forbes Magazine*, December 14, 2014, *https://www.forbes.com/ sites/alicegwalton/2014/12/11/study-is-sugar-worse-for-blood-pressure-than- salt/?sh=78 997fc525d3.*

106. Sara Gottfried, The Hormone Cure: Reclaim Balance, Sleep, Sex Drive, and Vitality Naturally with the Gottfried Protocol (New York: Scribner, 2013) 101.

107. William Davis, Wheat Belly: Lose the Wheat, Lose the Weight, and Find Your Path Back to Health (London: Harper Thorsons, 2015), 25.

108. Ibid.

109. Ibid.

110. Ibid.

111. John Douillard, "5 Things You Never Knew about Gluten ... But Should," John Douillard's LifeSpa, September 24, 2016, accessed March 8, 2019, *https://lifespa.com/5-things-never-knew-gluten-but-should/.*

112. William Davis, Wheat Belly Slim Guide: The Fast and Easy Reference for Living and Succeeding on the Wheat Belly Lifestyle (Emmaus, PA: Rodale, 2017), 4.

113. Ibid.

114. William Davis, Wheat Belly Slim Guide: The Fast and Easy Reference for Living and Succeeding on the Wheat Belly Lifestyle (Emmaus, PA: Rodale, 2017), 70.

115. David Perlmutter, Grain Brain: The Surprising Truth about Wheat, Carbs, and Sugar – Your Brain's Silent (New York, NY: Hodder & Stoughton, 2014), 67.

116. William Davis, Wheat Belly Slim Guide: The Fast and Easy Reference for Living and Succeeding on the Wheat Belly Lifestyle (Emmaus, PA: Rodale, 2017), 70.

117. Kimberly Holland, edited by Timothy Legg, "The Connection between Sugar and Depression," Healthline Media, February 11, 2020, *https://www.healthline.com/health/depression/sugar-and-depression#carbohydrates-and-depression*.

118. John Douillard, "Do Low-Gluten Diets Increase Type 2 Diabetes Risk?" John Douillard's LifeSpa, May 31, 2017, accessed March 08, 2019, *https://lifespa.com/do-low-gluten-diets-increase-type-2-diabetes-risk/*.

119. Rob Thompson, The Glycemic Load Diet: a Powerful New Program for Losing Weight and Reversing Insulin Resistance (New York, NY: McGraw-Hill, 2006) 61–62.

120. Michael Peluso, "The Effect of Refined Carbohydrates on the Metabolism," Healthy Eating – SF Gate, December 20, 2018, *https://healthyeating.sfgate.com/effect-refined-carbohydrates-metabolism-5461.html*.

121. Shereen Lehman, "How Free Radicals Can Develop in Our Bodies," Verywell Fit, October 6, 2020, *https://www.verywellfit.com/free-radicals-2507225*.

122. Gabriele Pizzino, Natasha Irrera, Mariapaola Cucinotta, Giovanni Pallio, Federica Mannino, Vincenzo Arcoraci, Francesco Squadrito, Domenica Altavilla, and Alessandra Bitto, "Oxidative Stress: Harms and Benefits for Human Health," *Oxidative Medicine and Cellular Longevity* 2017 (July 2017): 1–13, https://doi.org/10.1155/2017/8416763. *https://www.ncbi.nlm.nih.gov/pmc/articles/PMC5551541/*.

123. Erica M. Schulte, Nicole M. Avena, and Ashley N. Gearhardt, "Which Foods May Be Addictive? The Roles of Processing, Fat Content, and Glycemic Load," PLOS one V. 10, no. 2 (February 2015), *https://doi.org/10.1371/journal.pone.0117959*.

124. "McDonald's Nutrition Calculator: Calories and More: McDonald's," McDonald's, January 2020, *https://www.mcdonalds.com/us/en-us/about-our-food/nutrition-calculator.html*.

125. Joe Leech, "What Are Trans Fats, and Are They Bad for You?" Healthline, July 30, 2019, *https://www.healthline.com/nutrition/why-trans-fats-are-bad*.

126. AJ, Chef, and Glen Merzer, The Secrets to Ultimate Weight Loss: a Revolutionary Approach to Conquer Cravings, Overcome Food Addiction, and Lose Weight without Going Hungry (Los Angeles, CA: Hail to the Kale Publishing, 2018), 43.

127. James DiNicolantonio and James H O'Keefe, "Good Fats versus Bad Fats: A Comparison of Fatty Acids in the Promotion of Insulin Resistance, Inflammation, and Obesity," *Missouri Medicine* vol. 114, no. 4 (2017): 303–307, *https://www.ncbi.nlm.nih.gov/pmc/articles/PMC6140086/*.

128. Douglas N. Graham, The 80/10/10 Diet: Balancing Your Health, Your Weight, and Your Life One Luscious Bite at a Time (Key Largo, FL: FoodnSport, 2010), 127.

129. Jessica A. Scott, "The Untold Truth of Baskin-Robbins," Mashed, December 19, 2019, *https://www.mashed.com/177683/ the-untold-truth-of-baskin-robbins/.*

130. Ibid.

131. Ibid.

132. John Robbins, "Diet for a New America," Talks at Google, YouTube video, June 4, 2013, *https://www.youtube.com/ watch?v=EyoXk1nAfh8&feature=emb_rel_end.*

133. Ibid.

134. Alisa Fleming, "It's Not You, It's Brie: Breaking Up with Cheese Addiction," Go Dairy Free – Fleming Marrs, Inc., October 23, 2015, *https://www. godairyfree.org/news/cheese-addiction.*

135. Ibid.

136. Ibid.

137. Robert Grillo, "Addicted to Cheese and Ice Cream? The Opiate Qualities of Dairy," Free From Harm, February 18, 2016, *https://freefromharm.org/ health-nutrition/addicted-to-cheese-and-ice-cream-the-opiate-qualities-of-dairy/.*

138. M. Shahbandeh, "Per Capita Consumption of Dairy Products in the U.S., 2019," Statista, October 5, 2020, *https://www.statista.com/statistics/183717/ per-capita-consumption-of-dairy-products-in-the-us-since-2000/.*

139. "The Hidden Dangers of the 'Milk and Cookie Disease,'" TEDx Wilmington, YouTube video, December 1, 2015, *https://www.youtube. com/watch?v=R2C6bBNWGp0&list=LLAmDXLiwUmYcuFhuGEW8QCg &index=300.*

140. Ibid.

141. Christian Løvold Storhaug, Svein Kjetil Fosse, and Lars T Fadnes, "Country, Regional, and Global Estimates for Lactose Malabsorption in Adults: a Systematic Review and Meta-Analysis," *The Lancet Gastroenterology & Hepatology* 2, no. 10 (July 2017): 738– 46, *https://doi.org/10.1016/ s2468-1253(17)30154-1.*

142. "Calcium," The Nutrition Source – Harvard TH Chan School of Public Health, October 19, 2020, *https://www.hsph.harvard.edu/nutritionsource/ what-should-you-eat/calcium-and-milk/calcium-full-story/.*

143. Beverly Merz, "How Well Does Calcium Intake Really Protect Your Bones?" Harvard Health Publishing, June 17, 2020, *https://www.health.harvard.edu/blog/how-well-does-calcium-intake-really-protect-your-bones-201509308384*.

144. T. Colin Campbell and Thomas M. Campbell, *The China Study* (Dallas, TX: BenBella Books, 2016), 195.

145. Randy Dotinga, "Number of Hip Replacements Has Skyrocketed, U.S. Report Shows," WebMD, February 12, 2015, *https://www.webmd.com/arthritis/news/20150212/number-of-hip-replacements-has-skyrocketed-us-report-shows*.

146. "Calcium," The Nutrition Source – Harvard TH Chan School of Public Health, October 19, 2020, *https://www.hsph.harvard.edu/nutritionsource/what-should-you-eat/calcium-and-milk/calcium-full-story/*.

147. M. Shahbandeh, "U.S. Milk Product Sales by Category, 2019," Statista, May 19, 2020, *https://www.statista.com/statistics/257290/us-milk-product-sales-by-category/*.

148. Ibid.

149. Merideth A. Addicott, "Caffeine Use Disorder: A Review of the Evidence and Future Implications," *Current Addiction Reports* 1, no. 3 (May 2014): 186–92, *https://doi.org/10.1007/s40429-014-0024-9*.

150. Ibid.

151. Merideth A. Addicott, "Caffeine Use Disorder: A Review of the Evidence and Future Implications," *Current Addiction Reports* 1, no. 3 (May 2014): 186–92, *https://doi.org/10.1007/s40429-014-0024-9*.

152. Kris Gunnars, "13 Health Benefits of Coffee, Based on Science," Healthline Media, September 20, 2018, *https://www.healthline.com/nutrition/top-13-evidence-based-health-benefits-of-coffee*.

153. Shawn Stevenson, Sleep Smarter: 21 Essential Strategies To Sleep Your Way to a Better Body, Better Health, and Bigger Success (New York, NY: Rodale Books, 2016), 111.

154. Gwyn Cready and Ted Kyle, "'Upper' Limits The Value of Caffeine in Weight-Loss," Obesity Action Coalition, October 1, 2011, *https://www.obesityaction.org/community/article-library/upper-limits-the-value-of-caffeine-in-weight-loss/*.

155. "Alcohol Facts and Statistics," National Institute on Alcohol Abuse and Alcoholism, accessed May 7, 2020, *https://www.niaaa.nih.gov/publications/brochures-and-fact-sheets/alcohol-facts-and-statistics*.

156. Amelia Lucas, "Fewer Americans Are Drinking Alcohol So Bars and Brewers Are Adapting," CNBC, June 1, 2019, *https://www.cnbc.com/2019/06/01/ fewer-americans-are-drinking-alcoholso-bars-and-brewers-are-adapting.html.*

157. Amy Smith, edited by Adrienne Seitz, "Red Wine: Benefits and Risks,", *Medical News Today*, April 21, 2020, *https://www.medicalnewstoday.com/ articles/265635.*

158. "Alcohol Facts and Statistics," National Institute on Alcohol Abuse and Alcoholism, accessed May 7, 2020, *https://www.niaaa.nih.gov/publications/ brochures-and-fact-sheets/alcohol-facts-and-statistics.*

159. Dean Ornish and Anne Ornish, *Undo It!: How Simple Lifestyle Changes Can Reverse Most Chronic Diseases* (New York, NY: Ballantine Books, 2019), 80.

160. "Alcohol and Cancer Risk Fact Sheet," National Cancer Institute, September 13, 2018, *https://www.cancer.gov/about-cancer/causes-prevention/risk/alcohol/ alcohol-fact-sheet.*

161. Atli Arnarson, "Alcohol and Health: The Good, the Bad, and the Ugly," *Healthline* (October 29, 2018): 4, 7, *https://www.healthline.com/nutrition/ alcohol-good-or-bad.*

162. Ibid.

163. "Drinking Alcohol," Breastcancer.org, September 11, 2020, *https://www. breastcancer.org/risk/factors/alcohol.*

164. Gregory Traversy and Jean-Philippe Chaput, "Alcohol Consumption and Obesity: An Update," *Current Obesity Reports* 4, no. 1 (January 2015): 122–30, *https://doi.org/10.1007/s13679-014-0129-4.*

165. Vera Ingrid Tarman, *Food Junkies: The Truth about Food Addiction* (Toronto, Canada: Dundurn, 2014), 24.

166. 165. K. J. Martires, P. Fu, A. M. Polster, K. D. Cooper, and E. D. Baron, "Factors That Affect Skin Aging: A Cohort-Based Survey on Twins," *Arch Dermatol*, 145, no 12 (December 2009):1375–1379, *doi:10.1001/ archdermatol.2009.303.*

167. Gary Taubes, *The Case Against Sugar* (New York, NY: Anchor Books, 2016).

168. Jack Trimpey, *Rational Recovery: The New Cure for Substance Addiction* (New York, NY: Pocket Books, 1996), 111 and 119.

169. "Deprivation," *Merriam-Webster's Dictionary*, accessed June 5, 2020, *https:// www.merriam-webster.com/dictionary/deprivation.*

170. Jack Trimpey, *Rational Recovery: The New Cure for Substance Addiction* (New York, NY: Pocket Books, 1996), *https://rational.org/index.php?id=1*, accessed February 13, 2020.

Chapter 23: Perform a Gluttonectomy, Stat – Battle # 2 – Overeating

1. Diagnostic and Statistical Manual of Mental Disorders: DSM-5 (Arlington, VA: American Psychiatric Association, 2017), 345.

2. Michael Greger, *How Not To Diet* (New York, NY: Flat Iron Books, 2019), 490.

3. University of Pennsylvania, "Binge Eating Linked to Weight-loss Challenges," ScienceDaily, accessed May 29, 2020, *www.sciencedaily.com/ releases/2017/12/171205115949.htm.*

4. "Glutton," *Merriam-Webster's Dictionary*, accessed March 3, 2021, *https:// www.merriam-webster.com/dictionary/glutton.*

5. Michael Atnip, "The Sin of Gluttony," The Heartbeat of the Remnant, January/February, 2012, *http://www.ephrataministries.org/remnant-2012-01-sin-of-gluttony.a5w.*

6. "The Power of Nutrition (Part 2): The Global Burden of Non-Communicable Diseases • PAN International." PAN International, December 3, 2020. *https://pan-int.org/the-power-of-nutrition-part-2/.*

7. Michael Atnip, "The Sin of Gluttony," The Heartbeat of the Remnant, January/February, 2012, *http://www.ephrataministries.org/remnant-2012-01-sin-of-gluttony.a5w.*

8. Frederica Mathewes-Green, "To Hell on a Creampuff," *Christianity Today*, August 29, 2000, *https://www.christianitytoday.com/ct/2000/augustweb-only/23.0c.html.*

9. Michael Atnip, "The Sin of Gluttony," The Heartbeat of the Remnant, January/February 2012, *http://www.ephrataministries.org/remnant-2012-01-sin-of-gluttony.a5w.*

10. Frederica Mathewes-Green, "To Hell on a Creampuff," *Christianity Today*, August 29, 2000, *https://www.christianitytoday.com/ct/2000/augustweb-only/23.0c.html.*

11. Atnip, 3.

12. "World Hunger Is Still Not Going Down after Three Years and Obesity Is Still Growing – UN Report," World Health Organization, July 15, 2019, *https://www.who.int/news/item/15-07-2019-world-hunger-is-still-not-going-down-after-three-years-and-obesity-is-still-growing-un-report.*

13. Alexandra Sifferlin, "Obesity: 30% of People in the World Are Obese or Overweight," *Time*, June 12, 2017, *https://time.com/4813075/ obesity-overweight-weight-loss/.*

14.   Michael Atnip, "The Sin of Gluttony," The Heartbeat of the Remnant, January/February, 2012, *http://www.ephrataministries.org/remnant-2012-01-sin-of-gluttony.a5w.*

15.   Ibid.

16.   Ibid.

17.   Ibid.

18.   "What Did You Expect?" DVD (USA: Paul Tripp Ministries, 2012).

19.   Glenn Livingston, "Survey Results: How Much Our Readers Spend on Binge Food," Psy Tech, April 28, 2020, email.

20.   Ibid.

21.   Megan Leonhardt, "Here's How Much Debt Americans Have at Every Age," CNBC, August 20, 2018, *https://www.cnbc.com/2018/08/20/how-much-debt-americans-have-at-every-age.html.*

22.   Julia Belluz, Eliza Barclay, and Javier Zarracina, "It's Easy To Become Obese in America: These 7 Charts Explain Why," Vox, August 31, 2016, *https://www.vox.com/2016/8/31/12368246/obesity-america-2018-charts.*

23.   Ibid.

24.   Ibid.

25.   Ibid.

26.   Ibid.

27.   Ibid.

28.   Tamar Haspel, "One Big Fat Truth," Discover (May 2018): 41.

29.   Jo Craven McGinty, "Why Women's Clothing Sizes Aren't What They Used to Be," *The Wall Street Journal*, May 24, 2019, *https://www.wsj.com/articles/why-womens-clothing-sizes-arent-what-they-used-to-be-11558690200.*

30.   Cheryl D. Fryar, Margaret D. Carroll, and Joseph Afful, "Prevalence of Overweight, Obesity, and Severe Obesity Among Adults Aged 20 and Over: United States, 1960–1962 Through 2017–2018," Centers for Disease Control – U.S. National Center for Health Statistics, accessed January 29, 2021, *http://www.publicnow.com/view/57BFCB292A6D12A9A3EE633921C052DED8F0D94B.*

31.   Youfa Wang, May A. Beydoun, Benjamin Caballero, and Shiriki K. Kumanyika, "Will All Americans Become Overweight or Obese?" *Estimating the Progression and Cost of the U.S. Obesity Epidemic* 16, no. 10 (October 2008): 54–54, *https://doi.org/10.14341/2071-8713-5324.*

32. "Adult Obesity Prevalence Maps," Centers for Disease Control and Prevention, September 21, 2020, *https://www.cdc.gov/obesity/data/prevalence-maps.html.*

33. S. S. Casagrande, A. M. Anderson, A. Dalcin, L. J. Appel, C. J. Jerome, F. B. Dickerson, J. V. Gennusa, and G. L. Daumit, "Dietary Intake of Adults with Serious Mental Illness, *Psychiatric Rehabilitation Journal* 35, no. 2 (December 2011): 137–140, *https://doi.org/10.2975/35.2.2011.137.140.*

34. Lyn Patrick, "Eating Disorders: a Review of the Literature with Emphasis on Medical Complications and Clinical Nutrition (Eating Disorders)," *Alternative Medicine Review* (June 2002): 184+, Gale Academic OneFile, accessed March 14, 2020.

35. Ibid.

36. "Eating Disorder Statistics: General & Diversity Stats: ANAD," National Association of Anorexia Nervosa and Associated Disorders, March 3, 2021, *https://anad.org/get-informed/about-eating-disorders/eating-disorders-statistics/.*

37. "What Are the Real Facts about Bulimia?" American Addiction Centers, November 7, 2018, *https://americanaddictioncenters.org/bulimia-treatment/facts-and-statistics.*

38. Ibid.

39. *Diagnostic and Statistical Manual of Mental Disorders: DSM-5* (Arlington, VA: American Psychiatric Association, 2017), 345.

40. Joel Yager, "Binge Eating Disorder: The Search for Better Treatments," *Focus* 7, no. 4 (October 2009): 499–501, *https://doi.org/10.1176/foc.7.4.foc499.*

41. Juliann Schaeffer, "Binge Eating Disorder: Statistics, Facts, and You," Healthline Media, December 19, 2016, *https://www.healthline.com/health/eating-disorders/binge-eating-disorder-statistics.*

42. Joel Yager, "Binge Eating Disorder: The Search for Better Treatments," *Focus* 7, no. 4 (October 2009): 499–501, *https://doi.org/10.1176/foc.7.4.foc499.*

43. *Diagnostic and Statistical Manual of Mental Disorders: DSM-5* (Arlington, VA: American Psychiatric Association, 2017), 351.

44. David Engstrom, "Obesity and Depression," Obesity Action Coalition, accessed March 19, 2019, *https://www.obesityaction.org/community/article-library/obesity-and-depression/.*

45. Roseann E. Perterson, Shawn J. Latendresse, Lindsay T. Bartholome, Cortney S. Warren, and Nancy C. Raymond, "Binge Eating Disorder Mediates Links between Symptoms of Depression, Anxiety, and Caloric Intake in Overweight and Obese Women." Journal of Obesity 2012 (June 18, 2012): 1–8, *https://doi.org/10.1155/2012/407103.*

46. Carlos M. Grilo, Marney A. White, and Robin M. Masheb, "DSM-IV Psychiatric Disorder Comorbidity and Its Correlates in Binge Eating Disorder," *International Journal of Eating Disorders* 42, no. 3 (October 2008): 228–34, *https://doi.org/10.1002/eat.20599.*

47. *Diagnostic and Statistical Manual of Mental Disorders: DSM-5* (Arlington, VA: American Psychiatric Association, 2017), 350.

48. Juliann Schaeffer, "Binge Eating Disorder: Statistics, Facts, and You." Healthline (December 18, 2016), *https://www.healthline.com/health/eating-disorders/binge-eating-disorder-statistics.*

49. "Binge Eating Disorder (BED): Symptoms, Signs, Causes & Articles," Eating Disorder Hope, February 18, 2021, *https://www.eatingdisorderhope.com/information/binge-eating-disorder.*

50. Paulo P. Machado, Sónia Gonçalves, and Hans W. Hoek, "DSM-5 Reduces the Proportion of Ednos Cases: Evidence from Community Samples," *International Journal of Eating Disorders* 46, no. 1 (July 2012): 60–65, *https://doi.org/10.1002/eat.22040.*

51. Glenn Livingston, *Me, My Pig, and I: My Life Battling My Inner Food Demon* (Fort Lauderdale, FL: Psy Tech, Inc., 2019).

52. *2017 Membership Survey Report* (Rio Rancho, NM: Overeaters Anonymous, 2018).

53. Carolyn Coker Ross, *Food Addiction Recovery Workbook – How To Manage Cravings, Reduce Stress* (Oakland, CA: New Harbinger Publications, 2017), 29.

54. Karol K. Truman, *Feelings Buried Alive Never Die* (Phoenix: Olympus Publishing Company, 2003), 265.

55. Lisa Morrone, *Overcoming Overeating* (Eugene, OR: Harvest House Publishers, 2009), 119.

56. Jendayi Harris, The Chubby Church: A Call To Break Free of Weight & Eating Bondage (Denver, CO: Whole & Free Press, 2019) 255.

57. Rob Thompson, The Glycemic Load Diet: a Powerful New Program for Losing Weight and Reversing Insulin Resistance (New York, NY: McGraw-Hill, 2006) 5.

58. Jayson Calton and Mira Calton, The Micronutrient Miracle: The 28-day Plan to Lose Weight, Increase Your Energy, and Reverse Disease (Melbourne, Victoria.: Black Books, 2016), 26, 90.

59. Chef AJ and Glen Merzer, The Secrets to Ultimate Weight Loss: a Revolutionary Approach to Conquer Cravings, Overcome Food Addiction, and Lose Weight without Going Hungry (Los Angeles, CA: Hail to the Kale Publishing, 2018), 49.

60. Victoria Wolk, "Cut Your Cravings 95% with These 6 Superfoods," *Prevention*, June 10, 2019, *https://www.prevention.com/weight-loss/a20467964/thylakoids-in-green-superfoods-reduce-cravings/*.

61. Ibid.

62. Karen R. Koenig, The Rules of "Normal" Eating: A Commonsense Approach for Dieters, Overeaters, Undereaters, Emotional Eaters, and Everyone in Between! (Carlsbad, CA: Gurze Books, 2005), 47.

63. Marion Nestle, "Why Does the FDA Recommend 2,000 Calories Per Day?" The Atlantic Media Company, August 4, 2011, *https://www.theatlantic.com/health/archive/2011/08/why-does-the-fda-recommend-2-000-calories-per-day/243092/*.

64. *Clinical Guidelines on the Identification Evaluation and Treatment of Overweight and Obesity in Adults*, National Heart, Lung, and Blood Institute (Bethesda, MD: National Institute of Health, 1998), 139–140.

65. Jack F. Hollis, Christina M. Gullion, Victor J. Stevens, Phillip J. Brantley, Lawrence J. Appel, Jamy D. Ard, Catherine M. Champagne, et al, "Weight Loss During the Intensive Intervention Phase of the Weight-Loss Maintenance Trial," *American Journal of Preventive Medicine* 35, no. 2 (August 2008): 118–26, *https://doi.org/10.1016/j.amepre.2008.04.013*.

66. "FAA Food Plan," Food Addicts Anonymous, accessed June 14, 2020, *https://www.foodaddictsanonymous.org/faa-food-plan*.

67. Pauline Ducrot, Caroline Méjean, Vani Aroumougame, Gladys Ibanez, Benjamin Allès, Emmanuelle Kesse-Guyot, Serge Hercberg, and Sandrine Péneau, "Meal Planning Is Associated with Food Variety, Diet Quality, and Body Weight Status in a Large Sample of French Adults," *International Journal of Behavioral Nutrition and Physical Activity* 14, no. 1 (February 2017): 12, *https://doi.org/10.1186/s12966-017-0461-7*.

68. *2017 Membership Survey Report* (Rio Rancho, NM: Overeaters Anonymous, 2018).

69. Ibid.

70. Ibid.

Chapter 24: Eww, Spit it Out, That Wasn't Food – Battle # 3 – Unclean Eating

1. Matthew Zampa, "99% of U.S. Farmed Animals Live on Factory Farms," Sentient Media, October 8, 2020, https://sentientmedia.org/u-s-farmed-animals-live-on-factory-farms/.

2. Doris Lin, "Is There a Way To End Inhumane Factory Farming Techniques?" ThoughtCo, October 2, 2019, https://www.thoughtco.com/why-do-we-have-factory-farming-127703.

3. Felicity Lawrence, "If Consumers Knew How Farmed Chickens Were Raised, They Might Never Eat Their Meat Again," The Guardian News and Media, April 24, 2016, *https://www.theguardian.com/environment/2016/apr/24/real-cost-of-roast-chicken-animal-welfare-farms.*

4. Christopher Walljasper, "Large Animal Feeding Operations on the Rise" Investigate Midwest, September 23, 2019, *https://investigatemidwest.org/2018/06/07/large-animal-feeding-operations-on-the-rise/.*

5. John Robbins, Diet for a New America: How Your Food Choices Affect Your Health, Your Happiness, and the Future of Life on Earth (Tiburon, CA: H J Kramer, 2012), 117.

6. Megan Durisin and Shruti Date Singh, "Americans' Meat Consumption Set To Hit a Record in 2018." *The Seattle Times,* January 2, 2018, *https://www.seattletimes.com/business/americans-meat-consumption-set-to-hit-a-record-in-2018/.*

7. Dr. Phil McGraw, "How's That Working for You?" The Self-Help Whisperer®, August 12, 2020, *https://theselfhelpwhisperer.com/2019/06/09/dr-phil-mcgraw-hows-that-working-for-you/.*

8. Brian Wendel, *Forks over Knives* (USA: Monica Beach Media, 2011).

9. Ibid.

10. M. Shahbandeh, "Per Capita Consumption of Dairy Products in the U.S., 2019." Statista, October 5, 2020, *https://www.statista.com/statistics/183717/per-capita-consumption-of-dairy-products-in-the-us-since-2000/.*

11. Tim Whitnall and Nathan Pitts, "Meat Consumption," Department of Agriculture, October 21, 2020, *https://www.agriculture.gov.au/abares/research-topics/agricultural-outlook/meat-consumption.*

12. Alex Thornton, "This Is How Many Animals We Eat Each Year," World Economic Forum, February 8, 2019, *https://www.weforum.org/agenda/2019/02/chart-of-the-day-this-is-how-many-animals-we-eat-each-year/.*

13. Yuval Harari, "About," Yuval Noah Harari, August 17, 2020, *https://www.ynharari.com/about/.*

14. John Robbins, Diet for a New America: How Your Food Choices Affect Your Health, Your Happiness, and the Future of Life on Earth (Tiburon, CA: H J Kramer, 2012), 121.

15. Noa Dalzell, "Dangerous Working Conditions on Factory Farms," Factory Farming Awareness Coalition, February 17, 2021, *https://www.ffacoalition. org/blog-posts/dangerous-conditions-factory-farms*.

16. "What Is Ag-Gag Legislation?" ASPCA, accessed June 5, 2020, *https://www. aspca.org/animal-protection/public-policy/what-ag-gag-legislation*.

17. Ibid.

18. Carrie Hribar, edited by Mark Schultz, *Understanding Concentrated Animal Feeding Operations and Their Impact on Communities* (Bowling Green, OH: National Association of Local Boards of Health, 2010),

19. John Robbins, Diet for a New America: How Your Food Choices Affect Your Health, Your Happiness, and the Future of Life on Earth (Tiburon, CA: H J Kramer, 2012), 346.

20. Carrie Hribar, edited by Mark Schultz, *Understanding Concentrated Animal Feeding Operations and Their Impact on Communities* (Bowling Green, OH: National Association of Local Boards of Health, 2010), 2.

21. Ibid.

22. Understanding Concentrated Animal Feeding Operations and Their Impact on Communities, 1.

23. *Right to Harm* (USA: Hourglass Films, 2020), *https://vimeo.com/ondemand/ righttoharm*.

24. Understanding Concentrated Animal Feeding Operations and Their Impact on Communities, 7.

25. John Robbins, Diet for a New America: How Your Food Choices Affect Your Health, Your Happiness, and the Future of Life on Earth (Tiburon, CA: H J Kramer, 2012), 347.

26. Understanding Concentrated Animal Feeding Operations and Their Impact on Communities, 6.

27. Hulda Regehr Clark, *The Cure for All Diseases* (Chula Vista, CA: New Century Press, 1995), 45.

28. Dick Heederik, Torben Sigsgaard, Peter S. Thorne, Joel N. Kline, Rachel Avery, Jakob H. Bønløkke, Elizabeth A. Chrischilles, et al, "Health Effects of Airborne Exposures from Concentrated Animal Feeding Operations," *Environmental Health Perspectives* 115, no. 2 (February 2007): 298–302, https://doi.org/10.1289/ehp.8835. *https://www.ncbi.nlm.nih.gov/pmc/articles/ PMC1817709/*.

29. "Methane-vs-co2-Graphic-New," Big Picture Vegan, February 12, 2016, *https://bigpicturevegan.com/2016/02/15/emissions-cars-vs-cattle/ methane-vs-co2-graphic-new/*.

30. Understanding Concentrated Animal Feeding Operations and Their Impact on Communities, 6.

31. Ibid.

32. NW Farms and Food, "Methane-vs-co2-Graphic-New," Big Picture Vegan, February 12, 2016, *https://bigpicturevegan.com/2016/02/15/ emissions-cars-vs-cattle/methane-vs-co2-graphic-new/.*

33. John Robbins, Diet for a New America: How Your Food Choices Affect Your Health, Your Happiness, and the Future of Life on Earth (Tiburon, CA: H J Kramer, 2012), 341.

34. "Ogallala Aquifer," Wikipedia, Wikimedia Foundation, November 10, 2020, *https://en.wikipedia.org/wiki/Ogallala_Aquifer.*

35. John Robbins, Diet for a New America: How Your Food Choices Affect Your Health, Your Happiness, and the Future of Life on Earth (Tiburon, CA: H J Kramer, 2012), 344.

36. Ibid.

37. Ibid.

38. "Ogallala Aquifer," Wikipedia, Wikimedia Foundation, November 10, 2020, *https://en.wikipedia.org/wiki/Ogallala_Aquifer.*

39. Bethany Wood, "Factory Farming: It's Impacting Your Health, Animal Welfare, and the Environment. What Can You Do?" Medium, July 2, 2019, *https://medium.com/@bethanywood.healthcoach/ factory-farming-its-impacting-your-health-animal-welfare-and-the-environment-what-can-you-do-88e7d47aac15.*

40. John Robbins, Diet for a New America: How Your Food Choices Affect Your Health, Your Happiness, and the Future of Life on Earth (Tiburon, CA: H J Kramer, 2012), 342.

41. Ibid, 343.

42. Smt. Maneka Sanjay Gandhi, "What Happens to Animal Blood in Slaughterhouses? *New Delhi Times*, March 15, 2017, *https://www. newdelhitimes.com/what-happens-to-animal-blood-in-slaughterhouses123/.*

43. Jack Ofori and Peggy Hsieh, "Blood-derived Products for Human Consumption," *Revelation Sci.* 1 (January 2011): 14–15.

44. Ibid.

45. Brad Plumer, "How Much of the World's Cropland Is Actually Used To Grow Food?" Vox, August 21, 2014, *https://www.vox. com/2014/8/21/6053187/cropland-map-food-fuel-animal-feed.*

46. Alexandra Sifferlin, "Ground Beef Contains Dangerous Bacteria, Study Finds" *Time*, August 24, 2015, *https://time.com/4007975/ ground-beef-bacteria/*.

47. Holly Watt, "How Much Does Big Pharma Make from Animal Antibiotics?" The Guardian News and Media, June 19, 2018, https://www.theguardian.com/environment/2018/jun/19/ how-much-does-big-pharma-make-from-animal-antibiotics.

48. Ibid.

49. Ibid.

50. Understanding Concentrated Animal Feeding Operations and Their Impact on Communities, 9.

51. Alexandra Sifferlin, "Ground Beef Contains Dangerous Bacteria, Study Finds," *Time*, August 24, 2015, https://time.com/4007975/ ground-beef-bacteria/.

52. Ibid.

53. Umhee Lin and Johanna Lampe, "TMAO, the Gut Microbiome, and Colorectal Cancer Risk in the Multiethnic Cohort," Grantome – NIH, May 1, 2016, *https://grantome.com/grant/NIH/R01-CA204368-01*.

54. Alicja Wolk, "Potential Health Hazards of Eating Red Meat," *Journal of Internal Medicine* 281, no. 2 (September 6, 2016): 106–22, *https://doi. org/10.1111/joim.12543*.

55. Alexandra Sifferlin, "Ground Beef Contains Dangerous Bacteria, Study Finds," *Time*, August 24, 2015, *https://time.com/4007975/ ground-beef-bacteria/*.

56. "Farm Animal Welfare," ASPCA, accessed June 18, 2020, *https://www.aspca. org/animal-cruelty/farm-animal-welfare*.

57. Dan Flynn, "Bigger Buffers between Leafy Greens and CAFOs Ready for New Growing Season," Food Safety News, January 14, 2019, *https://www.foodsafetynews.com/2018/10/ bigger-buffers-between-leafy-greens-and-cafos-ready-for-new-growing-season/*.

58. Ibid.

59. Lori Cuthbert, "What Are Zoonotic Diseases?" *Science National Geographic*, February 10, 2021, *https://www.nationalgeographic.com/science/article/how-do-animals-pass-dangerous-zoonotic-diseases-to-humans-zoonoses-coronavirus*.

60. Michael Greger, "The Last Coronavirus Pandemic May Have Been Caused by Livestock," NutritionFacts.org, June 10, 2020, *https://nutritionfacts.org/ video/the-last-coronavirus-pandemic-may-have-been-caused-by-livestock/*.

61. "Climate Change Evidence: How Do We Know?" NASA, January 22, 2021, *https://climate.nasa.gov/evidence/*.

62. Denis Lu and Christopher Flavelle, "Rising Seas Will Erase More Cities by 2050, New Research Shows," *The New York Times*, October 29, 2019, *https://www.nytimes.com/interactive/2019/10/29/climate/coastal-cities-underwater.html*.

63. Daisy Dunne, "Interactive: What Is the Climate Impact of Eating Meat and Dairy?" Carbon Brief, September 14, 2020, *https://interactive.carbonbrief.org/what-is-the-climate-impact-of-eating-meat-and-dairy/*.

64. John Robbins, Diet for a New America: How Your Food Choices Affect Your Health, Your Happiness, and the Future of Life on Earth (Tiburon, CA: H J Kramer, 2012), 365.

65. M. Shahbandeh, "Per Capita Consumption of Pork in the U.S., 2029," Statista, March 24, 2020, *https://www.statista.com/statistics/183616/per-capita-consumption-of-pork-in-the-us-since-2000/*.

66. "Trichinosis – How Common Is the Disease?" Broken Arrow Ranch, August 17, 2018, *https://www.brokenarrowranch.com/Articles/Trichinosis.htm*.

67. Denise Minger, "4 Hidden Dangers of Pork," Healthline, June 22, 2017, *https://www.healthline.com/nutrition/is-pork-bad*.

68. Dr. Josh Axe, "Tapeworms, Toxins, and More: The Truth about Your Pork," Dr. Axe, December 18, 2019, *https://draxe.com/nutrition/why-you-should-avoid-pork/*.

69. "Original Glazed®," Krispy Kreme – Original Glazed Doughnuts, accessed March 18, 2021, *https://www.krispykreme.com/menu/doughnuts/original-glazed-doughnut*.

70. "Fil-A Chicken Sandwich," accessed March 18, 2021, *https://www.chick-fil-a.com/menu-items/chick-fil-a-chicken-sandwich*.

71. Ibid.

72. Kimberly Hartke, "Violent Behavior Linked to Nutritional Deficiencies," *Well Being Journal* (January/February 2014): 33–34.

73. Becky Maes, "Is DATEM Bad For You?" – Here Is Your Answer, Is it Bad for You, March 6, 2016, *https://www.isitbadforyou.com/questions/is-datem-bad-for-you*.

74. Stacy Simon, "World Health Organization Says Processed Meat Causes Cancer," American Cancer Society, October 26, 2015, accessed January 27, 2019, *https://www.cancer.org/latest-news/world-health-organization-says-processed-meat-causes-cancer.html*.

75. Eric Pfeiffer, "McDonald's Confirms That It's No Longer Using 'Pink Slime' Chemical in Hamburgers," Yahoo! News, February 1, 2012, *https://www.yahoo.com/news/blogs/sideshow/mcdonald-confirms-no-longer-using-pink-slime-chemicals-171209662.html.*

76. Michael Greger, *How Not To Diet* (New York, NY: Flat Iron Books, 2019), 52.

77. Ibid.

78. Brian Wendel, *Forks over Knives* (USA: Monica Beach Media, 2011).

79. Jennifer R. Scott, "What Is the Volumetrics Diet?" Verywell Fit, March 19, 2020, *https://www.verywellfit.com/the-volumetrics-diet-what-you-need-to-know-3496210.*

80. "Vegetables and Fruits," The Nutrition Source, Harvard School of Public Health, March 3, 2021, *https://www.hsph.harvard.edu/nutritionsource/what-should-you-eat/vegetables-and-fruits/.*

81. Becky Bell, "Is Raw Food Healthier Than Cooked Food?" Healthline, January 24, 2017, *https://www.healthline.com/nutrition/raw-food-vs-cooked-food.*

82. Karen Knowler, *Raw Food Made Simple* (United Kingdom: Raw Food Coach Media, 2010), 25.

83. Karen Dina, Raw Foods Mastery Summit, May 2020, "Rosalind Graham Interview."

84. Marsha McColloch, "13 Proven Health Benefits of Walnuts," Healthline Media, July 9, 2018, *https://www.healthline.com/nutrition/benefits-of-walnuts#TOC_TITLE_HDR_11.*

85. George Mateljan, "Celery – WHFoods," The World's Healthiest Foods, The George Mateljan Foundation, accessed June 15, 2020, *http://www.whfoods.com/genpage.php?tname=foodspice&dbid=14.*

86. "Hippocrates," Wikipedia, Wikimedia Foundation, March 15, 2021, *https://en.wikipedia.org/wiki/Hippocrates.*

87. Denis E. Corpet, "Red Meat and Colon Cancer: Should We Become Vegetarians, or Can We Make Meat Safer?" *Meat Science* 89, no. 3 (2011): 310–16, *https://doi.org/10.1016/j.meatsci.2011.04.009.*

88. GBD 2017 Diet Collaborators, "Health Effects of Dietary Risks in 195 Countries, 1990–2017: A Systematic Analysis for the Global Burden of Disease Study 2017," The Lancet, April 2, 2019, doi: 10.1016/S0140-6736(19)30041-8, *http://www.healthdata.org/news-release/new-study-finds-poor-diet-kills-more-people-globally-tobacco-and-high-blood-pressure.*

89. "Factory Farming's Toll on Human Health," Farm Sanctuary, accessed March 18, 2021, *https://www.farmsanctuary.org/issue/public-health/*.

90. "Findings for Lifestyle, Diet & Disease," Adventist Health Study, accessed March 18, 2021, *https://adventisthealthstudy.org/studies/AHS-2/findings-lifestyle-diet-disease*.

91. Ibid.

92. Gabrielle Turner-McGrievy, Trisha Mandes, and Anthony Crimarco, "A Plant-Based Diet for Overweight and Obesity Prevention and Treatment," *Journal of Geriatric Cardiology* 15, no. 5 (May 2017): 369–74, *https://doi.org/10.11909/j.issn.1671-5411.2017.05.002*.

93. Michael Greger, *How Not To Diet* (New York, NY: Flat Iron Books, 2019), 207.

94. "IGF-1, Diet and Cancer," Viva! – The Vegan Charity, July 9, 2020, *https://viva.org.uk/health/healthy-vegan-diet/why-veganism-is-healthy/diet-and-cancer/igf-1-diet-and-cancer/*.

95. Morgan E. Levine, Jorge A. Suarez, Sebastian Brandhorst, Priya Balasubramanian, Chia-Wei Cheng, Federica Madia, Luigi Fontana, et al, "Low Protein Intake Is Associated with a Major Reduction in IGF-1, Cancer, and Overall Mortality in the 65 and Younger but Not Older Population," *Cell Metabolism* 19, no. 3 (March 2014): 407–17, *https://doi.org/10.1016/j.cmet.2014.02.006*.

96. Michael Greger, *How Not To Diet* (New York, NY: Flat Iron Books, 2019), 219.

97. Amanda M. Fretts, Jack L. Follis, Jennifer A. Nettleton, Rozenn N. Lemaitre, Julius S. Ngwa, Mary K. Wojczynski, Loanna Panagiota Kalafati, et al, "Consumption of Meat Is Associated with Higher Fasting Glucose and Insulin Concentrations Regardless of Glucose and Insulin Genetic Risk Scores: a Meta-Analysis of 50,345 Caucasians," *The American Journal of Clinical Nutrition* 102, no. 5 (September 2015): 1266–78, *https://doi.org/10.3945/ajcn.114.101238*.

98. Jessica Jones, "The Protein Myth: Why You Need Less Protein Than You Think," HuffPost, November 20, 2012, *https://www.huffpost.com/entry/protein-diet_b_1882372*.

99. Heather Moore, "Bacon Apologists Prove That Meat Is Addictive," PETA, November 20, 2015, *https://www.peta.org/blog/bacon-apologists-prove-that-meat-is-addictive/*.

100. Tabitha Brown, "Why I Became Vegan and Why I Started Doing Videos!" YouTube, January 5, 2020, *https://www.youtube.com/watch?v=zUch4L2yhko&feature=youtu.be.*

101. Michael Greger, *How Not To Diet* (New York, NY: Flat Iron Books, 2019), 203.

102. Matthew Zampa, "99% of U.S. Farmed Animals Live on Factory Farms," Sentient Media, October 8, 2020, *https://sentientmedia.org/u-s-farmed-animals-live-on-factory farms/.*

Chapter 25: Forgo Fleshy Fasting – Battle # 4 – Undereating

1. Stephanie Averkamp, "Diet and Weight Loss Statistics," fitnessforweightloss.com, accessed March 16, 2019, *http://www.fitnessforweightloss.com/diet-and-weight-loss-statistics/.*

2. Myrtis Smith, "10 reasons Christians Should Care about What they Eat," June 12, 2012, *https://www.amazon.com/dp/B008B1H9F4/ref=rdr_kindle_ext_tmb.*

3. Aaron Kandola, edited by Stacy Samson, "9 Signs and Symptoms You're Not Eating Enough," May 29, 2019, *https://www.medicalnewstoday.com/articles/322157.*

4. Ibid.

5. Laura Schoenfield, "Undereating & Training – How Eating Too Little Affects Training," Girls Gone Strong, July 21, 2020, *https://www.girlsgonestrong.com/blog/articles/undereating/.*

6. J. L. Locher, C. S. Ritchie, C. O. Robinson, D. L. Roth, D. Smith West, and K. L. Burgio, "A Multidimensional Approach to Understanding Under-Eating in Homebound Older Adults: The Importance of Social Factors," *The Gerontologist* 48, no. 2 (April 2008): 223–34, *https://doi.org/10.1093/geront/48.2.223.*

7. "How To Make an Interesting Art Piece Using Tree Branches: EHow: Saint Quotes Catholic, Early Church Fathers, Catholic Quotes," Pinterest, accessed June 20, 2020, *https://www.pinterest.com/pin/Aa-UZfjIvta8hyIKKynQ3viWOzHnGjgEVj7dUinzsiV1v_e1djz9ZRl/.*

8. "Athanasius of Alexandria," Wikipedia, Wikimedia Foundation, November 12, 2020, *https://en.wikipedia.org/wiki/Athanasius_of_Alexandria.*

9. "Athanasius of Alexandria on #Fasting #ChurchHistory #ChurchFathers #SpiritualDisciplines: Saint Quotes, Early Church Fathers, Spiritual Wisdom," Pinterest, Twenty-OneCenturies.com, accessed June 20, 2020, *https://www.pinterest.co.uk/pin/391179917628072133/.*

10. S. Demirci, K. H. Dogan, and S. Koc, Evaluation of Forensic Deaths during the Month of Ramadan in Konya, Turkey, between 2000 and 2009, Am J Forensic Med Pathol 34, no. 3 (September 2013): 267–270, DOI: *10.1097/PAF.0b013e3182a0a430.*

11. "Christian Dies during 40-Day Fast," Daily Mail Online, *Associated Newspapers,* October 4, 2006, *https://www.dailymail.co.uk/news/article-408554/Christian-dies-40-day-fast.html.*

12. Philip S. Mehler and Carrie Brown, "Anorexia Nervosa – Medical Complications," *Journal of Eating Disorders* 3, no. 1 (2015), *https://doi.org/10.1186/s40337-015-0040-8.*

13. James J. DiNicolantonio and James H. O'Keefe, "Good Fats Versus Bad Fats: A Comparison of Fatty Acids in the Promotion of Insulin Resistance, Inflammation, and Obesity," *Missouri medicine* 114, no. 4 (2017): 303–307.

14. Boity Banks, "South African Pastor Dies Following 30 Days Fasting To Beat Jesus," BuzzSouthAfrica, July 29, 2020, *https://buzzsouthafrica.com/south-african-pastor-dies-following-30-days-fasting/.*

15. Sheraz Malik, "The Benefits of Fasting #Infographic," Dream Creation: World's Best Infographics Place, August 21, 2019, *https://www.dreamcreationinfo.com/2019/08/the-benefits-of-fasting-infographic.html.*

16. Paul C. Bragg, *The Miracle of Fasting* (Los Angeles, CA: Health Science, 1983), 116.

17. Jason Fung and Jimmy Moore, The Complete Guide to Fasting: Heal Your Body through Intermittent, Alternate-Day, and Extended Fasting (Las Vegas, NV: Victory Belt Publishing, 2016), 137.

18. The Complete Guide to Fasting, 111.

19. Benjamin D. Horne, Heidi T. May, Jeffrey L. Anderson, Abdallah G. Kfoury, Beau M. Bailey, Brian S. McClure, Dale G. Renlund, et al, "Usefulness of Routine Periodic Fasting To Lower Risk of Coronary Artery Disease in Patients Undergoing Coronary Angiography," *The American Journal of Cardiology* 102, no. 7 (July 2008): 814–19, *https://doi.org/10.1016/j.amjcard.2008.05.021.*

20. Rachel Link, "8 Health Benefits of Fasting, Backed by Science," Healthline, July 30, 2018, *https://www.healthline.com/nutrition/fasting-benefits.*

21. The Complete Guide to Fasting, 61.

22. Fehime B. Aksungar, Aynur E. Topkaya, and Mahmut Akyildiz, "Interleukin-6, C-Reactive Protein and Biochemical Parameters during Prolonged Intermittent Fasting," *Annals of Nutrition and Metabolism* 51, no. 1 (March 2007): 88–95, *https://doi.org/10.1159/000100954.*

23. Nicola Bragazzi, Maha Sellami, Iman Salem, Rosalynn Conic, Mark Kimak, Paolo Pigatto, and Giovanni Damiani, "Fasting and Its Impact on Skin Anatomy, Physiology, and Physiopathology: A Comprehensive Review of the Literature," *Nutrients* 11, no. 2 (January 2019): 249, *https://doi.org/10.3390/nu11020249.*

24. Charles L. Goodrick, Donald K. Ingram, Mark A. Reynolds, John R. Freeman, and Nancy L. Cider, "Effects of Intermittent Feeding upon Growth and Life Span in Rats," *Gerontology* 28, no. 4 (December 1981): 233–41, *https://doi.org/10.1159/000212538.*

25. Rachel Link, "8 Health Benefits of Fasting, Backed by Science," Healthline, July 30, 2018, *https://www.healthline.com/nutrition/fasting-benefits.*

26. Ibid.

27. Andrea S. Blevins-Primeau, "Intermittent Fasting and Cancer," Cancer Therapy Advisor, March 12, 2019, *https://www.cancertherapyadvisor.com/home/tools/fact-sheets/intermittent-fasting-and-cancer/.*

28. Frédérique R. Smink, Daphne van Hoeken, and Hans W. Hoek, "Epidemiology of Eating Disorders: Incidence, Prevalence and Mortality Rates," *Current Psychiatry Reports* 14, no. 4 (May 2012): 406–14, *https://doi.org/10.1007/s11920-012-0282-y.*

29. "Anorexia Nervosa," Wikipedia, Wikimedia Foundation, March 16, 2021, *https://en.wikipedia.org/wiki/Anorexia_nervosa.*

30. "South Carolina Department of Mental Health," Eating Disorder Statistics, South Carolina Department of Mental Health, accessed October 15, 2020, *https://www.state.sc.us/dmh/anorexia/statistics.htm.*

31. Ibid.

32. C. Laird Birmingham, Jenny Su, Julia A. Hlynsky, Elliot M. Goldner, and Min Gao, "The Mortality Rate from Anorexia Nervosa," *International Journal of Eating Disorders* 38, no. 2 (2005): 143–46, *https://doi.org/10.1002/eat.20164.*

33. Suzanne Leigh, "Many Patients with Anorexia Nervosa Get Better, But Complete Recovery Elusive to Most," UC San Francisco, March 17, 2021, *https://www.ucsf.edu/news/2019/11/416006/many-patients-anorexia-nervosa-get-better-complete-recovery-elusive-most.*

34. *Diagnostic and Statistical Manual of Mental Disorders: DSM-5* (Arlington, VA: American Psychiatric Association, 2017), 339.

35. "Anorexia Nervosa," Mayo Clinic, Mayo Foundation for Medical Education and Research, February 20, 2018, *https://www.mayoclinic.org/diseases-conditions/anorexia-nervosa/symptoms-causes/syc-20353591.*

36. Ibid.

37. Jason Fung, The Obesity Code: Unlocking the Secrets of Weight Loss (Vancouver: Greystone Books, 2016), 120.

38. Jendayi Harris, The Chubby Church: A Call to Break Free of Weight & Eating Bondage (Denver, CO: Whole & Free Press, 2019), 141.

39. S. D. Anton, et al., "Flipping the Metabolic Switch: Understanding and Applying the Health Benefits of Fasting," *Obesity* 26, no. 2 (October 2017): 254–268, DOI: *10.1002/oby.22065*.

Chapter 26: Jump off the Body Shame Train – Battle # 5 – Body Shame

1. "How Body Image Disturbance Relates to Eating Disorders." Eating Disorder Hope, accessed April 5, 2019, *https://www.eatingdisorderhope.com/information/body-image/how-body-image-relates-to-eating-disorders*.

2. Ibid.

3. Tufan Nayir, Ersin Uskun, Mustafa Volkan Yürekli, Hacer Devran, Ayşe Çelik, and Ramazan Azim Okyay. "Does Body Image Affect Quality of Life?: A Population Based Study." PLOS ONE 11, no. 9 (September 20, 2016). *https://doi.org/10.1371/journal.pone.0163290*.

4. "Body Image," National Eating Disorders Collaboration, accessed March 21, 2021, *https://nedc.com.au/eating-disorders/eating-disorders-explained/body-image/*.

5. Renee Engeln, "An Epidemic of Beauty Sickness," TEDxUConn 2013," YouTube, October 21, 2013, *https://www.youtube.com/watch?v=63XsokRPV_Y*.

6. David Garner, "Body Image in America: Survey Results," Psychology Today, Sussex Publishers, February 1, 1997, *https://www.psychologytoday.com/us/articles/199702/body-image-in-america-survey-results.n*.

7. Ibid.

8. Ibid.

9. Ibid.

10. "Psychology: Body Image Graphic," InfographicNow.com, July 5, 2017, *https://infographicnow.com/psychology-infographics/psychology-body-image-graphic-3/*.

11. David Garner, "Body Image in America: Survey Results," Psychology Today, Sussex Publishers, February 1, 1997, *https://www.psychologytoday.com/us/articles/199702/body-image-in-america-survey-results*.

12. Ibid.

13. Ibid.

14. Tina Kelley, "'Am I Too Fat?" *The New York Times*, April 4, 2004, *https://www.nytimes.com/2004/04/04/nyregion/am-i-too-fat.html.*

15. Norwegian University of Science and Technology, "Feeling Fat May Make You Fat, Study Suggests," ScienceDaily, accessed March 20, 2020, *www.sciencedaily.com/releases/2012/08/120808121816.htm.*

16. Ibid.

17. Shelly Grabe, L. Monique Ward, and Janet Shibley Hyde. "The Role of the Media in Body Image Concerns among Women: A Meta-Analysis of Experimental and Correlational Studies." Psychological Bulletin 134, no. 3 (June 2008): 460–76, *https://doi.org/10.1037/0033-2909.134.3.460.*

18. Heather A. Hausenblas and Elizabeth A. Fallon, "Exercise and Body Image: A Meta-Analysis," *Psychology & Health* 21, no. 1 (March 2005): 33–47, *https://doi.org/10.1080/14768320500105270.*

19. Dr. Jake Linardon, "2021 Body Image Statistics: 40 Shocking Body Image Facts," Break Binge Eating, March 6, 2021, *https://breakbingeeating.com/body-image-statistics/.*

20. "Eating Disorder Statistics for Anorexia, Bulimia, Binge Eating," Eating Disorder Hope, February 10, 2021, *https://www.eatingdisorderhope.com/information/statistics-studies.*

21. Andri S. Bjornsson, Elizabeth R. Didie, and Katharine A. Phillips, "Body Dysmorphic Disorder," *Obsessive-Compulsive Spectrum Disorders* 12, no. 2 (June 2010): 221–32, *https://doi.org/10.31887/dcns.2010.12.2/abjornsson.*

22. Talltanic, "10 Craziest Stories of Plastic Surgery Obsessions," YouTube, February 2, 2017, *https://www.youtube.com/watch?v=k-NFfEAyfK4.*

23. Ibid.

24. "Jessica Alves," Wikipedia, Wikimedia Foundation, March 12, 2021, *https://en.wikipedia.org/wiki/Jessica_Alves.*

25. *Diagnostic and Statistical Manual of Mental Disorders: DSM-5* (Arlington, VA: American Psychiatric Association, 2017), 242.

26. Diagnostic and Statistical Manual of Mental Disorders: DSM-5, 243.

27. Letter to Jendayi Harris – Re: Please Approve This Quote from You for The Chubby Church Book 2 in Chapter 26/6 on Body Image, March 22, 2021.

28. John Eldredge and Staci Eldredge, *Captivating: Unveiling the Mystery of a Woman's Soul* (Nashville, TN: Thomas Nelson, 2021), 24.

29. "FastStats – Body Measurements," Centers for Disease Control and Prevention, January 14, 2021, *https://www.cdc.gov/nchs/fastats/body-measurements.htm.*

30. Ibid.

31. "Top 30 Quotes of Martha Beck – Famous Quotes and Sayings: Inspiringquotes.us," Inspiring Quotes, accessed March 20, 2021, *https://www.inspiringquotes.us/author/2349-martha-beck.*

32. Anna Carey. "Little Photoshop of Horrors." Independent.ie, (November 30, 2012), *https://www.independent.ie/style/beauty/little-photoshop-of-horrors-26650439.html.*

33. Myles Munroe, *Single, Married, Separated, and Life after Divorce* (Shippensburg, PA: Destiny Image Publishing, 2003), 44.

34. C. B. Taylor, S. Bryson, A. A. Celio Doyle, K. H. Luce, D. Cunning, L. B. Abascal, R. Rockwell, et al, "The Adverse Effect of Negative Comments about Weight and Shape from Family and Siblings on Women at High Risk for Eating Disorders," *Pediatrics* 118, no. 2 (2006): 731–38, *https://doi.org/10.1542/peds.2005-1806.*

35. David Garner, "Body Image in America: Survey Results," Psychology Today, Sussex Publishers, February 1, 1997, *https://www.psychologytoday.com/us/articles/199702/body-image-in-america-survey-results.*

36. Mary Inman, Erica Iceberg, and Laura McKeel, "Do Religious Affirmations, Religious Commitments, or General Commitments Mitigate the Negative Effects of Exposure to Thin Ideals?" *Journal for the Scientific Study of Religion* 53, no. 1 (March 2014): 38–55, *https://doi.org/10.1111/jssr.12089.*

37. "Dana Christmas Story," Campus Firewatch, YouTube video, September 12, 2006, *https://www.youtube.com/watch?v=WzpxaUCOccY.*

38. Dan Barry, "3 Killed in Fire at Seton Hall; Dozens of Students Are Hurt," *The New York Times*, January 20, 2000, *https://www.nytimes.com/2000/01/20/nyregion/3-killed-in-fire-at-seton-hall-dozens-of-students-are-hurt.html.*

39. Bessel van der Kolk, "The Body Keeps the Score: Memory and the Evolving Psychobiology of Posttraumatic Stress," *Harvard Review of Psychiatry*, 1, no. 5 (January 1, 1994): 253-65, *https://pubmed.ncbi.nlm.nih.gov/9384857/.*

40. Ana Sandoiu, "How Can Exercise Improve Body Image?" Medical News Today, MediLexicon International, June 18, 2017, *https://www.medicalnewstoday.com/articles/317958#Post-exercise-positive-effects-can-be-immediate-and-long-lasting.*

41. David Garner, "Body Image in America: Survey Results," Psychology Today, Sussex Publishers, February 1, 1997, *https://www.psychologytoday.com/us/ articles/199702/body-image-in-america-survey-results*.

42. Ibid.

43. Rheana Murray, "Where's the Least Body-Positive State in America? You Might Be Surprised," TODAY, May 8, 2018, *https://www.today.com/style/ social-media-affecting-way-we-view-our-bodies-it-s-t128500*.

44. Kay Lazar, "As Women Have Grown Larger, Victoria's Secret Models Have Shrunk," The Boston Globe, January 3, 2020, *https://www.bostonglobe.com/ metro/2020/01/02/women-have-grown-larger-victoria-secret-models-have-shrunk/CQKFwaYXg4jbNtAJoWKyBK/story.html*.

45. Carly Cardellino, "16 Surprising Things You Didn't Know about the Victoria's Secret Fashion Show," Cosmopolitan, October 8, 2017, *https://www.cosmopolitan.com/style-beauty/beauty/news/a5045/ things-you-didnt-know-about-the-victorias-secret-fashion-show/*.

46. "Female Promotional Model Averages Infographic," TSM Agency, April 23, 2017, *http://www.blog.tsmagency.com/ average-model-height-and-weight-requirements/*.

Chapter 27: Decline Dates with Icy Isolation – Battle #6 – Soul Shame

1. "Isolated," Vocabulary.com, accessed September 4, 2020, https://www. vocabulary.com/dictionary/isolated.

2. Dale Burden, "Why People with Mental Illness Isolate Themselves," Psychreg, July 21, 2020, *https://www.psychreg.org/ why-people-isolate-themselves/*.

3. "Isolation – Learn about Emotional and Social Isolation, Treatment for," GoodTherapy, August 20, 2018. *https://www.goodtherapy.org/ learn-about-therapy/issues/isolation*.

4. Ibid.

5. Paul D. Tieger and Barbara Barron-Tieger, *The Art of Speedreading People: How to Size People up and Speak Their Language* (Boston, MA: Little, Brown, 1999) 15–34.

6. Ibid.

7. "Shame," Dictionary.com, accessed September 4, 2020, *https://www. dictionary.com/browse/shame?s=t*.

8. Ibid.

9. Brown Brené, The Power of Vulnerability Teachings on Authenticity, Connection, & Courage (Audible Book) (Louisville, CO: Sounds True, 2012).

10. John Bradshaw, *Healing the Shame That Binds You* (Deerfield Beach, FL: Health Communications, Inc., 2005), 37.

11. Healing the Shame That Binds You, 134.

12. Douglas J. Bremner and Charles R. Marmar, *Trauma, Memory, and Dissociation,* (Washington, DC: American Psychiatric Press Inc., 2002).

13. Healing the Shame That Binds You, 45.

14. Healing the Shame That Binds You, 126.

15. Healing the Shame That Binds You, 168.

16. Byron Brown, Soul without Shame: A Guide to Liberating Yourself from the Judge Within (Boston, MA: Shambhala, 1999), 62.

17. Barbra E. Russell, *Yes! I Said No!* (Aurora, CO: Noble House Press, 2017), 23.

18. Henry Cloud and John Sims Townsend, *Boundaries* (Grand Rapids, MI: Zondervan, 2004), 35.

19. Boundaries, 29–50.

20. Ibid.

21. Jendayi Harris, The Chubby Church: A Call To Break Free of Weight & Eating Bondage (Denver, CO: Whole & Free Press, 2019), 210.

22. Wayne W. Dyer, Your Destiny: The Nine Spiritual Principles for Getting Everything You Want, (New York, NY: Harper, 2008).

23. Keith J. Patterson, Keith, J. Grenny, R. McMillan, and A. L. Switzler, *Crucial Conversation: Tools for Talking When Stakes Are High,* 2nd ed. (New York, NY: McGraw-Hill, 2012), 91.

Chapter 28: Resize Family Fat Genes – Battle #7 – Genetic Predispositions

1. "Products – Data Briefs – Number 360 – February 2020," Centers for Disease Control and Prevention, February 27, 2020, *https://www.cdc.gov/nchs/products/databriefs/db360.htm*

2. Ibid.

3. Martínez-Hernández, Alfredo, Luís Enríquez, María Jesús Moreno-Moreno, and Amelia Martí, "Genetics of Obesity," *Public Health Nutrition* 10, no. 10A (April 2007): 1138–44, https://doi.org/10.1017/s1368980007000626.

4. Michelle L. Brandt, "Obese Parents Increase Kids' Risk of Being Overweight," Stanford University, July 21, 2004, *https://news.stanford.edu/news/2004/july21/med-obesity-721.html*.

5. K. Boyse, "Guide to Obesity and Overweight," accessed May 24, 2010, *www.med.umich.edu/yourchild/topics/obesity.htm*.

6. Michelle L. Brandt, "Obese Parents Increase Kids' Risk of Being Overweight," Stanford University, July 21, 2004, https://news.stanford.edu/ncws/2004/july21/med obesity-721.html.

7. M. K. Serdula, D. Ivery, R. J. Coates, D. S. Freedman, D. F. Williamson, and T. Byers, "Do Obese Children Become Obese Adults? A Review of the Literature," *Preventive Medicine* 22, no. 2 (1993): 167–77, *https://doi.org/10.1006/pmed.1993.1014*.

8. Blanca M. Herrera and Cecilia M. Lindgren, "The Genetics of Obesity," *Current Diabetes Reports* 10, no. 6 (2010): 498–505, *https://doi.org/10.1007/s11892-010-0153-z*.

9. "Noncommunicable Diseases: Childhood Overweight and Obesity," World Health Organization, October 19, 2018, *https://www.who.int/dietphysicalactivity/childhood/en/*.

10. 10. "Products – Health E Stats – Overweight Prevalence among Children and Adolescents 2007–2008," Centers for Disease Control and Prevention, November 6, 2015, *https://www.cdc.gov/nchs/data/hestat/obesity_child_07_08/obesity_child_07_08.htm*.

11. Ibid.

12. Ibid.

13. Ibid.

14. Craig M. Hales, Margaret D. Carroll, Cheryl D. Fryar, and Cynthia L. Ogden, "Prevalence of Obesity among Adults and Youth: United States, 2015–2016," *NCHS Data Brief; US Department of Health and Human Services* 288, no. 288 (October 2017): 3, *https://www.cdc.gov/nchs/data/databriefs/db288.pdf*.

15. Joel Fuhrman and Robert B. Phillips, Fast Food Genocide: How Processed Food Is Killing Us and What We Can Do about It (New York, NY: HarperOne, 2018), 156.

16. Joseph Erbentraut, "People of Color Bear the Brunt of Fast-Food Explosion," HuffPost, April 29, 2017, *https://www.huffpost.com/entry/fast-food-minority-communities_n_59035fb5e4b02655f83c9999?guccounter=1*.

17. Jason P. Block, Richard A. Scribner, and Karen B. DeSalvo, "Fast Food, Race/Ethnicity, and Income: A Geographic Analysis," American Journal of Preventive Medicine, September 23, 2004, *https://www.sciencedirect.com/science/article/abs/pii/S0749379704001394.*

18. Lauren Cox, "Courts Charge Mother of 555-Pound Boy," ABC News Network, June 26, 2009, *https://abcnews.go.com/Health/WellnessNews/story?id=7941609.*

19. *Fed Up,* directed by Stephanie Soechtig (Burbank, CA: Radius-TWC, 2014), DVD.

20. Ibid.

21. Obesity Action Coalition, *Understanding Obesity Stigma* (Tampa, FL: Obesity Action Coalition, 2016).

22. Ibid.

23. Michael Greger, *How Not To Diet* (New York, NY: Flat Iron Books, 2019), 48–49.

24. Obesity Action Coalition, *Understanding Obesity Stigma* (Tampa, FL: Obesity Action Coalition, 2016).

25. Janet A. Lydecker, Elizabeth O'Brien, and Carlos M. Grilo, "Parents Have Both Implicit and Explicit Biases against Children with Obesity," *Journal of Behavioral Medicine* 41, no. 6 (May 4, 2018): 784–91, *https://doi.org/10.1007/s10865-018-9929-4.*

26. *Fed Up,* directed by Stephanie Soechtig (Burbank, CA: Radius-TWC, 2014), DVD.

27. Ibid.

28. Ibid.

29. Ibid.

30. "Statistics on the Purchasing Power of Women," Girlpower Marketing Unified Strategies Public Relations, May 16, 2017, *https://girlpowermarketing.com/statistics-purchasing-power-women/.*

31. Michael Greger, *How Not To Diet* (New York, NY: Flat Iron Books, 2019), 21.

32. Gary Taubes, *The Case Against Sugar* (New York, NY: Anchor Books, 2016), 221.

33. Ibid.

34. Michael Greger, *How Not To Diet* (New York, NY: Flat Iron Books, 2019), 21.

35. Ibid.

36. Ibid.

37. The Case Against Sugar, 222.

38. How Not To Diet, 22.

39. Arlene Weintraub, "Obesity: an Answer in Your Genes?" September 19, 2017, *https://health.usnews.com/health-care/patient-advice/articles/2017-09-19/obesity-an-answer-in-your-genes.*

40. Peter M. Schmid, Iris Heid, Christa Buechler, Andreas Steege, Markus Resch, Christoph Birner, Dierk H Endemann, Guenter A Riegger, and Andreas Luchner, "Expression of Fourteen Novel Obesity-Related Genes in Zucker Diabetic Fatty Rats," *Cardiovascular Diabetology* 11, no. 1 (July 13, 2012): 48, *https://doi.org/10.1186/1475-2840-11-48.*

41. George Mateljan, The World's Healthiest Foods: Essential Guide for the Healthiest Way of Eating (Seattle, WA: George Mateljan Foundation, 2007), 82.

42. Arlene Weintraub, "Obesity: an Answer in Your Genes?" September 19, 2017, *https://health.usnews.com/health-care/patient-advice/articles/2017-09-19/obesity-an-answer-in-your-genes.*

43. Ibid.

44. "DRD2 Polymorphism and Sensitivity to Losses during Value-Based Decision-Making," University of Pittsburg, YouTube video, May 1 2020, https://www.youtube.com/watch?v=PdxnlCk46C4&feature=emb_logo.

45. Z. Liu, Y. Xiang, and G. Sun, The KCTD Family of Proteins: Structure, Function, Disease Relevance, Cell & Bioscience 3, no. 1 (November 2013): 45, *https://doi.org/10.1186/2045-3701-3-45.*

46. A. Vidal-Puig, M. Jimenez-Liñan, B. B. Lowell, A. Hamann, E. Hu, B. Spiegelman, J. S. Flier, and D. E. Moller, "Regulation of PPAR Gamma Gene Expression by Nutrition and Obesity in Rodents," The Journal of Clinical Investigation American Society for Clinical Investigation, June 1, 1996, *https://www.jci.org/articles/view/118703.*

47. *Orig3n. Rep. Noom DNA Life Profile for Jendayi Harris* (Boston, MA: Orig3n CLIA Laboratories, 2020), 14, *https://web.noom.com/support/2019/12/dna-kit-faq/.*

48. Ibid, 17.

49. Ibid, 18.

50. Ibid, 19.

51. Peter M. Schmid, Iris Heid, Christa Buechler, Andreas Steege, Markus Resch, Christoph Birner, Dierk H. Endemann, Guenter A. Riegger, and Andreas Luchner, "Expression of Fourteen Novel Obesity-Related Genes in Zucker Diabetic Fatty Rats," Cardiovascular Diabetology 11, no. 1 (July 2012): 48, *https://doi.org/10.1186/1475-2840-11-48*.

52. "African American Health," Centers for Disease Control and Prevention, July 3, 2017, *https://www.cdc.gov/vitalsigns/aahealth/index.html*.

53. Ibid.

54. Josh LaJaunie and Howard Jacobson, Sick to Fit: Three Simple Techniques That Got Me from 420 Pounds to the Cover of Runner's World, Good Morning America, and the Today Show (New Orleans, LA: WellStart Health, 2018), *https://joshlajaunie.com/*.

55. Michelle T. Adams, Family Strong: 7 Gifts for a Lasting Legacy (Aurora, CO: Legacy Heart Press, 2020), 72.

56. Jeanna Bryner, "Study: Obesity Is Socially Contagious," LiveScience, July 25, 2007, *https://www.livescience.com/4542-study-obesity-socially-contagious.html*.

57. Ibid.

58. Ibid.

Chapter 29: Keys to Whole & Free Health

1. Alina Petre, "Orthorexia: When Healthy Eating Becomes a Disorder," April 2, 2020, *https://www.healthline.com/nutrition/orthorexia-nervosa-101*.

2. Ibid.

3. AJ, Chef, and Glen Merzer, The Secrets to Ultimate Weight Loss: a Revolutionary Approach to Conquer Cravings, Overcome Food Addiction, and Lose Weight without Going Hungry (Los Angeles, CA: Hail to the Kale Publishing, 2018), 49.

4. Douglas and Alan Goldhamer, The Pleasure Trap: Mastering the Hidden Force That Undermines Health & Happiness (Summertown, TN: Healthy Living Publications, 2006),71.

5. Ibid.

6. Jamie Locher and Owen Moritz, "Eating While Driving Causes 80% of All Car Accidents, Study Shows," New York Daily News, January 11, 2019, *https://www.nydailynews.com/new-york/eating-driving-80-car-accidents-study-shows-article-1.427796*.

7.   "Dr. Seuss Quotes and Facts," EasyBib, January 1, 2021, *https://www.easybib.com/guides/quotes-facts-stats/dr-seuss/*.

Victory Morsels

1.   Nancy Appleton, *Lick the Sugar Habit*, (Garden City Park, NY: Avery Publishing Group, 1996), 68–72, *www.lickthesugarhabit.com*.

2.   "FAA's Promises." Food Addicts Anonymous. Accessed November 30, 2020. *https://www.foodaddictsanonymous.org/promises*.

3.   Annie Hall, "What the Average American Eats Infographic." Nature's Sunshine, June 2020. *https://blog.naturessunshine.com/en/what-are-we-eating/*.

Made in the USA
Monee, IL
28 March 2022

93673501R00240